Maternal and Infant Deaths: Chasing Millennium Development Goals 4 and 5

RCOG
PRESS

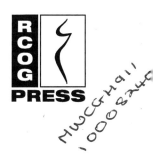

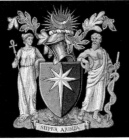

Since 1973 the Royal College of Obstetricians and Gynaecologists has regularly convened Study Groups to address important growth areas within obstetrics and gynaecology. An international group of eminent clinicians and scientists from various disciplines is invited to present the results of recent research and to take part in in-depth discussions. The resulting volume, containing enhanced versions of the papers presented, is published within a few months of the meeting and provides a summary of the subject that is both authoritative and up to date.

SOME PREVIOUS STUDY GROUP PUBLICATIONS AVAILABLE

Menopause and Hormone Replacement
Edited by Hilary Critchley, Ailsa Gebbie and Valerie Beral

Disorders of the Menstrual Cycle
Edited by PMS O'Brien, IT Cameron and AB MacLean

Infection and Pregnancy
Edited by AB MacLean, L Regan and D Carrington

Pain in Obstetrics and Gynaecology
Edited by A MacLean, R Stones and S Thornton

Incontinence in Women
Edited by AB MacLean and L Cardozo

Maternal Morbidity and Mortality
Edited by AB MacLean and J Neilson

Lower Genital Tract Neoplasia
Edited by Allan B MacLean, Albert Singer and Hilary Critchley

Pre-eclampsia
Edited by Hilary Critchley, Allan MacLean, Lucilla Poston and James Walker

Preterm Birth
Edited by Hilary Critchley, Phillip Bennett and Steven Thornton

Implantation and Early Development
Edited by Hilary Critchley, Iain Cameron and Stephen Smith

Contraception and Contraceptive Use
Edited by Anna Glasier, Kaye Wellings and Hilary Critchley

Multiple Pregnancy
Edited by Mark Kilby, Phil Baker, Hilary Critchley and David Field

Heart Disease and Pregnancy
Edited by Philip J Steer, Michael A Gatzoulis and Philip Baker

Teenage Pregnancy and Reproductive Health
Edited by Philip Baker, Kate Guthrie, Cindy Hutchinson, Roslyn Kane and Kaye Wellings

Obesity and Reproductive Health
Edited by Philip Baker, Adam Balen, Lucilla Poston and Naveed Sattar

Renal Disease in Pregnancy
Edited by John M Davison, Catherine Nelson-Piercy, Sean Kehoe and Philip Baker

Cancer and Reproductive Health
Edited by Sean Kehoe, Eric Jauniaux, Pierre Martin-Hirsch and Philip Savage

Reproductive Ageing
Edited by Susan Bewley, William Ledger and Dimitrios Nikolaou

Reproductive Genetics
Edited by Sean Kehoe, Lyn Chitty and Tessa Homfray

Maternal and Infant Deaths: Chasing Millennium Development Goals 4 and 5

Edited by

Sean Kehoe, James P Neilson and Jane E Norman

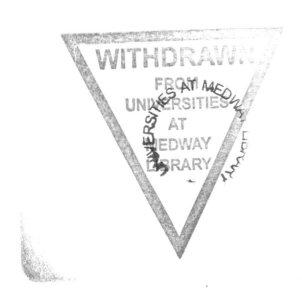

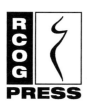

RCOG PRESS

Sean Kehoe MD FRCOG
Convenor of Study Groups, Lead Consultant in Gynaecological Oncology, Oxford Gynaecological Cancer Centre, John Radcliffe Hospital, Headington, Oxford OX3 9DU

James P Neilson MD FRCOG
NIHR Dean for Training and Professor of Obstetrics and Gynaecology, School of Reproductive and Developmental Medicine, University of Liverpool, University Department, 1st floor, Liverpool Women's Hospital, Crown Street, Liverpool L8 7SS

Jane E Norman MD FRCOG
Professor of Maternal and Fetal Health, University of Edinburgh Centre for Reproductive Biology, The Queen's Medical Research Institute, 47 Little France Crescent, Edinburgh EH16 4TY

Published by the **RCOG Press** at the Royal College of Obstetricians and Gynaecologists, 27 Sussex Place, Regent's Park, London NW1 4RG

www.rcog.org.uk

Registered charity no. 213280

First published 2010

© 2010 The Royal College of Obstetricians and Gynaecologists

ISBN 978-1-906985-30-1

A machine-readable catalogue record for this publication can be obtained from the British Library [www.bl.uk/catalogue/listings.html]

Front cover image courtesy of Jacqui Hill: 'The photograph was taken in the north of Afghanistan in the village of Pas-Pul in the district of Badakhshan. There was no school building at all so the boys were meeting under canvas set up by UNICEF and the girls, as pictured here, in the building used as the mosque. The teachers were not particularly qualified but at least the desire for education was there and the understanding that girls should be educated. The village leader was well educated and progressive. We were there as part of the Medair team, helping to establish both a health centre and a school in the village."

RCOG Editor: Andrew Welsh
Original design by Karl Harrington, FiSH Books, London
Typesetting by Andrew Welsh
Index by Jan Ross (Merrall-Ross International Ltd)
Printed by Henry Ling Ltd, The Dorset Press, Dorchester DT1 1HD

Contents

SECTION 3   CLINICAL PROBLEMS AND SOLUTIONS – NEONATAL

SECTION 4   TRAINING AND DEVELOPMENT

SECTION 5   SPECIFIC CHALLENGES IN SPECIFIC COUNTRIES

SECTION 6   CONSENSUS VIEWS

Participants

Stephen Allen
Professor of Paediatrics and International Health, Room 314, Grove Building, School of Medicine, Swansea University, Singleton Park, Swansea SA2 8PP, UK.

Zulfiqar Bhutta
Head, Division of Women & Child Health, The Aga Khan University, Stadium Road, Karachi 74800, Pakistan.

Oona Campbell
Professor in Epidemiology and Reproductive Health, London School of Hygiene & Tropical Medicine, Keppel Street, London WC1E 7HT, UK.

Anthony Costello
Director, UCL Institute for Global Health and the UCL Centre for International Health and Development, Institute of Child Health, 30 Guilford Street, London WC1N 1EH, UK.

Frances Day-Stirk
Director of Learning Research and Practice Development, International Office, Royal College of Midwives, 15 Mansfield Street, London W1G 9NH, UK.

Soo Downe
Professor of Midwifery Studies, Research in Childbirth and Health (ReaCH) group, Room 116, Brook Building, University of Central Lancashire, Preston PR1 2HE, UK.

Anthony Falconer
Senior Vice President, RCOG, and Consultant Gynaecologist, Derriford Hospital, Plymouth PL6 8DH, UK.

Kate Grady
Consultant Anaesthetist, Department of Anaesthetics, University Hospital of South Manchester NHS Foundation Trust, Southmoor Road, Manchester M23 9LT, UK.

Wendy Graham
Professor of Obstetric Epidemiology, Immpact, Health Sciences Building, University of Aberdeen, Foresterhill, Aberdeen AB25 2ZD, UK.

Jacqueline Hill
Consultant Obstetrician/Gynaecologist and Director of Physician Training, Education and Research, Oasis Hospital, PO Box 1016, Al Ain, United Arab Emirates.

Julia Hussein
Senior Clinical Research Fellow, Immpact, University of Aberdeen, Health Sciences Building, Foresterhill, Aberdeen AB25 2ZD, UK.

Sean Kehoe
Convenor of Study Groups, Lead Consultant in Gynaecological Oncology, Oxford Gynaecological Cancer Centre, John Radcliffe Hospital, Headington, Oxford OX3 9DU, UK.

Joy E Lawn
Director, Global Evidence and Policy, Saving Newborn Lives/Save the Children, Cape Town, South Africa.

Gwyneth Lewis OBE
International Clinical Lead for Maternal Health and Maternity Services, Department of
Health, Wellington House, Waterloo Road, London SE1 8UG, UK.

James McIntyre
Executive Director, Anova Health Institute, 12 Sherborne Road, Parktown,
Johannnesburg 2193, South Africa.

Stephen Munjanja
Senior Lecturer, Department of Obstetrics and Gynaecology, College of Health
Sciences, University of Zimbabwe, PO Box A178, Avondale, Harare, Zimbabwe.

James P Neilson
NIHR Dean for Training and Professor of Obstetrics and Gynaecology, School of
Reproductive and Developmental Medicine, University of Liverpool, University
Department, 1st floor, Liverpool Women's Hospital, Crown Street, Liverpool L8 7SS, UK.

Jane E Norman
Professor of Maternal and Fetal Health, University of Edinburgh Centre for
Reproductive Biology, The Queen's Medical Research Institute, 47 Little France
Crescent, Edinburgh EH16 4TY, UK.

Robert Pattinson
Director, MRC Maternal and Infant Health Care Strategies Research Unit, University
of Pretoria, Klinikala Building, PO Box 667, Pretoria 0001, South Africa.

Harshalal Seneviratne
Dean and Senior Professor of Obstetrics and Gynaecology, Faculty of Medicine,
University of Colombo, Kynsey Road, Colombo 08, Sri Lanka.

Nynke van den Broek
Head, Maternal and Newborn Health Unit and Director, LSTM–RCOG International
Partnership, Liverpool School of Tropical Medicine, Pembroke Place, Liverpool
L3 5QA, UK.

Andrew Weeks
Senior Lecturer, School of Reproductive and Developmental Medicine, Liverpool
Women's Hospital, Crown Street, Liverpool L8 7SS, UK.

Beverly Winikoff
President, Gynuity Health Projects, 15 East 26th Street, Suite 801, New York,
NY 10016, USA.

Additional contributors

Noureen Afzal
Fellow, Department of Paediatrics and Child Health, The Aga Khan University, Stadium
Road, Karachi 74800, Pakistan.

Jacqueline Bell
Research Fellow, Immpact, Health Sciences Building, University of Aberdeen,
Foresterhill, Aberdeen AB25 2ZD, UK.

Catriona Connolly
Consultant Anaesthetist, Department of Anaesthesia, Ninewells Hospital, Dundee
DD1 9SY, UK.

Christabel Enweronu-Laryea
Consultant Neonatologist, Korle Bu Hospital and Legon University, Accra Ghana.

Ann Fitzmaurice
Medical Statistician, Immpact, Health Sciences Building, University of Aberdeen, Foresterhill, Aberdeen AB25 2ZD, UK.

Nevine Hassanein
Consultant Obstetrician and Gynaecologist and Public Health Specialist, Office 1, 14 Waguih Pacha Street, Genaklees, Alexandria, Egypt.

Jan Hofman
Lecturer in Sexual and Reproductive Health, Liverpool School of Tropical Medicine, Pembroke Place, Liverpool L3 5QA, UK.

G Justus Hofmeyr
Director, Effective Care Research Unit, Eastern Cape Department of Health, University of the Witwatersrand, University of Fort Hare; East London Hospital Complex, PB X9047, East London 5201, South Africa.

Kate Kerber
Specialist, Africa Region, Newborn Health, Saving Newborn Lives/Save the Children, Cape Town, South Africa.

Karima Khalil
Egypt Team Coordinator, Choices and Challenges in Changing Childbirth Research Network, Al Galaa Hospital, Cairo, Egypt.

Zoë Matthews
Research Fellow, Centre for Global Health, Population Poverty and Policy, School of Social Sciences, Murray Building, University of Southampton, University Road, Southampton, UK.

Lauren Foster Mustardé
Research Fellow, London School of Hygiene & Tropical Medicine, Department of Epidemiology and Population Health, Keppel Street, London WC1E 7HT, UK.

Sarah Neal
Research Associate, Centre for Global Health, Population Poverty and Policy, School of Social Sciences, Murray Building, University of Southampton, University Road, Southampton, UK.

Siti Nurul Qomariyah
Researcher, Immpact, Center for Family Welfare, Faculty of Public Health, University of Indonesia, Indonesia.

Christina Pagel
Senior Research Fellow, Clinical Operational Research Unit, University College London, 4 Taviton Street, London WC1H 0BT, UK.

Audrey Prost
Lecturer, UCL Centre for International Health and Development, Institute of Child Health, 30 Guilford Street, London WC1N 1EH, UK.

Carine Ronsmans
Professor in Epidemiology, Infectious Diseases Epidemiology Unit, London School of Hygiene & Tropical Medicine, Keppel Street, London WC1E 7HT, UK.

Saad Seth
Fellow, Department of Paediatrics and Child Health, The Aga Khan University, Stadium Road, Karachi 74800, Pakistan.

Caitlin Shannon
Senior Program Associate, Gynuity Health Projects, 15 East 26th Street, Suite 801, New York, NY 11222, USA.

Eric Sinclair
Executive Vice President and Chief Operating Officer, Oasis Hospital, PO Box 1016, Al Ain, United Arab Emirates.

Leighton Walker
Research Assistant, Immpact, University of Aberdeen, Health Sciences Building, Aberdeen AB25 2ZD, UK.

Preface

The Millennium Development Goals (MDGs), created under the auspices of the United Nations, presented an opportunity for political, financial, medical and civil society leaders to focus on the huge disparities in global health provision. MDGs 4 and 5, which focus on child and maternal outcomes respectively, have proved more challenging than others to deliver. There are only 4 years left for these challenges to be realised.

The Royal College of Obstetricians and Gynaecologists, the Royal College of Midwives, the Royal College of Paediatrics and Child Health and the Royal College of Anaesthetists, although principally responsible for UK-based healthcare issues, are aware of their global responsibilities to women's and children's health.

This Study Group was designed to focus on the excellence that these institutions can deliver. The speakers from all four disciplines were selected as outstanding contributors in this area of global health. Midwives, obstetricians, paediatricians and anaesthetists have provided a review that will act as a scholastic resource but also as an immensely useful reference for those involved in advocacy on behalf of women and children.

The RCOG's global network has enabled us to draw examples from countries as diverse as Afghanistan and Egypt. Such illustrations demonstrate the required elements for success.

We hope that this work will prove a useful adjunct to those trying to tackle the issues of delivering MDGs 4 and 5 within the next 4 years.

Anthony Falconer
Senior Vice President, RCOG

The Millenium Development Goals

At the 2000 UN Millennium Summit, world leaders from rich and poor countries alike committed themselves – at the highest political level – to a set of eight time-bound targets that, when achieved, will end extreme poverty worldwide by 2015.

The eight Millennium Development Goals set out by the year 2015 to:

1. **end hunger and extreme poverty**
   - halve, between 1990 and 2015, the proportion of people whose income is less than one dollar a day
   - achieve full and productive employment and decent work for all, including women and young people
   - halve, between 1990 and 2015, the proportion of people who suffer from hunger

2. **universal education**
   - ensure that, by 2015, children everywhere, boys and girls alike, will be able to complete a full course of primary schooling

3. **gender equity**
   - eliminate gender disparity in primary and secondary education, preferably by 2005, and in all levels of education no later than 2015

4. **child health**
   - reduce by two-thirds, between 1990 and 2015, the under-five mortality rate

5. **maternal health**
   - reduce by three-quarters, between 1990 and 2015, the maternal mortality ratio
   - achieve, by 2015, universal access to reproductive health

6. **combat HIV/AIDS and other diseases**
   - have halted by 2015 and begun to reverse the spread of HIV/AIDS
   - achieve, by 2010, universal access to treatment for HIV/AIDS for all those who need it
   - have halted by 2015 and begun to reverse the incidence of malaria and other major diseases

7. **environmental sustainability**
   - integrate the principles of sustainable development into country policies and programmes and reverse the loss of environmental resources
   - reduce biodiversity loss, achieving, by 2010, a significant reduction in the rate of loss
   - halve, by 2015, the proportion of people without sustainable access to safe drinking water and basic sanitation
   - by 2020, to have achieved a significant improvement in the lives of at least 100 million slum dwellers

8. **global partnership**
   - develop further an open, rule-based, predictable, non-discriminatory trading and financial system (includes a commitment to good governance, development and poverty reduction – both nationally and internationally)
   - address the special needs of the least developed countries (includes: tariff- and quota-free access for the least developed countries' exports; enhanced programme of debt relief for heavily indebted poor countries (HIPC) and cancellation of official bilateral debt; and more generous ODA for countries committed to poverty reduction
   - address the special needs of landlocked developing countries and small island developing states (through the programme of action for the sustainable development of small island developing states and the outcome of the twenty-second special session of the general assembly)
   - deal comprehensively with the debt problems of developing countries through national and international measures in order to make debt sustainable in the long term
   - in cooperation with pharmaceutical companies, provide access to affordable essential drugs in developing countries
   - in cooperation with the private sector, make available the benefits of new technologies, especially information and communications.

Section 1

The size of the problem

Chapter 1

The geography of maternal death

Wendy Graham, Jacqueline Bell, Ann Fitzmaurice, Sarah
Neal, Siti Nurul Qomariyah and Zoë Matthews

Introduction

> The great blot on public health administration[1]

By 1905, the majority of deaths during pregnancy and childbirth in England and
Wales were registered officially and the maternal mortality ratio (MMR) was around
420 deaths per 100 000 live births.[2] Lack of progress in reducing this mortality during
the period up to the mid-1930s was a cause of great concern and indeed shame to
health authorities, as indicated in the quotation above from the then Minister of
Health. Awareness of this stalled progress also contributed to a wider public outrage
over the poor state of maternal and infant welfare.[3]

By 2005, at least 75% of maternal deaths in the developing world went unrecorded
and the estimated magnitude was 450 deaths per 100 000 live births.[4] The outcry
against this modern-day disgrace has become louder since 2000, when the Millennium
Declaration pledged wide-scale reductions in maternal mortality as one of eight
Millennium Development Goals (MDGs) agreed by an unprecedented concord of
198 nation states. Further momentum has gathered through national and international
advocacy for safe motherhood, such as through the White Ribbon Alliance[5] and the
Partnership for Maternal, Newborn and Child Health.[6]

The similarities between the contemporary movement to prevent maternal deaths
and the lay committees set up in Britain in the 1930s to lobby for greater attention
are striking in many ways. However, there are also major differences, some of which
highlight bleak prospects for achieving MDG 5. One such obstacle is the continuing
lack of essential, credible data on deaths, and indeed births, at subnational and national
levels in the poorest regions of the world – in the very places where the problem is
greatest. There is ample historical evidence to show the leverage that is achieved
through counting deaths and communicating the outrage that high mortality provokes
locally and nationally.[7] Today's champions for achieving MDG 5 must grapple with
the dilemma of making a powerful case for action while also appealing for better data
to inform and ultimately to judge progress: a challenge shared with five other MDGs
that require data on births and deaths.[8] The current heightened attention to MDG 5
as the most 'off-track' of the MDGs provides an opportunity to renew the imperative
to count maternal deaths and thus act – recognising that 'what you count is what

you do'.[9] The purpose of this chapter is to highlight the importance of a key, yet often neglected, aspect of counting and acting – where women die, or what we have termed the 'geography of maternal death'.

Understanding the spatial or geographical distribution of a problem is one of the most basic tenets of public health, confronting and aiding decision makers at all levels to act.[10] Numerous examples exist, both historical and contemporary, of the power of showing the location of health burdens, such as the outbreak of cholera and the location of contaminated water pumps in 1850s London, and the recent global maps showing malarial endemicity.[11,12] Besides the intuitive appeal for advocacy purposes of presenting data on where vital events occur, there are aspects to the geography of maternal death that have significant policy and programmatic implications. Comparing place of residence and place of death can, for example, help pinpoint areas for geographical targeting and prompt questions on barriers and facilitators to access to services as well as on quality of care. Investigating spatial patterns at various levels of magnitude illuminates social and economic inequities in the risk of maternal death between and within countries – in other words, revealing who is dying where. Crucially, the search for patterns also invariably reveals data gaps or blind spots, such as the absence of information on maternal deaths outside the health system – those dying at home or on the way to care. Understanding where and why women are missing from routine health statistics and care systems is thus important to achieving and demonstrating progress towards MDG 5.

This chapter seeks to raise awareness of these and other reasons for studying the geography of maternal death and to make the case for wider adoption of such a perspective. The first section summarises the principal challenges in identifying maternal deaths and deriving reliable mortality patterns in developing countries, including by place of death. The second section presents an aggregate perspective on the location of maternal deaths in the world. This is complemented in the third part by individual-level analyses to investigate key co-variates of place of death using selected data from published sources and from primary material available from Immpact, a research initiative on evidence to reduce maternal mortality.[13] Box 1.1 describes the search terms and methods used to access and categorise relevant published resources. The concluding section highlights the policy, programme and research and development implications of the geography of maternal death.

How are maternal deaths identified in developing countries?

All health problems present some generic and some specific challenges for measurement regardless of the setting – community or health facility, developed or developing country.[14] There is a long history of initiatives that have sought to strengthen the capture and use of data to improve health, yet Finagle's Laws still prevail: 'the data we have are not the data we want; the data we want are not the data we need; the data we need are not available'. It is thus a global imperative to continue to improve health measurement methods and systems.[15] In terms of mortality data, it is widely accepted that vital registration is the optimal source, yet serious investment in the development and sustainability of these systems for capturing births as well as deaths, particularly in developing countries, is inadequate.[9] It is estimated that only 25% of all deaths are recorded by vital registration, and in the poorest countries the figure is closer to 5–10%.[16] In the face of weak routine information systems, including health services data, other *ad hoc* sources and approaches have emerged to fill data gaps, such as household surveys, surveillance and special studies using mixed methods and record

Box 1.1	Literature search strategy

Two searches were undertaken, one focusing specifically on place of maternal death and the other on place of all types of death in developing countries. The electronic databases used were Popline, PubMed, Pubmed Central, Science Direct and the University of Aberdeen's Metalibrary, which includes OVID, MEDLINE and JSTOR. The period was restricted to the past 5–10 years depending on the database, and references were limited to the English language. For the first search, the terms and strings used were:

- 'place of death'/'location of death' and 'maternal mortality'
- 'place'/'location' and death and maternal
- 'place'/'location' and death and 'maternal mortality'.

For the second search, the terms and strings used were:

- 'place of death'/'location of death' and 'developing countries' (also used 'less developed countries' OR 'low income countries'
- 'place'/'location' and death and 'developing countries'.

This was then repeated using 'infant mortality'/'child mortality'/'adult mortality'/'cause of death'/'geograph*' (depending on database and the original number of hits).

The first search yielded 68 hits and the second 209. The abstracts for these articles were then scanned by the authors for relevance to the four categories of co-variates of place of death used in the paper – sociodemographic, economic, physical accessibility, and obstetric need and care. Forty-six full papers deemed relevant from the abstracts were retrieved and read. Not all of these articles are cited in the paper but the references are available on request.

linkage. For maternal deaths, this diversity is a positive development since studies have shown repeatedly that relying on single sources invariably leads to underestimation, in both developed and developing countries.[17,18] A study in Accra,[19] for instance, showed that 44% of maternal deaths would be missed if only official reports were used. A menu of measurement options is thus essential to enable diverse settings to meet diverse needs for information, such as monitoring the magnitude of maternal mortality, identifying socio-economic determinants or assessing substandard clinical care.[20]

Finding deaths

As for all cause-specific categories of death, identifying maternal cases involves two distinct steps:

1. finding deaths – among women of reproductive age, usually defined as 15–49 years
2. ascertaining the cause – in this case, causes associated with pregnancy and childbirth.

Much has been written about these two steps and the challenges they present, and several guides have been developed.[21–23] In terms of finding all deaths among women of reproductive age, the key distinction is between population-based versus health services-based sources. The former category includes vital registration, censuses, surveys and surveillance; the latter category includes the health management information system (including patient and administrative registers) and individual case records. While population-based sources can, in theory, capture all deaths regardless of where they occur using relatively simple questions to relatives and community members, health services-based sources, by definition, are essentially limited to deaths that are known to the health system, usually occurring in or brought to health facilities. In practice, however, both groups of sources have some level of selection bias that means particular deaths tend to be omitted. Such exclusion may be on the basis of cause of death (for example, abortion-related), place of usual residence (for example, immigrants), place of death (for example, *en route* to health care) or characteristics of the deceased (for example, poorest women). The challenge in many developing countries is being able to identify and adjust for such biases since reliable and representative comparator data sets are often lacking. A variety of proxy methods for assessment of bias, many from demography, have evolved since the 1960s and new ones continue to emerge, such as the approach developed by the Institute of Health Metrics and Evaluation.[24]

Identifying maternal deaths

Once the death of a woman of reproductive age is identified, a process for establishing and classifying the cause and the timing in relation to pregnancy is applied. The current International Classification of Diseases (ICD-10) definition of maternal death requires sufficient information to enable inclusion of causes 'related to or aggravated by pregnancy or its management' but exclusion of accidental or incidental causes and deaths beyond 42 days postpartum.[25] In recent years, the category of 'late maternal deaths' has also been used in some countries: these are deaths occurring between 42 days and 12 months postpartum. For those data sources that include medical certification (or at least where physician diagnosis is recorded), cause-specific identification of maternal deaths is possible. An estimated half of all countries in sub-Saharan Africa and South Asia do not have cause data for any types of death.[9] Moreover, research and special enquiries have shown high levels of misclassification even where cause data are available. In Mozambique, for instance, a retrospective analysis published in 2009[26] of maternal deaths in Maputo Central Hospital using autopsy as the gold standard found major clinical diagnostic errors in 40% of cases.

In population-based data sources such as household surveys there are typically two bases on which maternal deaths are identified among all deaths in women of reproductive age: time of death in relation to history of pregnancy, and cause of death. Given the difficulty of capturing reliable cause data for deaths outside of health facilities, an alternative definition has arisen: 'pregnancy-related deaths' defined on the basis of occurring during the interval from onset of pregnancy to 42 days postpartum, irrespective of the medical cause of death. These pregnancy-related deaths are typically what are captured by most population-based data sets in developing countries, although the term 'maternal death' still tends to be used. The 'sisterhood method', for example, asks siblings about the survival of their adult sisters and then ascertains time of death in relation to pregnancy status.[27] The pregnancy-related definition differs from ICD-10 by including accidental or incidental causes, but these additional deaths are generally regarded as representing a small proportion of the total and thus their inclusion produces minimal errors in estimates relative to the greater likelihood of missing deaths.[23] In the absence of physician verification of cause of death, particularly for events in the community, verbal autopsies (VA) are commonly used in surveys, surveillance or special studies. Here relatives or those in attendance close to the time of death report signs and symptoms. These data are then assigned to a probable medical cause of death using physician panels or computer-based algorithms, such as InterVA-M.[28,29]

Identifying place of maternal death

There are clearly significant challenges to finding deaths and determining whether they are maternal, many of which are common to other health outcomes. Nevertheless, with adequate resources and the application of suitable approaches, it is possible – indeed essential – for developing countries to have relevant data to plan, implement and monitor programmes to reduce maternal deaths. Efficient data capture implies that key associated factors, which might help to explain any variations found, are acquired concurrently. The alternative sources and methods used to capture and classify maternal deaths described above vary considerably in terms of being able to construct a useful picture of one of the most basic of variables, place of death. While most vital registration systems and death certificates include place of residence and place of death, these data are often not readily available in an aggregated form, in some situations for reasons of confidentiality. Health services data, on the other hand, often do not routinely report place of usual residence for deaths or pattern of referral, so that issues of access to care cannot be explored. Household surveys, surveillance or special studies may ascertain these details through questions to relatives, although one of the major sources for developing countries, the Demographic and Health Surveys (DHS), does not usually ascertain place of maternal death or usual residence in their use of the sisterhood method.[30]

Drawing on existing frameworks for investigating geospatial patterns of health outcomes, two main perspectives on place of maternal death are used in this chapter: geographical and categorical.[31] The former focuses on describing where maternal deaths occur in relation to political–administrative boundaries, such as world regions or districts. The latter categorises 'place' by type of venue, such as home or health facility, and relates this to other key co-variates such as cause and socio-economic status.

Where in the world do maternal deaths happen?

The simple answer to this question is everywhere. Maternal deaths have yet to be eliminated in any country, despite the oft-quoted World Health Organization (WHO) figure of 88–98% being preventable with timely and effective intervention.[32] These deaths are, however, extremely rare in many developed countries, to the point where the commonly used statistic, the MMR, fluctuates wildly on an annual basis. In such settings, debates rage about shifting from using maternal deaths to inform policy and practice to using 'near misses' (life-threatening complications) and about creating cross-national estimates, such as for the European Union.[33,34]

Global distribution of maternal deaths

International estimates of maternal mortality are co-produced by agencies of the United Nations and the most recent figures available at the time of writing are for 2005.[4] These figures, together with other relevant maternal health indicators, have featured prominently in several international documents, such as the 2008 UNICEF *Report Card on Maternal Mortality*.[35] The stark concentration of maternal mortality in the poorest countries is seen clearly in Figure 1.1. This presents the estimated lifetime risk, essentially the probability of a woman dying of maternal causes during her reproductive life. The difference between the highest lifetime risk of 1 in 7 for Niger and the lowest of 1 in 48 000 for Ireland reveals maternal mortality as the area of public health exhibiting the greatest gap between developing and developed countries.[4] At a global level, and given the vastly different sizes of country populations,

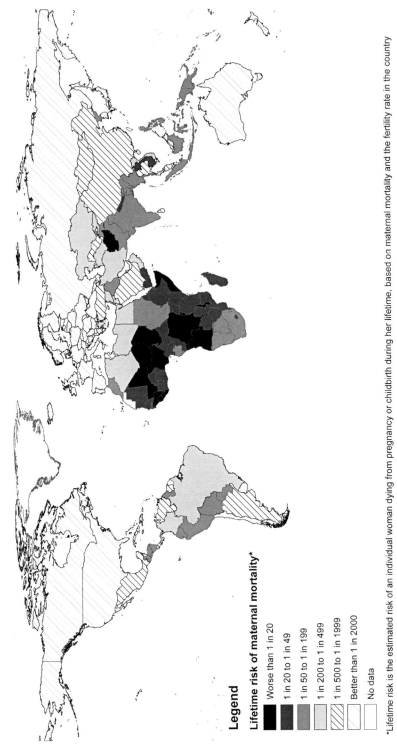

Legend

Lifetime risk of maternal mortality*

- Worse than 1 in 20
- 1 in 20 to 1 in 49
- 1 in 50 to 1 in 199
- 1 in 200 to 1 in 499
- 1 in 500 to 1 in 1999
- Better than 1 in 2000
- No data

*Lifetime risk is the estimated risk of an individual woman dying from pregnancy or childbirth during her lifetime, based on maternal mortality and the fertility rate in the country

Figure 1.1 Estimated lifetime risk of maternal death in 2005; data from World Health Organization[4]

relative measures of maternal mortality such as rates, ratios and proportions are crucial. However, for advocacy purposes, the estimated number of deaths paints a powerful picture. In 2005, just ten countries accounted for almost two-thirds of the estimated annual total of 536 000 maternal deaths. This geographic clustering reflects countries with large populations and high birth rates, such as India, and some also with high levels of obstetric risk, such as Ethiopia. A number of mapping initiatives, such as Gapminder and Worldmapper, provide alternative and novel forms of visual presentation of these and other health-related data.[36,37] However, given the data constraints mentioned earlier, it is also important to recognise the crude nature of global pictures of the magnitude of maternal mortality, as is apparent in Figure 1.2, which shows the high proportion of countries without any empirical estimates.

Efforts to understand or explain the geographical distribution of maternal deaths, as for other mortality outcomes, have tended to rely on correlational analyses of varying degrees of sophistication.[38,39] The overall degree of explanatory power of variance in national levels of maternal mortality of such exercises is generally poor, with the inability to allow adequately for confounding between variables and problems of data reliability often being cited as the main reasons for this. Moreover, some analyses reveal significant outliers, for example when the MMR is correlated with national income levels or the percentage of deliveries with health professionals present. One angle for further investigating these and other associations is to look for geographical patterns within countries.

Patterns of maternal mortality at subnational levels

Robust population-based estimates of maternal mortality at subnational levels are lacking in many parts of the world. Even in countries with complete civil registration and good attribution of cause of death, estimates are often released only for major geopolitical areas, in part owing to small numbers. Of the 106 developing countries regarded as without vital registration in 2005, only about 16% had data that could yield reasonably stable subnational estimates of maternal mortality.[40] Table 1.1 illustrates the wide range of MMR within selected countries. Expressed in this way, the estimates not only emphasise the need for tailored subnational plans but also highlight the limitations of relying on crude national averages. For example, India and Ghana appear different in terms of their national MMRs, with non-overlapping confidence intervals to the estimates. Yet some states of India appear to experience a similar magnitude of maternal mortality to some regions of Ghana. Once again, some words of caution are needed regarding data reliability and the stability of estimates at subnational levels.[41] Nevertheless, such geographically specific information has been found to act as an effective prompt for further investigation and action as seen historically, for example, with the panels set up in the 1930s in Britain and more recently with the local area maternal mortality committees in Brazil in the late 1990s.[2,42] Indeed, interest in rights-based approaches to maternal mortality reduction and reporting has been catalysed in part by the availability of local-level data on deaths combined with powerful information on the location and quality of health services.[43]

The use of geographic information systems (GIS) to map burdens and foci of care has been an important public health development in developing countries. As yet, this has had comparatively limited application in the maternal and newborn health arena, particularly in relation to mortality. The Service Provision Assessment and Service Availability Mapping initiatives of DHS and WHO, respectively, have provided useful planning data in selected countries but have not typically been linked to health

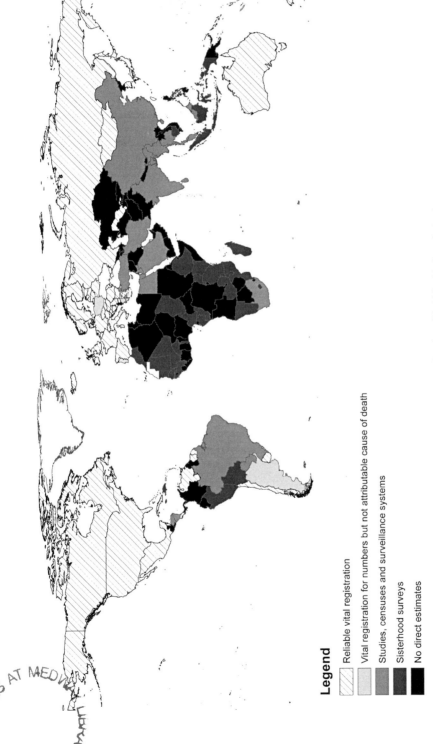

Legend

Reliable vital registration

Vital registration for numbers but not attributable cause of death

Studies, censuses and surveillance systems

Sisterhood surveys

No direct estimates

Figure 1.2   Sources of data used for national estimates of maternal mortality; data from World Health Organizat on[4]

Table 1.1 National and subnational estimates of maternal mortality for selected countries

Country	Reference year(s) for deaths	Data source	Level	Range	MMR[a] (95% CI)	National urban MMR[a] (95% CI)	National rural MMR[a] (95% CI)
Bangladesh[74]	1998–2001	Household survey of deaths in the previous 3 years	National Division	– Lowest (Rajshahi) Highest (Sylhet)	322 (253–391) 223 (96–351) 471 (259–682)	262 (62–463)	326 (251–401)
Egypt[66]	2000	RAMOS	National Region	– Lowest (Metropolitan) Highest (Frontier)	84 (80–89) 48 (40–56) 120 (78–161)	N/A	N/A
Ghana[75]	1997–2007	Household survey using direct sisterhood method[b]	National Region[c]	– Lowest (Ashanti) Highest (Eastern)	416 (313–420) 308 (113–503) 594 (302–885)	464 (265–662)	354 (244–463)
India[76]	2004–06	Sample registration system	National State	– Lowest (Kerala) Highest (Assam)	254 (239–269) 95 (45–145) 480 (355–606)	N/A	N/A
South Africa[77]	2000–01	Demographic census (10% microsample)	National Province	– Lowest (Western Cape) Highest (Kwazulu Natal)	551 (505–601) 245 (161–372) 772 (659–905)	505 (446–572)	604 (535–682)

CI = confidence interval; MMR = maternal mortality ratio; RAMOS = reproductive age mortality survey

[a] All estimates of MMR are derived from the same data source for that country

[b] Place of residence of reported maternal deaths is based on respondents' place of residence (siblings of deceased)

[c] Separate estimates are available for three of ten regions and a combined estimate for the remaining seven regions

outcomes.[44,45] An illustration of the potential from mapping deaths is provided by the work of Immpact in south-east Burkina Faso.[28] Here a complete enumeration of all deaths in women aged 15–49 years from 2001 to 2006 was conducted in two districts, Ouargaye and Diapaga, and verbal autopsies were gathered and processed using InterVA-M. Personal digital assistants (PDAs) were used to record GPS coordinates for all households visited, so enabling maps to be drawn showing the place of residence of women who had died and the location of health facilities.[46] For the district of Diapaga, which covers an area of about 14 780 km² and had a population of just over 250 000 in 2001, 300 maternal deaths were identified and mapped, as illustrated in Figure 1.3.[47] The Kulldorff spatial scan statistic was used to test for clusters using the *SaTScan* version 2.1 software package.[48,49] The analysis revealed three statistically significant clusters of higher maternal mortality in different geographic locations. Further possible steps in investigating these patterns would be to adjust for potential risk factors, such as distance to nearest health centre and wealth, and to relate place of residence to place of death.

What are the key differentials of place of maternal death?

The second perspective relating to place of death, categorical analysis, looks at categories of factors associated with maternal death that describe and help to explain place through individual-level analysis. In the literature searches for this paper, no

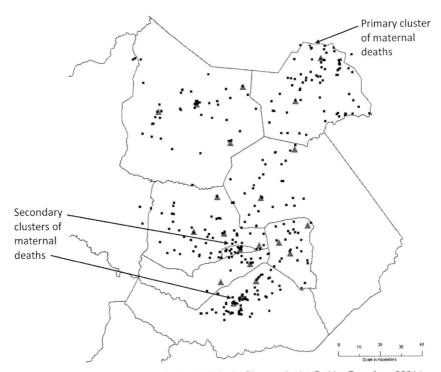

Figure 1.3   Map of maternal deaths (*n* = 300) in the Diapaga district, Burkina Faso, from 2001 to 2006; ■ = place of residence of maternal death; ▲ = health facility (one district hospital and 18 health centres); data from Immpact, University of Aberdeen

reviews were found specifically on place of maternal death nor, surprisingly, for other causes of death in developing countries (see Box 1.1). However, two structured reviews published in 2007 and 2009 focus on determinants of place of delivery, many of which are relevant to location of maternal death.[50,51] This is because an estimated half of all maternal deaths, and indeed 25–45% of neonatal deaths, occur during labour or the first 24 hours postnatal, and thus place of delivery is highly correlated with location of death,[52,53] as will be discussed later. The review by Gabrysch and Campbell[51] provides a useful framework that is adapted here to produce four main categories of co-variates: sociodemographic, economic, physical accessibility, and obstetric need and care. Our literature search focused on articles presenting reasonably large-scale studies and special enquiries on maternal deaths that included findings relevant to the four categories. Table 1.2 indicates the range of co-variates identified. Although several published series with place of death data were found, very few presented more than simple frequency distributions. Several appear also to have gathered information on some of the factors listed in Table 1.2 and thus may offer opportunities for further analysis.

Types of place of maternal death

The simplest differentiation of place is 'home' and 'health facility', reflecting the two main bases for capturing maternal deaths discussed earlier. In developing countries, typically only population-based sources of data can report on both types of place.

Table 1.2 Categorisation of co-variates of place of maternal death

Category	Co-variate
Sociodemographic	Maternal age
	Marital status
	Maternal education
	Ethnic group
	Women's autonomy
Economic	Wealth quintile
	Health insurance
	Occupation
Physical accessibility	Rural–urban residence
	Distance to health care (by type of place and functionality)
	Transport availability
Obstetric need and care	Parity
	Pregnancy status: pregnant, labour/delivery, postpartum
	Pregnancy wantedness
	Complications
	Cause of death (medical, lay, direct/indirect)
	Uptake of antenatal care
	Birth planning
	Place of delivery
	Attendant at delivery
	Awareness of danger signs
	Uptake of referral
	Care before death
	Length of stay (early discharge)

However, where all deaths are notified to health services regardless of where the death physically occurs (for example, Jamaica), potentially routine health service statistics could report on all places, although in practice this is unusual.[54] Table 1.3 shows proportional distributions of type of place of death using selected population-based sources. Notable findings are the wide overall range in the proportion of maternal deaths in health facilities (18–93%) but also the similarities in the proportion from data sets derived from very different country and health service contexts. The importance of context to understanding levels and patterns of health outcomes has been re-emphasised in several papers.[51,55]

For both 'home' versus 'facility' crude categories, further differentiation can provide useful insights. One complicating factor in terms of the 'home' category, for example, arises from patterns of migration close to the time of delivery when, in some cultures, women return to their parents' or parents-in-law's home.[56] This has relevance to continuity of care and health service provision since antenatal care may have been received elsewhere. Such migration can also affect local area statistics since women may be not be counted either at their place of origin or place of temporary residence, again contributing to the invisibility of some maternal deaths.[9] Place of death in health facilities can be further distinguished on the basis of, for example, public or private provision and level of care, as well as functionality in terms of ability to provide basic or emergency obstetric care. A further categorisation of facility-based maternal deaths is according to the ward or department. This can also be an important check on the completeness of recording, with the need for extra vigilance to capture maternal deaths on non-obstetric wards, such as emergency admission, medical wards and intensive care units. Work by Immpact, for example, found more than double the number of maternal deaths, compared with routine returns, by intensive searching of registers for all clinical areas of two hospitals in Banten Province.[57]

Are these patterns in the place of maternal death different from those for other causes of death? Some insights into this can be gained from data sources that ascertain deaths in women of reproductive age before identifying maternal causes. All reproductive age mortality surveys (RAMOS), for example, do this and so can variants of the sisterhood method when place of death is also asked. Figure 1.4 shows this breakdown from selected data sets and indicates that the proportion of maternal deaths in health facilities is consistently higher than that for non-maternal deaths. However there is a major confounding factor for this association, which is that women dying of maternal causes are more likely to be present in health facilities anyway owing to childbirth. One way to adjust for this would be to distinguish between women who attend the health facility because of a complication as opposed to those who attend for a normal delivery. Unfortunately, the data to enable such a distinction to be made are not widely available and this represents a key gap in information, as discussed further below.

Co-variates of place of maternal death

Having described the overall distribution of maternal deaths by place, the logical next line of enquiry is to look at explanatory factors. Table 1.2 proposed four categories of co-variates. Many of these are interrelated and hence multivariate analysis is preferable, with place of death as the dependent variable. To our knowledge, there are no published, large-scale studies or data series that provide this form of controlled analysis of place. The findings presented here are thus mainly from published univariate analyses.

Three of the four categories of co-variates of place of maternal death – sociodemographic, economic and physical accessibility – essentially operate as distal or

Table 1.3 Place of maternal death from large published series (close to or in excess of 100 maternal deaths)

Country	Level	Reference period	Number of maternal deaths	Place of maternal death						Deliveries in health facilities in the general population[a]
				Health facilities			Community		Unknown/ other	
				Hospital	Health centre	All facilities	Home	In transit		
Bangladesh[78]	National	1998–2001 (3 years)	131	–	–	18%	73%	5%	4%	8%
Burkina Faso[73]	Subnational (rural district – Ouargaye)	2002–06 (5 years)	99	21.2%	46.5%	67.7%	30.3%	–	2%	46%[80]
Egypt[66]	National	2000 (1 year)	580	–	–	62%	29%	9%	0	48%[81]
Ghana[73]	Subnational (districts in central region)	2000–05 (5 years)	93	57%	4.3%	61.3%	31.2%	3.2%	4.4%	63.6%[82]
Ghana[19]	Subnational (city – Accra)	2002 (1 year)	179	60%	–	60%	40% at home or in unspecified health facility		1%	79.3% (Greater Accra)[76]
India[82]	Subnational (three remote/rural districts in two states, Orissa and Jharkhand)	2004–06 (~2 years)	103	–	–	28.2%	60.2%	10.7%	1%	15%
Indonesia[60]	Subnational (two mixed rural and urban districts in Banten Province)	2004–05 (2 years)	455	31.6%	1.8%	33.6%	67.4%	–	–	17%[84]
Jamaica[54]	National	2001–03 (3 years)	130	93%	–	93%	7% (all deaths not in facilities)	–	–	~99%
Pakistan[84]	Subnational (major city – Faisalabad)	1989–1993 (4 years)	215	67.4%	–	67.4%	32.6%	–	–	N/A
Zimbabwe[62]	National (11 representative districts)	2006 (1 year)	243	34%	2.1%	38.2%	45.1%	4.1%	12.3%	68.9%

[a] Percentage of deliveries in facilities reported by living women for same reference period and data source, unless indicated otherwise

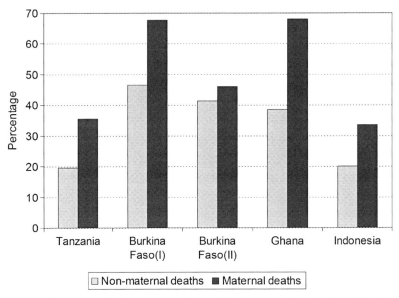

Figure 1.4   Percentage of deaths to women of reproductive age occurring in health facilities by maternal or non-maternal causes; all data sets are subnational, each with more than 200 deaths to women of reproductive age (all causes); sources: Tanzania[72], Burkina Faso I and II[73], Ghana[73] and Indonesia[60]

intermediate determinants of the uptake of care related to pregnancy and childbirth, be this for preventive or curative reasons. Uptake of care, in turn, influences survival prospects in the presence of a problem and thus explains the place of some deaths in health facilities. Sociodemographic factors include those related directly to the risk of complications (for example, age) as well as those affecting decision making for care (for example, a woman's educational level or autonomy).[58] Data on sociodemographic factors are widely available from international survey programmes such as the DHS, which also provide information on uptake of maternity care. Economic factors that may help explain place of maternal death are correlated with sociodemographic factors and also tend to operate through influencing uptake of care. The most common economic factor used in studies of uptake is household poverty. This affects ability to pay for care as well as to reach care promptly and so contributes to both the second and third delays in the McCarthy and Maine conceptual model of the determinants of maternal mortality.[59] There are several published analyses showing a clear association between poverty and risk of maternal death, one reporting a greater than six-fold higher risk in the poorest versus richest groups.[52] The interpretive challenge is to link these patterns with the third category of explanatory factors, physical accessibility to care.

Uptake is related directly and indirectly to the presence of care and carers, whether this is based at a facility or at home. In the presence of severe obstetric complications, it is the second referral level of district hospitals that is most likely to be needed. Physical access to care is typically considered in terms of place of residence, distance and transport availability. Rural or urban residence is a common differential for levels of maternal mortality, with a higher burden usually found in rural areas. Table 1.1 included levels for selected countries and, although there are differences between the rural and urban estimates, the confidence intervals overlap. The proportion of deaths in facilities might be expected to be high in urban areas owing to the availability of care, higher average income and education levels and a possible propensity to deliver in institutions, in part because of a lack of privacy in crowded urban homes and to the absence of relatives nearby to attend. Several studies, however, have found surprisingly high levels of maternal mortality in urban areas, with significant proportions both of deaths among adolescents and deaths arising from unsafe abortions.[19,60] Financial rather than physical barriers to emergency care have emerged as key explanatory factors for deaths, particularly as women may not have ready access to relatives to help cover costs (for example, for caesarean section).[61] Estimation for populations with high mobility, as found in urban areas, is, however, particularly problematic. Here the number of deaths and births may be inflated by women who migrate to town to stay with relatives close to the time of delivery in order to have better access to referral facilities or, conversely, deflated by women who return to their rural place of origin, as noted earlier. Robust description and understanding of these migratory patterns around the time of delivery is generally lacking and warrants further research to help inform service planning.

In rural areas, physical inaccessibility to emergency care has been reported as a risk factor for maternal death in numerous studies.[50,62] Combined with higher poverty levels and thus lack of finance, physical distance contributes to lack of seeking any care or to major delays. Studies also show, however, that distance is mediated by transport considerations, both in terms of state of the roads, in general and seasonally, and the availability of vehicles or other modes for transport when there is an emergency.[63] Problems of transport and access are reflected in maternal deaths in transit, as shown for selected studies in Table 1.3, and are highlighted in a 2009 paper[64] that compared maternal deaths with near misses. This found higher ratios of near misses to deaths in urban areas and the converse in remote rural areas.

The fourth category of co-variates of place of maternal death indicated in Table 1.2 reflects obstetric need and care. In terms of place and cause of death, a number of studies have shown distinctly different patterns between home and facilities. Generally speaking, proportional distributions show indirect deaths to be more common in facilities than at home, although this may vary according to the dominant cause and the definition of maternal death used. For example, in populations with high prevalence of AIDS, there may be a tendency for all deaths due to this cause to take place at home and, where a 90-day or late maternal death definition is adopted, the proportional contribution from this cause is particularly marked.[65] Figure 1.5 provides an illustration of different patterns of cause by place. This large data set from West Java shows a statistically significant difference (Pearson $\chi^2 = 27.325$; $P = 0.011$) between home and facility maternal deaths in terms of causes and provides valuable insights for local-level planning of services. The cause showing the largest difference by place of death was chronic non-infectious disease, constituting 11% of deaths at home and 21% in health facilities.

Indicators of obstetric risk, such as parity, and of quality of care, such as timely and appropriate use of life-saving surgery, provide further insights into place of maternal death. Findings from confidential enquiries as well as routine audits of maternal and newborn deaths show poor quality of obstetric care to be a major predictor of deaths in facilities.[33,66,67] This factor is, however, complex to define and measure. Moreover, disentangling iatrogenic from essentially unpreventable deaths owing to, for example, poor state of the woman on admission to a facility is also complex. The apparently higher risks of death among deliveries in facilities and with skilled attendants noted earlier, and identified by several studies, also reflects the limitations of analysis that has

(a)

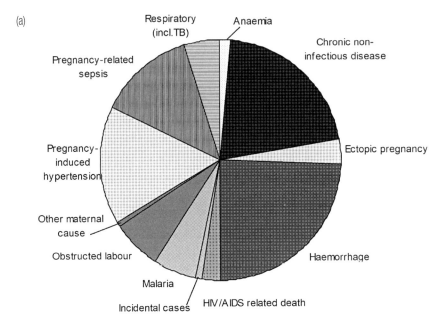

(b)

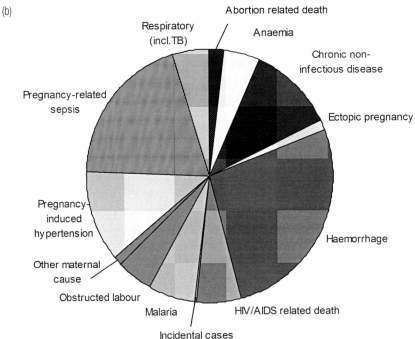

Figure 1.5   Cause and place of maternal deaths, Serang and Pandeglang districts, Banten Province, Indonesia 2004–05 (26 deaths omitted owing to missing information on place and/or cause): (a) maternal deaths in health facilities ($n=152$), which includes deaths in hospitals, health centres (puskesmas), maternity homes (polindes) and en route between facilities; (b) maternal deaths at home ($n=296$); data from Immpact Indonesia[60]

not been able to adjust for predisposing factors such as complication on admission and absence of or poor quality of prior contact with services.[54,68] The complex relationship between place of death and place of delivery warrants further investigation. Table 1.3 suggests a crude relationship at the population level between the proportions of maternal deaths and deliveries occurring in facilities, with the former typically higher than the latter. This supports the logic that women are generally more likely to seek facility care for delivery when there is a complication than when there is not. However, the relationship is not consistent in Table 1.3, with the series from Zimbabwe showing a reverse pattern, and this highlights the ecological fallacy of such aggregate-level analysis.

A step forward in understanding place of death and place of delivery can be achieved with individual-level analysis. Table 1.4 shows this for three data series from different country contexts relating place of death and place of birth. For two of the series, odds ratios derived from simple bivariate analysis show place of delivery to have a significant association with place of death, with women delivering at home having a higher relative odds of dying at home than in facilities compared with women delivering in facilities, with an odds ratio of 15 in the Indonesian series. Although this individual level of analysis is an improvement over crude correlations, as noted earlier, ideally multivariate analysis is needed to adjust for confounding factors. A preliminary indication of the potential of this approach can be given using the Immpact data from Indonesia. This not only enables bivariate analysis of several of the co-variates of place of death flagged in Table 1.2 but also multivariate (adjusted) logistic regression.

Table 1.4   Place of death and place of delivery from three selected data sets

Country	Source details	Place of delivery	Place of death[a] Home	Facility	In transit[b]	Unadjusted OR[a] (95% CI)
Egypt[66]	National, reference period 1 year (2000), 580 maternal deaths	Home	55 (48.2%)	42 (14.8%)	17	5.37 (3.28–8.78)
		Facility	59 (51.8%)	242 (85.2%)	21	
		In transit[b]	0	0	1	
		Undelivered	55	76	12	
India[83]	Subnational (three remote/rural districts in two states, Orissa and Jharkhand), ~2 year reference period (2004–06), 103 maternal deaths	Home	42[c] (100%)	14 (64%)	2	N/A
		Facility	0 (0%)	8 (36%)	1	
		In transit[b]	0	0	0	
		Undelivered	21	7	2	
Indonesia[60,d]	Subnational (two districts in Banten Province), ~2 year reference period (2004–05), 467 maternal deaths	Home	189 (87.5%)	33 (31.7%)	6	15.06 (8.46–26.82)
		Facility	27 (12.5%)	71 (68.3%)	0	
		In transit[b]	0	0	0	
		Undelivered	86	48	7	

OR = odds ratio

[a] Percentages and odds ratios exclude women undelivered and in transit

[b] Refers to in transit to a health facility

[c] Includes one death in the community but not at home

[d] Deaths in facilities include in hospitals, health centres (puskesmas), maternity homes (polindes) and en route between facilities

Table 1.5 shows that statistically significant crude or unadjusted odds ratios were found for place of death with maternal education, wealth, residence, insurance, antenatal care, skilled attendant at delivery and place at delivery. For example, women living in the remotest areas were nearly five times more likely to die at home than in a facility, whereas urban women were twice as likely to die in a facility (a relative odds ratio for remote women dying at home of about 9). Table 1.6 presents the adjusted analysis and reveals that only two variables – presence of a health facility in the village and place of delivery – remain statistically significant predictors of death at home versus in a health facility after allowing for all other variables in the model. Women delivering at home, for example, were nine times more likely to die at home than in health facilities. These illustrative findings emphasise the potential of controlled analysis for unpacking complex interrelationships between factors determining place and risk of death.[64]

Conclusion

Levels of maternal mortality in the poorest parts of the world today remain high and apparently resistant to progress. There have been similar moments in the history of developed countries when these avoidable deaths have not responded to intervention, which is seen as a 'great blot on public health administration'.[1] These so-called dark periods in history have been overturned in comparatively short intervals of time and with multiple interventions. In parts of the UK, for instance, the MMR fell by over 75% between 1935 and 1950, and indeed by 44% over the 5 years from 1940, during a time of international conflict.[2,69] Five years is the period now left for the MDGs to be delivered. MDG 5 may indeed be achieved for some parts of the developing world such as South Asia but remains a distant prospect for other regions such as sub-Saharan Africa.[40] Data on who is dying, where and why have been fundamental ingredients in the successful reduction of maternal mortality in the distant past and in more recent times in transitional countries such as Jamaica and Malaysia.[54,70] Ensuring the availability of such data should be seen as an investment and as part of the essential package of interventions to achieve MDG 5. The 'where, who and why' of maternal deaths are inextricably linked. This chapter has emphasised the 'where' and sought to show the power and potential of the geography of maternal death for informing policies and programmes.

Maternal death is not a random event in space or time but clusters in certain areas and among certain women. A major policy implication is the importance of targeting care to match need. Such targeting is particularly challenging when marginalised and vulnerable groups of women remain outside the health system and beyond the reach of routine data sources. The poorest women, for example, are most likely to die at home and without trace, and a similar invisibility exists in specific geographic circumstances such as fragile states. Tracking deaths in relation to place thus not only reveals excluded or vulnerable populations but also provides a marker of the functioning of the wider health system. New initiatives, such as removing financial barriers to emergency delivery care, may produce shifts in place of death that reflect the success of the scheme. Geographically presented data, such as maps of deaths, also have value for advocacy purposes as well as for local-level planning and programming. Place of death is a relatively simple and unambiguous data item to gather, it can prompt a cascade of questions when integrated into routine audits and it can be added to major survey programmes where maternal mortality is ascertained. Deaths outside of facilities after contact with the health system, for example, may point to inappropriate early discharge policies as well as raise questions on the quality of care.

Table 1.5   Univariate analysis of place of maternal death by key variables, Serang and Pandeglang districts, Banten Province, Indonesia, 2004–05

Theme	Variable	Place of death		P value	Unadjusted OR of dying at home versus in a facility (95% CI)
		Facility[a] (maximum n = 153)	Home (maximum n = 302)		
Sociodemographic	Education (n = 447)			0.01	
	No schooling	7 (26%)	20 (74%)		1.00
	Primary	93 (30%)	216 (70%)		2.43 (0.95–6.21)
	Secondary or higher	51 (46%)	60 (54%)		1.97 (1.27–3.09)
	Age (n = 455)			0.11	
	20–34 years	84 (30%)	196 (70%)		1.00
	< 20 years	16 (41%)	23 (59%)		0.62 (0.31–1.23)
	≥ 35 years	53 (39%)	83 (61%)		0.67 (0.44–1.04)
Economic	Wealth (n = 445)			<0.001	
	Poorest	17 (19%)	74 (81%)		5.16 (2.61–10.19)
	Poor	23 (24%)	73 (76%)		3.76 (1.99–7.11)
	Middle	22 (26%)	62 (74%)		3.34 (1.74–6.40)
	Rich	42 (46%)	49 (54%)		1.38 (0.76–2.51)
	Richest	45 (54%)	38 (46%)		1.00
	Insurance (n = 455)			<0.001	
	Self-paid	108 (29%)	264 (71%)		4.40 (1.44–13.43)
	Poor insurance	36 (52%)	33 (48%)		1.65 (0.50–5.43)
	Private insurance	9 (64%)	5 (36%)		1.00
Physical accessibility	Residence (n = 455)			<0.001	
	Urban	45 (65%)	24 (35%)		1.00
	Rural	91 (32%)	194 (68%)		3.40 (2.30–7.00)
	Remote	17 (17%)	84 (83%)		9.27 (4.51–19.02)
Obstetric need and care	Parity (n = 416)			0.86	
	0	11 (37%)	19 (63%)		0.77 (0.34–1.78)
	1	36 (32%)	78 (68%)		0.97 (0.56–1.68)
	2–3	39 (31%)	87 (69%)		1.00
	≥ 4	51 (35%)	95 (65%)		0.84 (0.50–1.39)
	Time of death (n = 455)			0.25	
	While pregnant	40 (38%)	65 (62%)		1.00
	During labour and delivery	44 (37%)	76 (63%)		1.06 (0.62–1.83)
	Postpartum	69 (30%)	161 (70%)		1.44 (0.89–2.33)
	Antenatal care (n = 440)			<0.001	
	No antenatal care	20 (17%)	98 (83%)		3.40 (2.00–5.78)
	Antenatal care with health provider	132 (41%)	190 (59%)		1.00
	Skilled birth attendant (n = 455)			<0.001	
	Skilled birth attendant	82 (60%)	55 (40%)		1.00
	No skilled birth attendant	23 (12.5%)	161 (87.5%)		10.44 (6.00–18.17)
	No delivery	48 (36%)	86 (64%)		2.67 (1.63–4.37)
	Place of delivery (n = 454)			<0.001	
	Health facility	71 (72%)	27 (28%)		1.00
	At home	33 (15%)	189 (85%)		15.06 (8.46–26.82)
	No delivery	48 (36%)	86 (64%)		4.71 (2.67–8.30)

OR = odd ratio

[a] Deaths in facilities include in hospitals, health centres (puskesmas), maternity homes (polindes) and en route between facilities

Table 1.6   Multivariate analysis of place of maternal death by key variables, Serang and Pandeglang districts, Banten Province, Indonesia, 2004–05

Theme	Variable	P value	Adjusted OR of dying at home versus in a facility[a] (95% CI)
Sociodemographic and economic	Wealth[b] and education	0.4	
	Poor, no secondary schooling		1.96 (0.89–4.32)
	Poor, with secondary schooling		2.17 (0.39–12.01)
	Middle, no secondary schooling		1.74 (0.75–4.06)
	Middle, with secondary schooling		2.60 (0.41–16.67)
	Rich, no secondary schooling		1.02 (0.48–2.17)
	Rich, with secondary schooling		1.00
	Age group	0.12	
	20–34 years		1.00
	< 20 years		0.49 (0.19–1.24)
	≥ 35 years		0.61 (0.32–1.16)
Economic	Insurance	0.41	
	Self paid		0.69 (0.18–2.60)
	Poor insurance		0.46 (0.11–1.94)
	Private insurance		1.00
Physical accessibility	Residence	0.13	
	Rural		2.01 (0.98–4.13)
	Remote		2.42 (0.91–6.38)
	Urban		1.00
Obstetric need and care	Parity	0.88	
	0		1.57 (0.51–4.79)
	1		1.03 (0.50–2.15)
	2–3		1.00
	≥ 4		0.85 (0.43–1.69)
	Unknown		1.14 (0.45–2.85)
	Time of death	0.50	
	Delivery		1.11 (0.40–3.10)
	Postpartum		1.61 (0.51–5.09)
	While pregnant		1.00
	Antenatal care	0.19	
	Antenatal care with a provider		1.57 (0.80–3.06)
	No antenatal care		1.00
	Place of delivery	<0.001	
	At home		9.23 (4.69–18.20)
	No delivery		3.70 (1.27–10.78)
	Health facility		1.00
	Health facility available in village	0.04	
	No		1.79 (1.04–3.08)
	Yes		1.00
	Health provider resident in village	0.36	
	No		1.45 (0.77–2.72)
	Not known		0.97 (0.42–2.21)
	Yes		1.00

[a] Deaths in facilities include in hospitals, health centres (puskesmas), maternity homes (polindes) and en route between facilities

[b] Wealth quintiles regrouped into three: poor and poorest, middle, rich and richest

Similarly, deaths occurring at home in urban areas where physical availability of care is not a major barrier can illuminate obstacles of cost, confidence in service and other restrictions on women's movements.

As a field of study, the geography of maternal death has several issues warranting further research and development. In terms of data gaps, for example, there is a need to improve the capture of the variable 'place' in both routine and population-based data sources, for deaths as well as births. Studies are needed that enable individual-level investigation of associations between place of delivery and place of death, and that also help to build a better understanding of women's migration around the time of delivery. Stronger conceptual and analytical frameworks need to be developed as well as indicators that capture key contextual factors. Finally, a number of new technologies for gathering and presenting data have great potential for improving the availability as well as the robustness of information on vital events and their place of occurrence. Mobile phones to report deaths and births, for example, may speed up reporting processes and reduce omissions, and can be linked to GIS technology to locate events.[11] Similarly, interactive maps and model-based geostatistics have yet to be widely applied to the area of maternal mortality and lessons should be learnt from other fields already using these techniques.[12] These devices, however, also raise new questions on the confidentiality of information and may require extra safeguards for families as well as ethical procedures for release of data. Ultimately, the invisibility of maternal deaths in the poorest countries must be tackled if progress towards lower mortality is to be achieved and shown to be achieved – in other words, for history to repeat itself.

Acknowledgements

The authors would like to thank colleagues in Immpact, particularly David Braunholtz, for commenting on an earlier version of this chapter, and Lisa Davidson for assistance with the references. The chapter draws heavily on previously unpublished data from Immpact and thus the original funders should be acknowledged: the Bill & Melinda Gates Foundation, the UK Department for International Development and USAID. The authors were stimulated to work on this chapter by a continuing collaborative project – The Birth Atlas – involving the White Ribbon Alliance (Brigid McConville and Katy Woods), the University of Southampton and Immpact at the University of Aberdeen, funded by the Norwegian Government. The views expressed herein are solely those of the authors.

References

1.   Wood K. Quotation by Sir Kingsley Wood, Minister of Health, Great Britain. 1935. In: Loudon I. *Death in Childbirth: An International Study of Maternal Care and Maternal Mortality 1800–1950*. New York: Oxford University Press; 1992. p. 211.

2.   Loudon I. *Death in Childbirth: An International Study of Maternal Care and Maternal Mortality 1800–1950*. New York: Oxford University Press; 1992. p. 543.

3.   *The Times*. Maternal mortality. 23 June 1934. p. 13.

4.   World Health Organization. *Maternal Mortality in 2005. Estimates Developed by WHO, UNICEF, UNFPA and the World Bank*. Geneva: WHO; 2007.

5.   The White Ribbon Alliance for Safe Motherhood [www.whiteribbonalliance.org].

6.   The Partnership for Maternal, Newborn & Child Health [www.who.int/pmnch/en].

7.   Van Lerberghe W, De Brouwere V. Of blind alleys and things that have worked: history's lessons on reducing maternal mortality. In: Van Lerberghe W, De Brouwere V, editors. *Safe Motherhood*

Strategies: a Review of the Evidence. Studies in Health Services Organisation and Policy 17. Antwerp: ITG; 2001. p. 7–33.

8. Graham WJ, Hussein J. The right to count. *Lancet* 2004;363:67–8.

9. Setel PW, MacFarlane SB, Szreter S, Mikkelsen L, Jha P, Stout S, *et al.* A scandal of invisibility: making everyone count by counting everyone. *Lancet* 2007;370:1569–77.

10. Szreter S. The population health approach in historical perspective. *Am J Public Health* 2003;93:421–431.

11. Porter R. *The Greatest Benefit to Mankind. A Medical History of Humanity from Antiquity to the Present.* London: Fontana Press; 1992. p. 413.

12. Hay SI, Guerra CA, Gething PW, Patil AP, Tatem AJ, Noor AM, *et al.* A world malaria map: *Plasmodium falciparum* endemicity in 2007. *PLoS Med* 2009;6:e1000048.

13. Immpact (Initiative for Maternal Mortality Programme Assessment) [www.immpact-international. org].

14. Murray CJ, Frenk J. Health metrics and evaluation: strengthening the science. *Lancet* 2008;371:1191–9.

15. Boerma T, Stansfield S. Health statistics now: are we making the right investments? *Lancet* 2007;369:779–86.

16. Murray CJ. Towards good practice for health statistics: lessons from the Millennium Development Goal health indicators. *Lancet* 2007;369:862–73.

17. Horon IL. Underreporting of maternal deaths on death certificates and the magnitude of the problem of maternal mortality. *Am J Public Health* 2005;95:478–82.

18. Songane FF, Bergstrom S. Quality of registration of maternal deaths in Mozambique: a community-based study in rural and urban areas. *Soc Sci Med* 2002;54:23–31.

19. Zakariah AY, Alexander S, van Roosmalen J, Buekens P, Kwawukume EY, Frimpong P. Reproductive age mortality survey (RAMOS) in Accra, Ghana. *Reprod Health* 2009;6:7.

20. Maternal Mortality Measurement Resource [www.maternal-mortality-measurement.org].

21. Graham WJ, Ahmed S, Stanton C, Abou-Zahr CL, Campbell OM. Measuring maternal mortality: An overview of opportunities and options for developing countries. *BMC Med* 2008;6:12.

22. World Health Organization. *Beyond the Numbers: Reviewing Maternal Deaths and Complications to Make Pregnancy Safer.* Geneva: WHO; 2004.

23. Hill K, El Arifeen S, Koenig M, Al-Sabir A, Jamil K, Raggers H. How should we measure maternal morality in the developing world? A comparison of household deaths and sibling history approaches. *Bull World Health Organ* 2006;84:173–180.

24. Murray CL, Lopez A, Barofsky J, Bryson-Cahn C, Lozano R. Estimating population cause-specific mortality fractions from in-hospital mortality: validation of a new method. *PLoS Med* 2007;4:e326.

25. World Health Organization. *International Statistical Classification of Diseases and Related Health Problems.* Tenth revision. Geneva: WHO; 1992.

26. Ordi J, Ismail MR, Carrilho C, Romagosa C, Osman N, Machungo F, *et al.* Clinico-pathological discrepancies in the diagnosis of causes of maternal death in sub-Saharan Africa: Retrospective analysis. *PLoS Med* 2009;6:e1000036.

27. Graham WJ, Brass W, Snow RW. Estimating maternal mortality: the sisterhood method. *Stud Fam Plann* 1989;20:125–35.

28. Fottrell E, Byass P, Ouedraogo TW, Tamini C, Gbangou, A, Sombie I, *et al.* Revealing the burden of maternal mortality: a probabilistic model for determining pregnancy-related causes of death from verbal autopsies. *Popul Health Metr* 2007;5:1.

29. Chandromahan D, Rodrigues LC, Muade GH, Hayes RJ. The validity of verbal autopsies for assessing causes of institutional maternal deaths. *Stud Fam Plann* 1998;29:414–22.

30. Stanton C, Abderrahim N, Hill K. *DHS Maternal Mortality Indicators: an Assessment of Data Quality and Implications for Data Use.* DHS analytical report no. 4. Calverton, MD: Macro International; 1997.

31. Lawson AB. *Statistical Methods in Spatial Epidemiology.* Chichester: John Wiley and Sons; 2001.

32. World Health Organization. *The World Health Report 2005: Make Every Mother and Child Count.* Geneva: WHO; 2005.

33. Lewis G, editor. *Saving Mothers' Lives: Reviewing Maternal Deaths to Make Motherhood Safer 2003–2005. The Seventh Report on Confidential Enquiries into Maternal Deaths in the United Kingdom.* London: CEMACH; 2007.

34. Keirse MJ. Maternal mortality: stalemate or stagnant? *BMJ* 1994;308:354–5.

35. UNICEF. *Progress for Children. A Report Card on Maternal Mortality.* No. 7. New York: UNICEF; 2008.

36. Gapminder [www.gapminder.org].

37. Worldmapper [www.worldmapper.org].

38. Graham W, Bell J, Bullough C. Can skilled attendance at delivery reduce maternal mortality in developing countries? In: De Brouwere V, Van Lerberghe W, editors. *Safe Motherhood Strategies: A Review of the Evidence.* Studies in Health Service Organisation and Policy 17. Antwerp: ITG; 2001. p. 97–130.

39. Shah IH, Say L. Maternal mortality and maternity care from 1990 to 2005: uneven but important gains. *Reprod Health Matters* 2007;15:17–27.

40. Hill K, Thomas K, AbouZahr C, Walker N, Say L, Inoue M, *et al.* Estimates of maternal mortality worldwide between 1990 and 2005: and assessment of valid data. *Lancet* 2007;370:1311–19.

41. ICDDR-B. Selected maternal health indicators obtained by geographical reconnaissance. *Health Sci Bull* 2006;4:12–17.

42. Valongueiro Alves S. Maternal mortality in Pernambuco, Brazil: what has changed in ten years? *Reprod Health Matters* 2007;15:134–44.

43. Hawkins K, Newman K, Thomas D, Carlson C. *Developing a Human Rights Based Approach to Addressing Maternal Mortality: Desk review.* London: DFID Health Resource Centre; 2005.

44. Demographic and Health Surveys Service Provision Assessment [www.measuredhs.com/aboutsurveys/spa/start.cfm].

45. World Health Organization. *Service Availability Mapping.* Geneva: WHO; 2009 [www.who.int/healthinfo/systems/serviceavailabilitymapping/en/index.html].

46. Byass P, Hounton S, Ouedraogo M, Some H, Diallo I, Fottrell E. Direct data capture using hand-held computers in rural Burkina Faso: experiences, benefits and lessons learnt. *Trop Med Int Health* 2008;13 Suppl 1:25–30.

47. Bell JS, Ouedraogo M, Ganaba R, Sombie I, Byass P, Baggaley RF, *et al.* The epidemiology of pregnancy outcomes in rural Burkina Faso. *Trop Med Int Health* 2008;13 Suppl 1:21–43.

48. Kulldorff M. A spatial scan statistic. *Commun Stat Theory Methods* 1997;26:1481–96.

49. Kulldorff M, Rand K, Gherman G, Williams G, DeFrancesco D. *SatSCan – Software for the Spatial and Space-time Scan Statistics.* Version 2.1. Bethesda: National Cancer Institute; 1998.

50. Say L, Raine R. A systematic review of inequalities in the use of maternal health care in developing countries: examining the scale of the problem and the importance of context. *Bull World Health Organ* 2007;85:812–19.

51. Gabrysch S, Campbell OM. Still for far to walk: literature review of the determinants of delivery service use. *BMC Pregnancy Childbirth* 2009;9:34.

52. Ronsmans C, Graham WJ; Lancet Maternal Survival Series steering group. Maternal mortality: who, when, where, and why. *Lancet* 2006;368:1189–200.

53. Lawn JE, Cousens S, Bhutta ZA, Darmstadt GL, Martines J, Paul V, *et al.* Why are 4 million newborn babies dying each year? *Lancet* 2004;364:399–401.

54. McCaw-Binns A, Lindo JLM, Lewis-Bell KN, Ashley DEC. Maternal mortality surveillance in Jamaica. *Int J Gynaecol Obstet* 2008;100:31–6.

55. Stephenson R, Baschieri A, Clements S, Hennink M, Madise N. Contextual influences on the used of health facilities for childbirth in Africa. *Am J Public Health* 2006;96:84–94.

56. Magadi M, Diamond I, Rodrigues RN. The determinants of delivery care in Kenya. *Soc Biol* 2000;47:164–88.

57. Qomariyah SN, Bell JS, Pambudi ES, Anggondowati T, Latief K, Achadi E, *et al.* A practical approach to identifying maternal deaths missed from routine hospital reports; lessons learned from Indonesia. *Global Health Action* 2009.

58. Geubbels E. Epidemiology of maternal mortality in Malawi. *Malawi Med J* 2006;18:206–25.

59. McCarthy J, Maine D. A framework for analyzing the determinants of maternal mortality. *Stud Fam Plann* 1992;23:23–33.

60. Ronsmans C, Scott S, Qomariyah SN, Achadi,E, Braunholtz D, Marshall T, *et al.* Professional assistance during birth and maternal mortality in two Indonesian districts. *Bull World Health Organ* 2009;87:416–23.

61. Chowdhury RI, Islam MA, Gulshan J, Chakraborty N. Delivery complications and healthcare-seeking behaviour: the Bangladesh Demographic and Health Survey 1999–2000. *Health Soc Care Community* 2007;15:254–64.

62. Munjanja S. *Zimbabwe Maternal and Perinatal Mortality Study 2007.* Zimbabwe: Ministry of Health and Child Welfare; 2009.

63. Fawcus S, Mbizvo M, Lindmark G, Nyström L. A community-based investigation of avoidable factors for maternal mortality in Zimbabwe. *Stud Fam Plann* 1996;27:319–27.

64. Ronsmans C, Scott S, Adisasmita A, Deviany P, Nandiaty F. Estimation of population-based incidence of pregnancy-related illness and mortality (PRIAM) in two districts in West Java, Indonesia. *BJOG* 2009;116:82–90.

65. South Africa Every Death Counts Writing Group, Bradshaw D, Chopra M, Kerber K, Lawn JE, Bamford L, *et al.* Every death counts: use of mortality audit data for decision making to save the lives of mothers, babies, and children in South Africa. *Lancet* 2008;371:1294–304. Erratum in: *Lancet* 2008;372:1150.

66. Ministry of Health and Population, Egypt. *National Maternal Mortality Study 2000.* Cairo: MHP; 2001.

67. Graham WJ. Criterion-based clinical audit in obstetrics: bridging the quality gap? *Best Pract Res Clin Obstet Gynaecol* 2009;23:375–88.

68. Altabe F, Bergel E, Cafferata ML, Gibbons L, Ciapponi A, Alemán A, *et al.* Strategies for improving the quality of health care in maternal and child health in low- and middle-income countries: an overview of systematic reviews. *Paediatr Perinat Epidemiol* 2008;22 Suppl 1:42–60.

69. Ensor T, Cooper S, Davidson L, Fitzmaurice A, Graham WJ. *Do Recessions Kill? The Impact of Economic Downturn on Maternal and Infant Mortality During the 20th Century.* Aberdeen: Immpact, University of Aberdeen; 2009.

70. Ministry of Health, Malaysia. *Evaluation of Implementation of the Confidential Enquiries into Maternal Deaths in the Improvement of Maternal Health Services.* Kuala Lumpur: Ministry of Health; 1998.

71. Vital Wave Consulting. *mHealth for Development: The opportunity of mobile technology for healthcare in the developing world.* Washington, DC and Berkshire, UK: UN Foundation–Vodafone Foundation Partnership; 2009.

72. Bicego G, Curtis S, Raggers H, Kapiga S, Ngallaba S. *Sumve Survey on Adult and Child Mortality, Tanzania 1995.* Calverton, MD: Macro International; 1997.

73. Immpact, University of Aberdeen. Sampling-at-service–sites (SSS). Module 4, Tool 1. In: *Immpact Toolkit: a Guide and Tools for Maternal Mortality Programme Assessment.* Aberdeen: University of Aberdeen; 2007 [www.immpact-international.org/toolkit].

74. National Institute of Population Research and Training (NIPORT), ORC Macro, Johns Hopkins University and ICDDR-B. *Bangladesh Maternal Health Services and Maternal Mortality Survey 2001.* Dhaka: NIPORT; 2003.

75. Ghana Statistical Service (GSS), Ghana Health Service (GHS), Macro International. *Ghana Maternal Health Survey 2007.* Calverton, MD: GSS, GHS, Macro International; 2009.

76. Office of the Registrar General of India. *Special Bulletin on Maternal Mortality in India 2004–2006. Sample Registration System.* New Delhi: ORG; 2009 [www.censusindia.gov.in/vital_statistics/srs_bulletins/mmr-bulletin-april-2009.pdf].

77. Garenne M, McCaa R, Nacro K. Maternal mortality in South Africa in 2001: from demographic census to epidemiological investigation *Popul Health Metr* 2008;6:4.

78. Koblinsky M, Anwar I, Mridha MK, Chowdhury ME, Botlero R. Reducing maternal mortality and improving maternal health: Bangladesh and MDG 5. *Health Popul Nutr* 2008;26:280–94.

79. Hounton S, Ouedraogo M, Some H, Diallo I, Fottrell E. Direct data capture using hand-held computers in rural Burkina Faso: experiences, benefits and lessons learnt. *Trop Med Int Health* 2008;13 Suppl 1:25–30.

80. EDHS. *Egypt Demographic and Health Survey 2000. Final Report.* Cairo: Ministry of Health and Population, National Population Council, Macro International; 2001.

81. Armar-Klemesu M, Arhinful D, Aikins M, Asante F, Bosi W, Deganus S, *et al. An Evaluation of Ghana's Policy of University Fee Exemption for Delivery Care. Final Report.* Noguchi Memorial Institute for Medical Research, Immpact (University of Aberdeen) and London School of Hygiene and Tropical Medicine; 2006.

82. Barnett S, Nair N, Tripathy P, Borghi J, Suchitra Rath S, Costello A. A prospective key informant surveillance system to measure maternal mortality – findings from indigenous populations in Jharkhand and Orissa, India. *BMC Pregnancy Childbirth* 2008;8:6.

83. Achadi E, Scott S, Pambudi ES, Makowiecka K, Marshall T, Adisasmita A, *et al.* Midwifery provision and uptake of maternity care in Indonesia. *Trop Med Int Health* 2007;12:1490–7.

84. Bashir A, Aleem M, Mustansar M. A 5-year study of maternal mortality in Faisalabad City, Pakistan. *Int J Gynaecol Obstet* 1995;50 Suppl 2:S93–6.

Chapter 2

Delivering on neonatal survival to accelerate progress for Millennium Development Goal 4

Joy E Lawn, Kate Kerber and Christabel Enweronu-Laryea

Introduction

The enormous burden of almost 3.6 million neonatal deaths remains relatively invisible because of gaps in data or ineffective use of existing data, the perceived complexity and expense of solutions, and societal norms for seclusion of newborns and acceptance of neonatal deaths.

The data for action for neonatal survival highlight many commonalities with maternal survival and indeed mothers and their babies are intimately linked. Stillbirths are not mentioned in Millennium Development Goal (MDG) 4 or 5, yet they are largely preventable with the same solutions. Previous false dichotomies in advocacy and programmes for maternal and newborn survival have not been helpful in accelerating progress. An integrated call for action would be more likely to increase global visibility and national action. Health professionals and policy makers need to link numbers for mothers, newborns and stillbirths together, and to work together to implement the highest impact solutions that save women and babies.

This chapter reviews the progress for MDG 4 (child survival), with a focus on neonatal survival and on highlighting linkages with MDG 5 (maternal survival). Priorities for programmatic action based on the data are identified.

Progress for neonatal and child survival

The MDGs are the most widely ratified health and development targets ever. Nearly every nation has agreed to reach these eight interlinking goals that address poverty, hunger, education and health by 2015. Multiple reports have been published and many commitments have been agreed but is progress being made? Are fewer mothers and children dying? Is access to essential health care improving for the poor?

The target of MDG 4 is a two-thirds reduction in under-five mortality between 1990 and 2015 (Figure 2.1). Remarkable progress was achieved before 1990, with a halving in risk of death for children under five between 1960 and 1990. Since 1990, the global under-five mortality rate has declined by 28% and the total number of under-five deaths is under 9 million for the first time.[1] However, progress towards MDG 4 must increase six-fold between now and 2015 in order to reach the target.

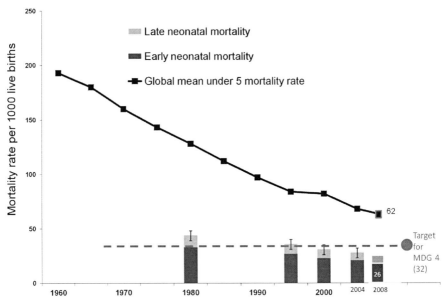

Figure 2.1   Progress towards MDG 4 for child survival showing the increasing proportion of under-five deaths that occur in the neonatal period (up to 28 days of life) and the lack of progress for deaths in the early neonatal period (first 7 days); based on Lawn *et al.*[3] and updated for progress up to 2008 using UN data

A number of Latin American and Asian countries have made substantial progress and are on track to meet the goal.[2] In Africa, progress has been slower but there are signs of accelerated action. Malawi has recently been declared on track to meet MDG 4, and is one of only six countries in sub-Saharan Africa with this status. While not yet officially on track to meet the goal, other large countries in the region, such as Ethiopia, Ghana, Uganda and Tanzania, have also made significant progress.[3]

One important barrier to progress for MDG 4 is the failure to reduce neonatal deaths (deaths in the first 4 weeks of life). Child survival programmes have primarily focused on important causes of death after the first 4 weeks of life – pneumonia, diarrhoea, malaria and vaccine-preventable conditions.[4] However, in the past few years it has become obvious that deaths during the first weeks of life account for an increasing proportion of under-five deaths and have not seen similar rates of decline. Globally, over 41% of under-five deaths occur during the neonatal period.[3] Particularly striking is the lack of any measurable progress over the past decade to reduce deaths in the first week of life or the early neonatal period (Figure 2.2).

At the same time, maternal health programmes have often focused primarily on the mother and do not always include the highest impact interventions to reduce newborn deaths and stillbirths. Yet newborn deaths, and especially deaths in the first week, can be reduced by strengthening care within existing maternal and child health programmes. To accelerate progress towards MDGs 4 and 5 in the short time before 2015, action must be taken to reduce neonatal deaths now, with a focus on maternal and neonatal survival.

A critical cornerstone for progress is to make better use of existing data, to improve the data and to connect these data to selecting and implementing the 'best buys.'

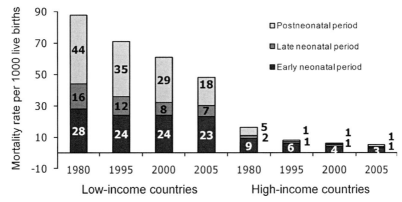

Figure 2.2 Progress for reducing infant deaths showing the rates for early neonatal (first week), late neonatal (weeks 1–3) and postneonatal (weeks 4–52) and contrasting progress between high- and low-income countries; based on Lawn *et al.*[39] and updated for progress up to 2005

Available information is often not used effectively to strengthen existing programmes, especially at district level, or to present the case for more investment.[5]

Data to inform programmatic action

Where do newborns die?

Over two-thirds of the world's maternal and neonatal deaths occur in sub-Saharan Africa and South Asia. The variation in neonatal mortality rate (NMR) and maternal mortality ratio (MMR) within regions is wide (Tables 2.1 to 2.3).[6,7] Some low-income countries, such as Thailand and Sri Lanka, have managed to achieve NMRs under 10 per 1000 live births.[8] Five countries account for just over 2 million deaths (over half the total newborn deaths) and ten countries account for two-thirds of the total. Because of their large populations, these same countries also have high numbers

Table 2.1 Neonatal and maternal mortality by region; data from UNICEF[6] and WHO[7]

Region	Neonatal mortality rate per 1000 live births (2008)	Annual number of neonatal deaths	Maternal mortality ratio per 100 000 live births (2005, adjusted)	Annual number of maternal deaths
Sub-Saharan Africa	41	1 230 000	920	278 972
Middle East and North Africa	21	209 000	210	20 425
South Asia	37	1 571 000	500	189 930
East Asia and Pacific	13	346 000	150	44 660
Latin America and Caribbean	11	117 000	130	14 795
Central and Eastern Europe and the Commonwealth of Independent States	12	66 000	46	2 558
High-income	4	44 000	8	882
Middle-income	26	2 382 000	450	550 197
Low-income	37	1 149 000	870	252 961

Table 2.2 The ten countries with the highest number of neonatal deaths, with associated maternal deaths and national plans and situation analysis of relevance; data from UNICEF,[6] WHO,[7] Countdown to 2015[40] and Save the Children[41]

Countries and territories	Neonatal mortality rate per 1000 live births (2008);	Annual number of neonatal deaths	Maternal mortality ratio per 100 000 live births (2005)	Annual number of maternal deaths	National MNCH plan[40]	National newborn situation analysis[41]
India	37	1 004 000	450	122 000	Yes	Yes
Nigeria	49	298 000	1100	66 000	Yes	Yes
Pakistan	53	284 000	320	14 000	Yes	Yes
China	11	206 000	45	8 000	Yes	–
DR Congo	56	163 000	1100	34 000	Yes	–
Ethiopia	39	122 000	720	23 000	Child only	–
Bangladesh	33	114 000	570	23 000	Neonatal only	Yes
Indonesia	19	80 000	420	18 000	No	–
Afghanistan	50	63 000	1800	24 000	Yes	Yes
Tanzania	33	59 000	950	15 000	Yes	Yes
Total number (percentage of the global total)		2 393 000 (67%)		347 000 (64%)		

MNCH = maternal, newborn and child health

Table 2.3 The ten countries with the highest neonatal mortality rates, showing the maternal mortality ratio and numbers of maternal deaths; data from UNICEF[6] and WHO[7]

Countries and territories	Neonatal mortality rate per 1000 live births (2008)	Annual number of neonatal deaths	Maternal mortality ratio per 100 000 live births (2005)	Annual number of maternal deaths
Somalia	61	24 000	1400	5 000
DR Congo	56	163 000	1100	34 000
Pakistan	53	284 000	320	14 000
Mali	52	28 000	970	6 000
Afghanistan	50	63 000	1800	24 000
Nigeria	49	298 000	1100	66 000
Myanmar	48	49 000	380	3 000
Central African Republic	47	7 000	980	2 000
Angola	47	36 000	1400	11 000
Guinea-Bissau	45	3,000	1100	1 000

of maternal deaths. While maternal mortality is difficult to measure and there are wide uncertainties around the estimates, efforts are continuing to improve assessment of the burden.[9] Many of the ten countries with the highest risk of newborn death are countries that have experienced recent war or other disasters and there is limited information to guide newborn survival programming in such settings.

Poverty and the ill health of newborns are closely linked. While the newborn health gap between rich and poor countries is unacceptably high, ranging from an NMR of 1 in Japan (gross national income, GNI, per capita = US$37,670) to 61 in Somalia (GNI per capita = US$140),[6,7] some countries are making progress despite their low-income status. Similarly, the list of countries with highest risk also includes some such as Nigeria, which has relatively much higher GNI per capita compared with other African countries with lower NMRs. Low-income countries that have achieved major reductions in maternal and neonatal mortality have also reached high coverage of skilled attendance during childbirth.[8] For the most part, however, human resources for health are grossly inequitable. Figure 2.3 demonstrates the inverse relationship between human resources for health and mortality burden. In the maps in Figure 2.3, from the Worldmapper website,[10] the area of each country is directly proportional to the measure indicated, which dramatically portrays the heavy burden of neonatal mortality in these regions and the disproportionate distribution of human resources for health. These maps show clearly that the highest density of neonatal deaths is concentrated in sub-Saharan Africa and South Asia and coincides with the greatest burden for maternal deaths and also for stillbirths. Yet these are also the places suffering from the most desperate shortage of physicians, with a near absence of physicians and a dearth of midwives.[10]

There is also inequitable distribution within countries, with an unacceptably large gap between rich and poor. An analysis of 13 African Demographic and Health Surveys (DHS) data sets with a relative index of economic status indicates that families in the poorest quintile experience, on average, 68% higher neonatal mortality than the richest quintile.[11] Among countries with these recent asset indices calculated from household surveys, the largest disparity is in Nigeria, with an NMR of 23 per 1000 among the richest quintile compared with 59 per 1000 in the poorest

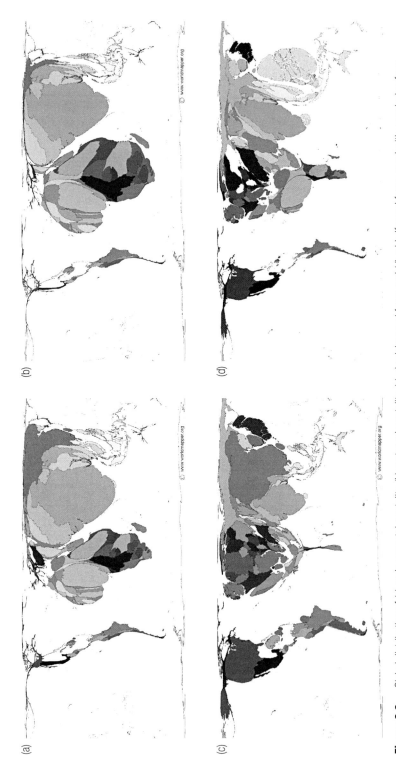

Figure 2.3 Global distribution of (a) early neonatal mortality, (b) maternal mortality, (c) physician workforce and (d) midwife workforce; used with permission from www.worldmapper.org (map numbers 260, 258, 219 and 215, respectively); © Copyright 2006 SASI Group (University of Sheffield) and Mark Newman (University of Michigan)

quintile, representing a gap of 156%.[12] If all of Nigeria experienced an NMR of 23 per 1000 live births, 133 000 fewer babies would die each year. Similarly, the doctor-to-population ratio in urban areas in India is 1.3 per 1000 population, whereas it is just 0.33 in rural areas. Mothers and newborns in poor families are at increased risk of illness and face more challenges in accessing timely, high-quality care compared with wealthier families. More systematic policy and support for implementation to benefit the poorest families, with equity-based tracking, is required. Governments should be held accountable for reducing and eliminating inequities in health outcomes.

For 22 countries in Africa with DHS published during the 5 years up to 2009, the NMR was, on average, 42% higher among rural families. While babies born to families living in rural areas are at greater risk of death than babies born to families living in urban areas,[3] a matter of increasing concern in the developing world is the urban poor. However, data on neonatal outcomes for the urban and peri-urban poor are lacking. More than half of the newborn babies who die do so at home. In Bangladesh, for example, as few as 15% of babies are born or die in a hospital. In northern Ghana, only 13% of neonatal deaths are in hospital.[13] For the 60 million women giving birth at home each year, physical distance is often a barrier. In many cases, there are also cultural norms that keep pregnancy hidden and preclude care-seeking outside the home at the time of birth or in the postnatal period.[14]

When do newborns die?

The birth of a baby should be a time of celebration yet, during the entire human lifespan, the day of birth is the day of greatest risk of death. In total, over 2 million deaths occur every year during childbirth (Figure 2.4).[15] The risk of dying during the first day of life is close to 10 per 1000 live births (1%). In fact, this is likely to be

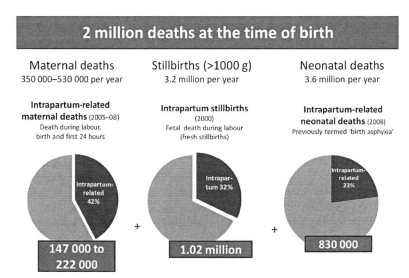

Figure 2.4   Care at birth is critical – the proportion of maternal deaths, stillbirths and neonatal deaths that are intrapartum related; based on Lawn et al,[42] data sources: maternal deaths: Hogan et al,[9] Hill et al,[43] Li et al,[44] stillbirths: Stanton et al,[45] Lawn et al,[20] neonatal deaths: WHO;[7] intrapartum-related neonatal deaths based on CHERG/WHO estimates[17] updated for 2009 using neonatal mortality and revised neonatal cause-specific estimates for Black et al.[19] based on methods from Lawn et al.[17]

an underestimate of the true proportion of deaths in the first 24 hours because of inconsistencies in recording the 24 hour period after birth. These deaths are closely linked to lack of adequate maternal and neonatal care at this critical time. Globally, an estimated 42% of maternal deaths are intrapartum related, defined as during birth or the first day after birth. For mothers who die of an intrapartum cause, it is rare for the baby to survive. Maternal morbidity and 'near miss' maternal deaths are also closely linked to adverse fetal and neonatal outcomes.[15] Recognition of the importance of reaching mothers and newborns in this crucial early period resulted in a UN statement in 2009 on home visits for newborn care.[16]

Delivering solutions for the main causes of neonatal death

In all regions, deaths in children under 5 years of age that are due to neonatal causes represent the biggest proportion of deaths, ranging from 26% to 64% of under-five deaths. Most neonatal deaths in Africa and Asia are due to conditions that are rarely seen in high-income countries and, when they are seen, would not be likely to result in death. The three major causes of neonatal death are the same for all high-mortality settings and account for 81% of all newborn deaths globally (Figure 2.5). These are:

▓ neonatal infection – 972 000 newborn deaths globally, not including tetanus

▓ intrapartum-related neonatal deaths – 828 000 newborn deaths globally

▓ preterm birth complications – 1 044 000 newborn deaths globally.

However, the relative proportions of these three causes vary between and even within countries, as shown in Figure 2.6. For settings with very high NMR (greater than 45 neonatal deaths per 1000 live births), around half of neonatal deaths are due to infections, including tetanus. In low-mortality settings (NMR less than 15), approximately 15% of deaths are due to infections and solutions will require more complex inputs. Hence, paradoxically, the populations with the highest neonatal mortality can achieve the most feasible reductions. Rapid reductions in mortality, with the greatest effect on equity, are possible as conditions such as neonatal tetanus almost

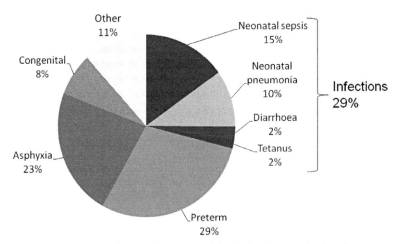

Figure 2.5 Causes of death for 3.6 million neonatal deaths, for 192 countries based on cause-specific mortality data and multi-cause modelled estimates; detailed methods in Lawn *et al*,[17] data from Black *et al.*[18]

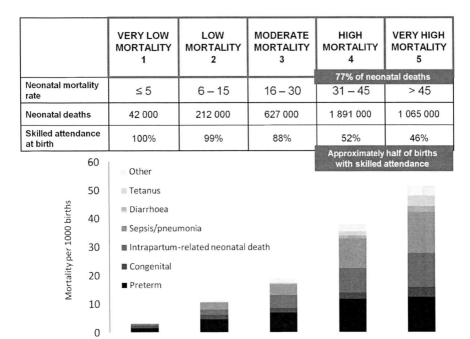

	VERY LOW MORTALITY 1	LOW MORTALITY 2	MODERATE MORTALITY 3	HIGH MORTALITY 4	VERY HIGH MORTALITY 5
				77% of neonatal deaths	
Neonatal mortality rate	≤ 5	6 – 15	16 – 30	31 – 45	> 45
Neonatal deaths	42 000	212 000	627 000	1 891 000	1 065 000
Skilled attendance at birth	100%	99%	88%	52%	46%

Figure 2.6 Variation of cause-specific neonatal mortality across 193 countries organised according to five levels of neonatal mortality; based on Lawn et al,[15] data sources: new analysis of 193 countries grouped by level of NMR adapted from Lawn et al.[3] and updated for 2008 using neonatal mortality and revised neonatal cause-specific estimates for Black et al.[19] based on methods from Lawn et al,[17] skilled birth attendance data from UNICEF[6]

exclusively affect the poorest families.[15] Table 2.4 gives an overview of the global burden and potential solutions to the top five causes of newborn deaths estimated for 192 countries[17–19] together with the percentage of lives that could be saved.

Neonatal infection – 972 000 newborn deaths globally

The most preventable killer of newborns is neonatal infection, particularly sepsis, pneumonia and meningitis. Prevention is mainly dependent on maternal health programmes such as antenatal care, hygienic care during childbirth and the postnatal period, and early and exclusive breastfeeding. Treatment is possible through existing child health programmes, particularly integrated management of childhood illness (IMCI) and referral care in hospitals. Adding antibiotic treatment of newborn infections further increases the number of potential lives that can be saved. The scaling up of case management to date has probably contributed to some reduction of deaths from infection in the late neonatal period.[13] Adding a new algorithm for care of babies in the first week of life to IMCI has provided a further opportunity to reduce neonatal and under-five mortality.

Tetanus – 72 000 newborn deaths globally

Tetanus was not a major killer of babies in the industrialised world, even before the tetanus toxoid vaccine was developed. Traditional practices such as putting harmful

Table 2.4 Interventions and estimated potential lives saved with essential maternal, newborn and childcare interventions according to the most common causes of newborn death; adapted from Lawn and Kerber[11] with permission; data sources: neonatal deaths from WHO[7] and Black et al,[19] neonatal lives saved for Africa and South Asia from Darmstadt et al.[46]

Cause of death	Estimated deaths globally	Timing of deaths	Prevention solutions	Treatment solutions	Potential lives saved	Feasibility
Neonatal infections (sepsis, meningitis, pneumonia and diarrhoea)	972 000	Sepsis and meningitis: first week Pneumonia and diarrhoea: increases towards end of first month	• Treating maternal infections • Clean childbirth practices and hygienic care, especially cord care • Breastfeeding	• Case management as an outpatient, inpatient care with full case management but coverage is very low owing to physical and cultural barriers to access in the first month of life • In countries with integrated management of childhood illness, adding neonatal illness case management is an important opportunity • Enabling policies for what to give and where and by whom, e.g. 'gold standard' regimen (7–10 days injectable antibiotics, usually in hospital) may block community-based treatment	47–82%	• Highly feasible through routine increased skilled attendance, postnatal care, integrated management of childhood illness and improved hospital care of sick newborns
Intrapartum-related deaths ('birth asphyxia')	828 000	First day of life	• Antenatal care, especially to identify/manage hypertension in pregnancy and pre-eclampsia • Skilled attendance, including use of partograph • Emergency obstetric care for complications (e.g. obstructed labour, haemorrhage)	• Resuscitation • Care of babies with neonatal encephalopathy • Lack of capacity and staff with necessary skills for resuscitation, even in countries where more births are in health facilities • Lack of supplies, e.g. bag and mask	39–71%	• Feasible with more commitment to scaling upskilled attendance during childbirth and emergency obstetric care and adequate referral and transport
Complications of preterm birth	1 044 000	First week for many (in the absence of intensive care) but continuing increased risk, especially from infections	• Treating maternal infections • Iron/folic acid supplements • Preventing malaria in pregnancy • Antenatal steroids	• Resuscitation at birth • Improved breastfeeding practices • Kangaroo mother care • Early identification and treatment of complications, especially infections	37–71%	• Prevention feasible through antenatal care, especially with malaria prevention in endemic areas • Treatment feasible through existing facility care, especially kangaroo mother care and extra support for feeding • Improved coverage and quality of postnatal care
Tetanus	72 000	Peaks during days 4–9 of life	• Tetanus toxoid immunisation during pregnancy • Clean childbirth practices and cord hygiene	• Antibiotics • nti-tetanus globulin • Supportive care	–	• Highly feasible through routine antenatal care and immunisation outreach campaigns
Congenital abnormalities	288 000	First week of life for severe abnormalities	• Preconceptional folic acid to prevent neural tube defects • Preventing unwanted pregnancy for older women	• Supportive care, depending on type and severity	–	• Curative care is often complex and expensive • Reducing unwanted pregnancy for older women would reduce incidence of Down syndrome • Preconceptional folic acid may be cost-effective in low-resource settings, especially through food fortification

substances on the cord contribute to this burden. Investment in vaccine coverage has resulted in global coverage of maternal tetanus immunisation climbing to 81%. Since 2000, 14 countries and 15 states in India have been certified as having eliminated tetanus. Although tetanus is responsible for fewer newborn deaths each year, it is unacceptable that in the 21st century neonatal tetanus still accounts for so many preventable newborn deaths.

Intrapartum–related neonatal deaths – 828 000 newborn deaths globally

Babies born in the world's least developed countries have a very high risk of intrapartum-related injury (birth asphyxia) and of intrapartum stillbirth.[20] The most effective interventions for intrapartum-related newborn deaths involve prevention through improved antenatal care, and particularly through skilled attendance and emergency obstetric care.[21,22] Once obstructed labour or haemorrhage have resulted in severe intrapartum injury, the baby may be stillborn or have a high chance (30–50%) of dying on the first day of life.[20] Inclusion of neonatal resuscitation as a core skill for all skilled attendants is a critical missed opportunity: national service provision assessments in six African countries show that on average only one in four babies is delivered by an attendant trained in neonatal resuscitation and who has the simple equipment (bag and mask) required.

The only two published studies from low-income settings of long-term follow-up of severely asphyxiated babies are from hospital-based cohorts in South Africa[23] and Nepal.[24] The limited follow-up data from these studies suggest that initial mortality is very high, and survivors with disability are fewer than expected, but more data are required on long-term outcomes.

Preterm birth complications – 1 044 000 newborn deaths globally

At least half of newborn deaths in Africa are in preterm babies. However, the direct cause of death is only to be attributed to preterm birth if the death is in a severely preterm baby or results from complications specific to preterm birth. For example, if a moderately preterm baby has an infection and dies, the death is most appropriately attributed to infection; thus, many babies recorded as dying from infection are also preterm. Most preterm babies are born between 33 and 37 weeks of gestation. They should survive with careful attention to feeding, warmth and early treatment of problems, including breathing problems, infections and jaundice. Babies born before 33 weeks of gestation or with birth weight under 1500 g are more likely to need advanced care, especially for breathing problems and feeding. If possible, these very small babies should receive care in a referral hospital. Kangaroo mother care involves caring for small, particularly preterm, babies by having them strapped skin-to-skin to the mother's front. A new meta-analysis of three randomised controlled trials suggests a 51% reduction in mortality for newborns less than 2000 g.[25] Kangaroo mother care is simple and effective, empowers mothers, and can be feasibly introduced in most facilities in low-income settings where care for small babies is provided. In addition, extra care of small babies at home with skin-to-skin care and additional support for breastfeeding has great potential.[26] Preventing certain causes of preterm birth is also an effective strategy that is feasible through control of malaria in pregnancy and identification and treatment of sexually transmitted infections, since HIV/AIDS and malaria in pregnancy interact to greatly increase the risk of preterm birth. The use of antenatal steroids is a missed opportunity with the potential to reduce neonatal deaths by up to half a million per year.[27]

Small babies – big risk of death

Globally, an average of 14% of babies are born with low birth weight (LBW) – a weight at birth of less than 2500 g.[6] LBW babies account for the majority of neonatal deaths and may be due to preterm birth or term babies who are growth restricted, or a combination of the two. Preterm babies have a risk of death that is around 13 times higher than full-term babies.[28] Babies who are both preterm and growth restricted have an even higher risk of death.[28] The limited data available suggest that most LBW babies in Africa are preterm. This differs markedly from the situation in South Asia, where the LBW rate is almost twice that of Africa's but the majority of LBW babies are term babies who are small for gestational age. Babies in Africa are at higher risk of being born preterm – the regional estimate for preterm birth is around 12%, which is almost double the frequency of preterm birth in European countries and probably related to infections, particularly sexually transmitted infections, malaria and HIV/AIDS. Indeed, co-infection during pregnancy with HIV and malaria is more than 'double trouble': the two infections act synergistically, with serious consequences for maternal and newborn health, especially increasing the LBW rate.[29] To date, strategies to prevent LBW and preterm birth have not resulted in significant mortality reductions. However, identifying small babies and providing extra support for feeding, warmth and care has great potential to reduce NMR.

Girls and neonatal deaths

After controlling for other factors, baby girls are found to have a lower mortality rate than baby boys. In societies where care is equal for boys and girls, the ratio of neonatal mortality for boys to girls is usually at least 1.2. Analysis of DHS data for African countries does not show a loss of this advantage for girl babies, although DHS may not be sensitive enough to detect this difference. A number of studies from South Asia have reported reduced care-seeking for baby girls, and even female infanticide.

Addressing deadly delays in care-seeking

Delays in receiving appropriate care can be important for many conditions but delays of even a few hours in addressing an obstetric emergency around the time of birth can be significant. The 'classic' three delays were first described in relation to delay for women with obstetric emergencies.[30] These three delays are:

1. **Delay in recognition of the problem and the decision to seek care.** Physical distance and financial and cultural barriers to seeking care are compounded when there is a delay in recognising illness and making decisions to seek care. These delays, even if short, can be deadly since neonatal illness generally presents less obviously and progresses more quickly than in older infants.

2. **Delay to reach a health facility.** This involves a delay in reaching the first-level facility – often using public transport on bad roads – as well as transport to a higher level health facility when referred. In an IMCI study in Uganda,[31] fewer than 10% of newborns referred from the first-level facility actually went.

3. **Delay in receiving quality care at the facility.** For example, there may be a gap between those women who attend antenatal care and those whose risk condition (malpresentation, pre-eclampsia, diabetes) is identified and correctly managed.

Strategies to reduce these three delays are crucial to effectively link mothers and babies to skilled obstetric and newborn care, as depicted in Figure 2.7. The continuum from the home to first-level health clinic to referral hospital ensures effective linkages from

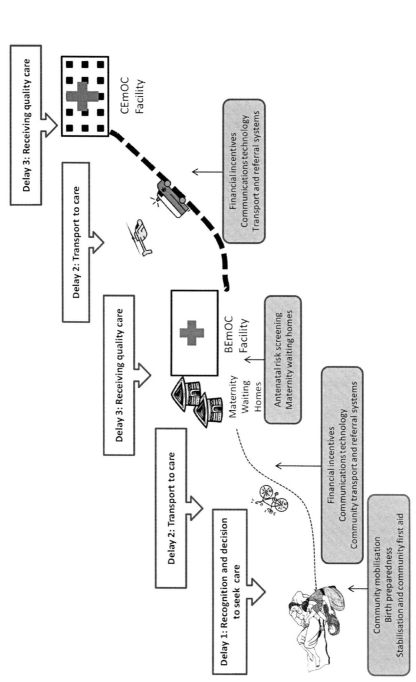

Figure 2.7 Reducing delays to emergency obstetric and neonatal care; BEmOC = Basic Emergency Obstetric Care; CEmOC = Comprehensive Emergency Obstetric Care; reproduced with permission from Lawn et al.[42]

all potential places of care-giving. Functional linkages to emergency obstetric care services are especially crucial for the 60 million women who deliver at home each year.[1] The continuum of care approach is a conceptual framework for integrated maternal, neonatal and child health that has been defined by the dimensions of time through the lifecycle and levels of care within the health system.[32] The solutions require community mobilisation and linkages with facilities, not community alone or facility interventions alone, across the continuum.

Coverage of care and current trends

Evidence-based strategies to save the lives of women and children include a wide range of interventions, which are usually provided through integrated service delivery packages along the timeline of the continuum of care,[32] notably:

- reproductive health services to provide contraceptive services
- antenatal care for pregnant women
- skilled attendance and emergency obstetric care during birth
- postnatal care services, including both preventive and curative interventions.

Global tracking mechanisms tend to collect information on the contact point but not always on the provision of effective care, although there is more information available on the numbers of visits and visit content for antenatal care than for intrapartum care or, especially, for postnatal care.

Nevertheless, coverage and trend data for these contact points provide valuable information. Contraceptive use, although one of the most cost-effective interventions for maternal, newborn and child health, appears to be stagnating, possibly related to lack of global prioritisation and funding.[33] Overall contact for women in low-income countries is much higher for antenatal care (64%) than for use of a modern contraceptive (29%), although it should be noted that the target for contraceptive prevalence is not 100% as for the other packages as not all women will need contraception. Another option for a reproductive health indicator is met need for contraception.

Data on trends in service coverage have limitations but it is clear that antenatal care has increased in all regions: indeed, in sub-Saharan Africa, 72% of women now have at least one visit, although fewer have four or more visits (42%). Antenatal care is one of the success stories in low-income settings, with high coverage and relatively equitable reach to poor and marginalised populations. However, the content of care does not always include the most effective interventions, nor is the service delivered with high quality. Given the high potential to save lives and the low cost and apparent feasibility in low-resource settings, the current low coverage of antenatal steroids represents a major missed opportunity.

There is a big decrease in coverage of women receiving care between pregnancy and childbirth, with only 32% of women in the 50 least developed countries having a skilled attendant present during childbirth. Except for eastern and southern Africa, all developing regions have increased their coverage of skilled delivery attendance during the past decade, with a particularly marked increase in the Middle East and North Africa. However, regional and country averages hide large inequities in care, especially for skilled attendance.[34] For example, while 6% of women in Ethiopia overall have a skilled attendant at birth, 25% of the wealthiest quintile do and only 1% of the poorest.[35] Similarly, rural mothers have much lower access to skilled birth attendance and caesarean section than mothers in urban areas.[33] The gap in coverage of skilled birth attendance is widest in sub-Saharan Africa and South Asia, where baseline coverage is lowest globally and progress to reaching universal skilled attendance is slow. Rates of increase of skilled birth attendance in these regions is less than 0.5% per year and, at current rates, by 2015 a skilled birth attendant will only reach one in two women in sub-Saharan Africa and South Asia.[15] This is a priority gap requiring substantial work to define potentially scalable approaches to reaching universal skilled birth attendance in varying contexts.

Postnatal care is also a critical yet neglected gap in low- and middle-income countries and its coverage is even lower than skilled birth attendance and much lower than antenatal care. Early contact with mothers and babies is critical, ideally within 24 or at most 48 hours of birth for the first visit (in addition to the more common visit 6 weeks after birth). Important new data from Bangladesh show that a visit in the first 2 days of life is associated with significantly lower neonatal deaths compared with those who did not receive a postnatal visit.[36] In the 68 priority Countdown countries, a median of only 21% of mothers received postnatal care within 48 hours of birth.[33] For babies and mothers facing complications such as neonatal sepsis or postpartum haemorrhage, a delay of even a few hours before receiving appropriate care can be fatal or result in long-term injuries or disability. This is also the crucial time for establishing healthy practices: evidence shows that effective breastfeeding support and counselling for mothers in the first days after birth directly increase rates of exclusive breastfeeding.[37] Other key behaviours during the neonatal period, such as hygienic cord care and keeping the baby warm, can make the difference between life and death, particularly for babies who are born preterm. In addition, evidence shows that active case-finding through routine home visits has a major effect on increasing treatment for neonatal sepsis and reducing mortality. However, in many countries the 6-week visit is the mother and baby's first interaction with the formal health system after birth. There is a clear need to better define the package of postnatal practices and also the delivery strategies in varying settings, and consensus is increasing.[6,16] The indicator measuring postnatal care for the global Countdown to 2015 for maternal, newborn and child health has changed to focus on care within 2 days of birth.[33] Large-scale surveys are changing to measure this indicator in more countries and communities.

Addressing research gaps

There are clear priorities from the data to drive the priorities for action. There are immediate opportunities to add or strengthen high-impact neonatal interventions within current maternal and child health programmes and to monitor and evaluate the effectiveness of such implementation.

Reducing the major gap for saving the lives of mothers and babies is not new science but innovation in implementation science – a better understanding of how to deliver effective care and reach the poorest families with high-impact interventions. New technology or improved existing technology may make a substantial difference for some priority areas (for example, by identifying fetal distress or preventing preterm labour). Often the key questions are 'who, where and how' regarding task shifting, supervision and management at scale. Much of the evidence to date has come from Asia. A new network of studies in eight African countries is examining nationally adapted packages and potentially scalable cadres of workers. Analysis of lives saved, costs and feasibility at scale will help guide policies and programmes to improve maternal and newborn care in varying settings.

Addressing data gaps

To effectively track progress, there are key actions required that could improve the quantity and quality of data in the short term (Box 2.1). Actions to build improved health information systems to capture maternal and newborn outcomes and especially quality of care are also critical.

Neonatal deaths, especially intrapartum-related stillbirths and neonatal deaths

Reliable coverage with vital registration systems is available for fewer than 3% of all neonatal deaths and are not generalisable to typical low- and middle-income country settings. Verbal autopsy methods (questionnaires used with family members after the death) are the only option for cause-of-death data for the majority of neonatal deaths and stillbirths. There have been advances in case definitions and algorithms for use in verbal autopsy but full consensus and consistent use is still lacking, particularly for hierarchical attribution if the baby died with signs suggestive of several possible causes of death. Neonatal deaths that occur in the first hours after birth or in small babies are less likely than other neonatal deaths to be reported. Additionally, recording an infant as stillborn may avoid a sense of blame for the family or birth attendant, or circumvent the need to fill out a death certificate.

Coverage

While some progress has been made on the package definition and delivery strategies for postnatal care, key gaps around implementation and data remain. The little information available on the timing of the first visit after birth and cadre of provider comes from mothers' responses in household surveys such as DHS or from research settings. Additional routine tracking is needed to inform the content and quality of postnatal visits, such as the number of visits, extra visits for small or sick babies, mothers who know newborn danger signs, breastfeeding, family planning, thermal care and hygienic practices.

Conclusion

Together, maternal, newborn and child deaths are a massive burden but more low-income countries are now progressing for MDG 4 and, with strategic investments, including more attention to neonatal deaths, MDG 4 is achievable for many countries. While uncertainties remain about the data, it is clear that there are huge numbers of maternal (between 340 000 and 540 000) and neonatal (3.6 million) deaths, also closely linked with stillbirths (3.2 million). For every mother that dies, at least 15 babies are stillborn or die in the first month of life. Often, however, maternal health documents and advocates do not include the neonatal outcomes, or vice versa, and stillbirths are not included in the MDG framework. These outcomes should be consistently linked as this will increase attention and action. Given the high proportion of maternal (at least 42%), neonatal (23%) and stillbirths (31%) that are directly related to care at birth, the data support the critical need to invest in care at birth and in the early postnatal period. Reaching 60 million home births must be a priority.

The political priority and investment for a given global health issue is not always directly correlated to the size of the problem but is determined by other factors such as consensus regarding practical solutions. There are also many common themes in the solutions for mothers and babies, particularly related to health systems issues,

Box 2.1	Improving the data for decision making for programmes at the time of birth and for stillbirth and neonatal outcomes; reproduced with permission from Lawn *et al.*[15]

Improved measurement of outcome data for stillbirths and neonatal deaths

Intrapartum stillbirths
- Improved measurement of the numbers/rates of stillbirths, especially in settings where most births occur at home and/or where stillbirths are normally a taboo subject
- Consistent definitions and classification systems to allow comparability of causes of death measurement across low- and high-income settings
- Tools to assess the causes of stillbirths, and to better distinguish intrapartum stillbirths versus antepartum stillbirths versus intrapartum-related neonatal deaths (for example, through verbal autopsy)
- Linking to other data collection mechanisms (for example, vital registration, household surveys, demographic surveillance systems)

Intrapartum-related neonatal deaths (previously called 'birth asphyxia')
- Improved measurement of intrapartum-related outcomes (mortality and morbidity)
- Consistent definitions and classification systems to allow comparability of measurement of intrapartum-related neonatal outcomes across low- and high-income settings
- Verbal autopsy tools and hierarchical methods to distinguish intrapartum-related neonatal deaths from other causes of very early death such as early-onset sepsis and preterm birth

Combined marker of intrapartum-related stillbirths and neonatal deaths, and/or intrapartum-related maternal deaths
- Validation of a composite indicator of quality of intrapartum care;[47] for example, intrapartum stillbirths plus first-day (or predischarge if earlier) neonatal deaths more than 2000 g as a surrogate for intrapartum-related neonatal deaths, consider addition of intrapartum-related maternal deaths
- Classification systems to cross-tabulate stillbirth and neonatal outcomes with maternal deaths, complications and risk factors

Impairment and disability
- Feasible case definitions for neonatal encephalopathy in low-income and community settings (for example, surrogate marker proposed is seizures in first 24 hours in neonate with birth weight above 2500 g)
- Screening methods (for example, application of surveillance or screening tool followed by definitive testing of screen positives) for identification of infants at high risk of disability or impairment and who may benefit from early intervention
- Feasible, sustainable instruments to measure disability that are validated at population level to ensure that improved newborn survival (from intrapartum-related or other conditions such as preterm birth or infection) is not contributing to an increase in disability rates

Improvement in measurement of service coverage data for care at birth

Obstetric care coverage indicators (refinement, consensus and consistent reporting)
- Attendance at birth
  - Skilled birth attendance coverage, monitoring of skills, competence, and procedures performed by skilled attendants
  - Place of delivery, and other birth attendants
  - Cross tabulation by rural/urban and by socio-economic status
- Emergency obstetric care services
  - Access, utilisation and met need for emergency obstetric care services, better determination of baseline marker of 'need' in different settings
  - Consistent definitions of maternal indications, complications and life-saving interventions
  - Caesarean sections as percentage of all births: specify those for maternal–fetal indications
- Indicators to track referral systems for obstetric and newborn care from community to facility and between facilities

Neonatal care coverage (refinement, consensus, and consistent reporting)
- Indicators of newborn care at birth – proportion of facilities with capacity for neonatal resuscitation (training and equipment), proportion of staff competent in neonatal resuscitation, neonates receiving neonatal resuscitation, validation of data collected through facility assessments or through retrospective surveys
- Routine postnatal care – timing, frequency, cadres and content of postnatal care visit in facility and at home, validation of data collected through retrospective surveys
- Emergency newborn care – proportion of facilities with capacity for continuing care for neonatal encephalopathy (neonatal intensive care, assisted ventilation, nutrition support and fluid management)

notably the need for rapid scale-up of skilled human resources to provide care at birth, increasing emergency obstetric care, solutions to address the gap for early postnatal care, and case management of ill newborns or mothers.

Given the short timeline until the target date of the MDGs in 2015 and the fact that there is not a 'magic bullet' for saving lives, it is critical that implementation priorities be set using data at national or subnational level, particularly at district level. Where possible, consideration should be given to using evidence-based mortality effect estimation tools to guide implementation priorities, based on local cause of death data, effect of interventions and local coverage of interventions.[38] Existing solutions to the largest burdens could save hundreds of thousands of lives each year.

While existing data are often underused for action, there are nevertheless major gaps. A shift in focus to measurement of pregnancies and pregnancy outcomes for mother, fetus and baby would benefit public health planning. Reliable stillbirth data are particularly lacking. There are also important gaps for coverage-of-care data, especially at the time of birth, and postnatal care and there are very limited data on quality of care at this crucial time for saving lives.

For research investments, the most effect on lives saved would come from a greater focus on implementation research – the 'how-to' questions – but still with as rigorous design as possible to better inform policy priority regarding cost and effect of various strategies to implement known interventions.

Investment in maternal and neonatal survival is increasing. Even given the limitations in the current data, the priorities are clear, especially for more investment immediately around the time of birth. The use of data to prioritise programmatic action has the potential to result in major changes for maternal and newborn survival in many countries and for the world's poorest families before 2015 – the question is are we using the data and will we act?

Acknowledgments

The authors thank Professor Jim Neilson for his support in commissioning and reviewing this chapter and Andrew Welsh for the editing.

References

1. You D, Wardlaw T, Salama P, Jones G. Levels and trends in under-5 mortality, 1990–2008. *Lancet* 2010;375:100–3.
2. UNICEF. *Progress for Children: A World Fit for Children Statistical Review*. New York: UNICEF; 2007.
3. Lawn JE, Cousens S, Zupan J; Lancet Neonatal Survival Steering Team. 4 million neonatal deaths: when? Where? Why? *Lancet* 2005;365:891–900.
4. Martines J, Paul VK, Bhutta ZA, Koblinsky M, Soucat A, Walker N, *et al*. Neonatal survival: a call for action. *Lancet* 2005;365:1189–97.
5. Lawn JE, Kerber K, Enweronu-Laryea C, Massee Bateman O. Newborn survival in low resource settings – are we delivering? *BJOG* 2009;116 Suppl 1:49–59.
6. UNICEF. *State of the World's Children 2009*. New York: UNICEF; 2009.
7. World Health Organization. Dataset for neonatal mortality in 2008 [www.who.int/healthinfo/statistics/mortality_neonatal/en/index.html].
8. Rohde J, Cousens S, Chopra M, Tangcharoensathien V, Black R, Bhutta ZA, *et al*. 30 years after Alma-Ata: has primary health care worked in countries? *Lancet* 2008;372:950–61.
9. Hogan MC, Foreman KJ, Naghavi M, Ahn SY, Wang M, Makela SM, *et al*. Maternal mortality for 181 countries, 1980–2008: a systematic analysis of progress towards Millennium Development Goal 5. *Lancet* 2010;375:1609–23.

10.   Newton M, Dorling D, Barford A, Wheeler B, Pritchard J, Allsopp G. Worldmapper [www. worldmapper.org].

11.   Lawn J, Kerber K, editors. *Opportunities for Africa's Newborns: Practical Data, Policy and Programmatic Support for Newborn Care in Africa.* Cape Town: PMNCH, Save the Children, UNFPA, UNICEF, USAID, WHO; 2006.

12.   National Population Commission (NPC) and ICF Macro. *Nigeria Demographic and Health Survey 2003.* Abuja: National Population Commission and ICF Macro; 2004.

13.   Baiden F, Hodgson A, Adjuik M, Adongo P, Ayaga B, Binka F. Trend and causes of neonatal mortality in the Kassena-Nankana district of northern Ghana, 1995–2002. *Trop Med Int Health* 2006;11:532–9.

14.   Lawn JE, Yakoob MY, Haws RA, Soomro T, Darmstadt GL, Bhutta ZA. 3.2 million stillbirths: epidemiology and overview of the evidence review. *BMC Pregnancy Childbirth* 2009;9 Suppl 1:S2.

15.   Lawn JE, Kinney M, Lee AC, Chopra M, Donnay F, Paul VK, et al. Reducing intrapartum-related deaths and disability: Can the health system deliver? *Int J Gynaecol Obstet* 2009;107:S123–42.

16.   World Health Organization, USAID, Save the Children. *WHO-UNICEF Joint Statement on Home Visits for the Newborn Child: A Strategy to Improve Survival.* Geneva: WHO; 2009.

17.   Lawn JE, Wilczynska-Ketende K, Cousens SN. Estimating the causes of 4 million neonatal deaths in the year 2000. *Int J Epidemiol* 2006;35:706–18.

18.   Bryce J, Boschi-Pinto C, Shibuya K, Black RE. WHO estimates of the causes of death in children. *Lancet* 2005;365:1147–52.

19.   Black RE, Cousens S, Johnson HL, Lawn JE, Rudan I, Bassani DG, et al; for the Child Health Epidemiology Reference Group of WHO and UNICEF. Global, regional and national causes of child mortality in 2008: a systematic review. *Lancet* (in press).

20.   Lawn J, Shibuya K, Stein C. No cry at birth: global estimates of intrapartum stillbirths and intrapartum-related neonatal deaths. *Bull World Health Organ* 2005;83:409–17.

21.   Adam T, Lim SS, Mehta S, Bhutta ZA, Fogstad H, Mathai M, et al. Cost effectiveness analysis of strategies for maternal and neonatal health in developing countries. *BMJ* 2005;331:1107.

22.   Darmstadt GL, Bhutta ZA, Cousens S, Adam T, Walker N, De Bernis L. Evidence-based, cost-effective interventions: how many newborn babies can we save? *Lancet* 2005;365:977–88.

23.   Thompson CM, Puterman AS, Linley LL, Hann FM, van der Elst CW, Molteno CD, et al. The value of a scoring system for hypoxic ischaemic encephalopathy in predicting neurodevelopmental outcome. *Acta Paediatr* 1997;86:757–61.

24.   Ellis M, Manandhar N, Shrestha PS, Shrestha L, Manandhar DS, Costello AM. Outcome at 1 year of neonatal encephalopathy in Kathmandu, Nepal. *Dev Med Child Neurol* 1999;41:689–95.

25.   Lawn JE, Mwansa-Kambafwile J, Horta BL, Barros FC, Cousens S. 'Kangaroo mother care' to prevent neonatal deaths due to preterm birth complications. *Int J Epidemiol* 2010;39(Suppl 1):i44–54.

26.   Darmstadt GL, Kumar V, Yadav R, Singh V, Singh P, Mohanty S, et al. Introduction of community-based skin-to-skin care in rural Uttar Pradesh, India. *J Perinatol* 2006;26:597–604.

27.   Mwansa-Kambafwile J, Cousens S, Hansen T, Lawn JE. Antenatal steroids in preterm labour for the prevention of neonatal deaths due to complications of preterm birth. *Int J Epidemiol* 2010;39(Suppl 1):i122–33.

28.   Yasmin S, Osrin D, Paul E, Costello A. Neonatal mortality of low-birth-weight infants in Bangladesh. *Bull World Health Organ* 2001;79:608–14.

29.   ter Kuile FO, Parise ME, Verhoeff FH, Udhayakumar V, Newman RD, van Eijk AM, et al. The burden of co-infection with human immunodeficiency virus type 1 and malaria in pregnant women in sub-saharan Africa. *Am J Trop Med Hyg* 2004;71(2 Suppl):41–54.

30.   Rosenfield A, Maine D. Maternal health in Third World. *Lancet* 1987;1:691.

31.   Nsungwa-Sabiiti J, Burnham G, Pariyo G; Uganda IMCI documentation team. Implementation of a national Integrated Management of Childhood Illness (IMCI) program in Uganda. *J Health Popul Dev Ctries* 2004:1–16.

32.   Kerber KJ, de Graft-Johnson JE, Bhutta ZA, Okong P, Starrs A, Lawn JE. Continuum of care for maternal, newborn, and child health: from slogan to service delivery. *Lancet* 2007;370:1358–69.

33.   Bryce J, Daelmans B, Dwivedi A, Fauveau V, Lawn JE, Mason E, et al. Countdown to 2015 for maternal, newborn, and child survival: the 2008 report on tracking coverage of interventions. *Lancet* 2008;371:1247–58.

34. Houweling TA, Ronsmans C, Campbell OM, Kunst AE. Huge poor–rich inequalities in maternity care: an international comparative study of maternity and child care in developing countries. *Bull World Health Organ* 2007;85:745–54.
35. Knippenberg R, Lawn JE, Darmstadt GL, Begkoyian G, Fogstad H, Walelign N, *et al.* Systematic scaling up of neonatal care in countries. *Lancet* 2005;365:1087–98.
36. Baqui AH, Ahmed S, El Arifeen S, Darmstadt GL, Rosecrans AM, Mannan I, *et al*; Projahnmo 1 Study Group. Effect of timing of first postnatal care home visit on neonatal mortality in Bangladesh: a observational cohort study. *BMJ* 2009;339:b2826.
37. Bhutta ZA, Ahmed T, Black RE, Cousens S, Dewey K, Giugliani E, *et al.* What works? Interventions for maternal and child undernutrition and survival. *Lancet* 2008;371:417–40.
38. Stover J, McKinnon R, Winfrey B. Spectrum: a model platform for linking impact of maternal and child survival interventions with AIDS, family planning and demographic projections. *Int J Epidemiol* 2010;39(Suppl 1): i7–10.
39. Lawn JE, Zupan J, Begkoyian G, Knippenberg R. Newborn survival. In: Jamison D, Measham A, editors. *Disease Control Priorities.* 2nd edition. The World Bank and the National Institutes of Health; 2006. p. 531–49.
40. Bryce J, Requejo JH. *Tracking Progress in Maternal, Newborn and Child Survival: The 2008 Report.* Countdown to 2015. New York: UNICEF; 2008.
41. Save the Children. *Saving Newborn Lives.* 2009 [www.savethechildren.org/savenewborns].
42. Lawn JE, Lee AC, Kinney M, Sibley L, Carlo WA, Paul VK, *et al.* Two million intrapartum-related stillbirths and neonatal deaths: Where, why, and what can be done? *Int J Gynecol Obstet* 2009;107:S5–19 [www.ijgo.org/issues/contents?issue_key=S0020-7292%2809%29X0010-X].
43. Hill K, Thomas K, AbouZahr C, Walker N, Say L, Inoue M, *et al.* Estimates of maternal mortality worldwide between 1990 and 2005: an assessment of available data. *Lancet* 2007;370:1311–19.
44. Li XF, Fortney JA, Kotelchuck M, Glover LH. The postpartum period: the key to maternal mortality. *Int J Gynecol Obstet* 1996;54:1–10.
45. Stanton C, Lawn JE, Rahman H, Wilczynska-Ketende K, Hill K. Stillbirth rates: delivering estimates in 190 countries. *Lancet* 2006;367:1487–94.
46. Darmstadt GL, Walker N, Lawn JE, Bhutta ZA, Haws RA, Cousens S. Saving newborn lives in Asia and Africa: cost and impact of phased scale-up of interventions within the continuum of care. *Health Policy Plan* 2008;23:101–17.
47. Fauveau V. New indicator of quality of emergency obstetric and newborn care. *Lancet* 2007;370:1310.

Chapter 3

Beyond the Numbers: reviewing maternal deaths and disabilities to make pregnancy safer

Gwyneth Lewis OBE

> Whose faces are behind the numbers? What were their stories? What were their dreams? They left behind children and families. They also left behind clues as to why their lives ended early.[1]

Introduction

This chapter briefly describes how maternal death or severe morbidity reviews, as described in the World Health Organization (WHO) publication *Beyond the Numbers: Reviewing Maternal Deaths and Disabilities to Make Pregnancy Safer* (BTN),[2] can save mothers' and newborns' lives as well as help to reduce severe maternal and neonatal morbidity. The purpose of the reviews is to assess and identify any underlying factors that may have contributed to mothers' deaths and to learn lessons from these to develop and promulgate recommendations to improve access to, and the quality of, maternity care in future. The methodologies can be used at national, regional, local or community level and take a number of forms. The technique chosen will depend on the specific local circumstances, the scope and scale of the proposed study, and the size of the population under review. Implementation of the guidelines and recommendations can improve access to, and the quality of, maternity care for all pregnant or recently delivered women and their infants.

Background

If governments are to redouble their efforts to make an impact on reducing their maternal death rates by 75% by 2015, as set out in the United Nations Millennium Development Goal 5 (MDG 5),[3] they need better information about exactly why and where their mothers are dying, who they are, and what might be done to remedy this. The role of this information-gathering process is similar to that of a doctor working through a difficult case where, before deciding on a management and treatment programme, it is first necessary to have reached a diagnosis, usually through using a case history review and various investigative measures. Additional diagnostic techniques are required for maternal death reviews as routinely collected data do not provide the whole story. The information to be collected needs to include basic demographic and clinical details but should also chart the course of the pregnancy, birth and postnatal period of each woman who died as well as identifying, at each step of her journey, any avoidable factors that impeded her access to safe and high-quality maternal care.

The maternal mortality ratio (MMR) is defined as the number of maternal deaths due to direct and indirect causes per 100 000 live births. It is the standard international tool used for benchmarking and for measuring changes in rates of maternal health overall. However, the MMR provides little information on the specific challenges faced within a country. Furthermore, they are only estimates, with a wide range of uncertainty between the lower and upper estimates in many resource-poor countries.[4] There may also be wide variations in death rates within a country, for example between women living in urban and rural areas, between rich and poor, and between different religious or ethnic groups. Using the UK as an example, *Saving Mothers' Lives*, the latest report of the Confidential Enquiry into Maternal Deaths (CEMD),[5] revealed that, behind the overall low and internationally comparable MMR of 7 deaths per 100 000 live births lay a more than ten-fold difference in maternal mortality (Figure 3.1). This variation was between unemployed single women and women in any type of employment. Although still worrying, this variation has actually narrowed in comparison with previous triennial reports, possibly as a result of action generated by earlier findings.[6] For example, Maternity Matters, a renewed national programme for maternity care in England, addresses the inequalities gaps and specifically targets mothers who find it hard to access or stay in touch with maternity services.[7]

The use of death certificate data to diagnose why mothers are dying carries little additional insight over the MMR. This is because, even if the coding of cause of death is correct (and data entry mistakes are common), death certificates provide little or no information on the real reasons why the women died. For example, a woman stated to have died from haemorrhage may have bled to death, unattended, at home or have received optimum care in a fully functioning tertiary referral unit. She may not

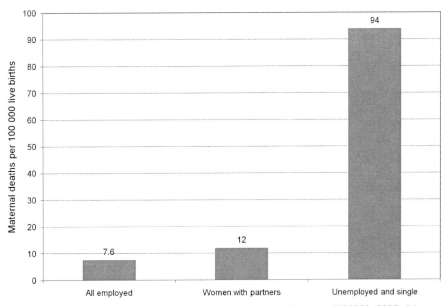

Figure 3.1   Maternal mortality ratio by employment and partnership status, UK 2003–2005; data from Lewis[5]

have understood the need to seek care, may have been subject to harmful traditional practices, may not have had money or access to transport, may have received inadequate clinical care or may have been treated in a facility without access to surgery or blood products. Many who work in the field of international women's health use the model of the 'three delays' to try to explain the barriers pregnant women face in receiving the care they really need.[8] These barriers may be in the family, the community or the healthcare system and are often interlinked:

- **Delay associated with the decision to seek care.** Were these women or their families unaware of the need for care or unaware of the warning signs of problems in pregnancy, or did financial, family or socio-cultural barriers prevent this?
- **A delay in arriving at a place of care.** Did the services exist? If so, how far away were they? Was there a lack of transport? Were they too expensive? Or were the facilities inaccessible for other reasons such as poor reputations or socio-cultural barriers?
- **A delay in the provision of appropriate care.** Was the facility equipped and staffed appropriately? Was the care the women received inadequate or actually harmful?

Beyond the Numbers

To help address the information gap and provide politicians, policy makers and health professionals with the information they require, in 2004 WHO published a maternal mortality review toolkit and programme, *Beyond the Numbers* (BTN).[2] The handbook and its accompanying CD-ROM describe the benefits and disadvantages of five possible approaches to maternal death or near miss review that are adaptable to any level and any setting. BTN also provides advice on how to choose and adapt the most suitable methodology for a given set of circumstances and then lists the practical steps to enable implementation and review.

The underlying philosophy is that every number in a statistical table should be recognised as a woman – a woman who died before her time, a mother, a member of a family, a member of a community – as the quote at the start of this chapter highlights so well.[1] The reviews go beyond counting numbers to tell the stories of the mothers who died, or survived life-threatening complications, to learn lessons that may save the lives of those who follow. The methodologies are facility-based deaths reviews, community-based death reviews (also known as verbal autopsies), confidential enquiries into maternal deaths (CEMDs), near miss reviews and criterion-based clinical audit. Although each of these approaches has different characteristics, they also have a number of key aims and objectives in common, as shown in Box 3.1.[9]

Box 3.1 Maternal death reviews: key points; reproduced with permission from Lewis[9]

The aims and objectives of maternal death or 'near miss' reviews are:
- to help save more women's and newborns' lives, to reduce deaths and complications and to improve the quality of maternity services for the benefit of all pregnant women and their babies
- through the use of guidelines and recommendations, to help ensure that all pregnant and recently delivered women receive the best possible care, delivered in appropriate settings in ways that takes account of, and meet, their individual needs
- to identify the wider non-health system barriers to maternity care and to take action or advocate for beneficial changes such as improved status of women, health education programmes and improved community transport.

The approaches can be used at community or healthcare facility or at regional or national level. Different approaches are appropriate for different circumstances and different levels of health service provision, and can review a number of different outcomes, not just death.

A continual audit cycle

The use of the maternal mortality or morbidity review, or audit cycle, as shown in Figure 3.2, is an essential component of any of these reviews. Completing the feedback, or audit, loop ensures that learning lessons and, most importantly, acting on the results is an integral part of any of these approaches. The process can also be modified, based on experience, to make it easier to use in future.

There is no point in committing valuable resources to collecting information that just gathers dust on shelves. The information must be used for action to help improve maternal health outcomes and empower healthcare professionals to examine their current practices or those of the facility in which they work. Because action is the ultimate goal of these reviews, it is important that those with the ability to implement the recommended changes fully participate in the process. Another crucial part of the surveillance cycle is that the implementation and outcome of any recommendations or changes in practice that have been implemented as a result of these reviews be audited and amended if necessary. Therefore, at the outset, it needs be agreed that

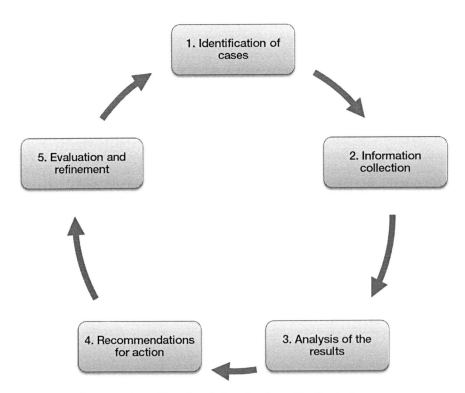

Figure 3.2 The maternal mortality audit cycle; based on *Beyond the Numbers*[2]

the information obtained will be used for action and this is why the involvement and support of the national or local ministry of health is so helpful.

The lessons learnt and guidelines and recommendations arising from them will almost certainly include raising the standards of clinical care, such as through the introduction of evidence-based guidelines or enhanced staff training. Other recommendations may relate to increasing resources, including addressing the manpower gaps, changes in the health system structure, communications or wider social or community issues, including education. In general, recommendations made should be simple, affordable, effective and widely disseminated. Most of the clinical recommendations likely to emerge will be very similar to the evidence-based guidelines already in existence, including those from the WHO Department for Making Pregnancy Safer,[10] the Royal College of Obstetricians and Gynaecologists[11] and a number of other organisations, which are suitable for local adaptation.

Confidentiality

Another common principle is the importance of a confidential, preferably anonymous, non-threatening environment in which to describe and analyse the results. Ensuring confidentiality leads to openness in reporting, which provides a more complete picture as to the precise sequence of events, including possible errors and omissions in the care of a woman. Participants, including healthcare and community workers and family members, need to be assured that the sole purpose of the study is to save lives and not to apportion blame. A prerequisite, therefore, is that strict confidentiality, or anonymity, must be maintained at all times – a principle of 'no name, no blame'. These reviews seek only to identify failures in the healthcare system, not to provide the basis for litigation, management sanctions or blame. This is particularly the case in the former Soviet countries where, even if a death was unavoidable, punishment and legal action are currently the norm, although the introduction of confidential enquiries has led to a softening of attitude in some states.[12]

Self-reflective learning

Participating in reviews such as those discussed here, whether by describing their own contribution to the care of a particular woman, extracting information from the case notes or by assessing the case anonymously, is itself a healthcare worker intervention. Experience has shown that the use of these approaches can have a major impact on those involved. Often those participating in the review are motivated to change their practice or service delivery, even before the formal publication of the results. These healthcare workers, who have seen for themselves the benefits from such relatively simple reviews, including the adoption of simple changes in local practice, become advocates for change. They can then motivate others to undertake similar work and to help spread evidence-based best practice guidance. In the UK, as long ago as 1954,[13] it was recognised that participating in such a study (in this case a confidential enquiry into maternal deaths) had a 'powerful secondary effect' in that 'each participant in these enquiries, however experienced he or she may be, and whether his or her work is undertaken in a teaching hospital, a local hospital, in the community or the patient's home must have benefited from their educative effect'.[14]

The methodologies

This chapter will briefly describe four of the five methodologies that are summarised in Table 3.1. Clinical audit is not considered further here as it is very different technique but all five are explained in full, together with examples, within the BTN document.[2]

Community-based death reviews (verbal autopsies)

These are useful when mothers die outside a health facility. In these reviews, specially trained workers visit the families and communities of women who have died at home and, through the use of semi-structured questionnaires, talk to their relatives and others about the circumstances of the death. These reviews are particularly helpful where the majority of women die at home and may be the only means of deciding a cause of death, although this is often dependent on the relatives' and assessor's interpretation of the story. They also enable both the contributory medical and nonmedical factors to be explored and the barriers to care documented, even where adequate services exist.[15] Verbal autopsies also provide useful information on the demographic and social characteristics of the women who died. Acting on the results can save lives not only through introducing or refocusing health education messages and improving community awareness and knowledge but also by adopting changes in clinical practice and reconfiguring local services to make them more acceptable, accessible and available. However, community-based death reviews can be resource-

Table 3.1 The five methodologies for maternal death or disability reviews described in *Beyond the Numbers*[2]

Approach	Definition
Community-based maternal death reviews (verbal autopsies)	A method of finding out the medical causes of death and ascertaining the personal, family or community factors that may have contributed to the deaths in women who died outside of a medical facility.
Facility-based maternal deaths review	A qualitative, in-depth investigation of the causes of and circumstances surrounding maternal deaths occurring at health facilities. Deaths are initially identified at the facility level but such reviews are also concerned with identifying the combination of factors at the facility and in the community that contributed to the death, and which ones were avoidable.
Confidential enquiries into maternal deaths	A systematic multidisciplinary anonymous investigation of all or a representative sample of maternal deaths occurring at an area, regional (state) or national level. It identifies the numbers, causes and avoidable or remediable factors associated with them.
Surveys of severe morbidity (near misses)	The identification and assessment of cases in which pregnant women survive obstetric complications. There is no universally applicable definition for such cases and it is important that the definition used in any survey be appropriate to local circumstances to enable local improvements in maternal care.
Clinical audit (not discussed further in this chapter)	Clinical audit is a quality improvement process that seeks to improve patient care and outcomes through systematic review of aspects of the structure, processes and outcomes of care against explicit criteria and the subsequent implementation of change. Where indicated, changes are implemented at an individual, team or service level and further monitoring is used to confirm improvement in healthcare delivery.

intensive and the results may lack reliability in ascertaining the medical cause of death. Also, the subjective assessment of the case notes by the review team may be problematic. There may also be over- or under-reporting of cases. For example, there is usually under-reporting of deaths in early pregnancy and over-reporting of deaths from other causes misclassified as being due to maternal reasons.

In a study in Mexico, the methodology identified two key barriers to be the relatives' inability to recognise the importance of symptoms and the need to seek skilled care, and the lack of transport. These findings led to the recommendation that antenatal care should also teach women to recognise and act on complications that require care, including understanding that there may be a possible need for emergency transport during labour and delivery.[16] In Garissa, northeast Kenya, local reviews revealed that women did not go to the local hospital because of a lack of privacy in the delivery room, a perceived lack of cleanliness and the culturally unacceptable presence of a male midwife. Providing curtains between beds, tiling the floors and walls, and the midwife himself voluntarily changing to a managerial position meant the institutional delivery rate rose from 8% to 45% within a year and the MMR declined significantly as a result.[17]

Facility-based maternal death review

It should be established good clinical practice to review each case of a maternal or perinatal death or serious unexpected incident occurring in any facility, at regular multidisciplinary team meetings. Such reviews are of fundamental importance as they offer an opportunity to identify where clinical care may have been below standard and to consider what lessons may be derived from the management of the case and how local procedures and protocols might be improved. However, to strengthen the findings and recommendations even further, it is very helpful to aggregate the findings from all of the cases over a defined period of time to look for factors and avoidable causes that may be common to a significant number of cases. The results of these more comprehensive reviews may point to the need for local guidelines or service reconfiguration, or even something as simple as knowing where the keys to the drug cabinet are at night or at weekends, or the access code to the labour ward if the door is locked. Those responsible for pre- or in-service training may also act on the findings by making changes in the curriculum, introducing more teaching and improving supervisory/feedback mechanisms. The head of obstetrics or midwifery may use the findings to persuade managers or policy makers about the resource needs (staffing, equipment and drugs) of the maternity service. Health managers at district, regional or national level could be provided with a summary of the findings to help them identify service needs and prioritise resources.

Facility-based reviews can be conducted at a single health facility or extended across several facilities as part of a city, district or even regional or national assessment. Many countries that aim to undertake a full-scale CEMD have found it easier to start by identifying and assessing the deaths of women who die in health facilities as they can be more readily identified and assessed. In facilities where maternal deaths are relatively few in number but where there is still a need to review cases to help identify areas for healthcare improvement, it may be helpful to include the more numerous cases of severe morbidity to strengthen the survey. Examples of these and a checklist for their planning and implementation is contained within BTN.[2] As well as a near miss component, it is sometimes also possible to include a verbal autopsy component in some of these reviews.

The most often cited impediment to starting these reviews is ensuring confidentiality for participating members of staff. Encouraging openness in reporting without fear of reprisal or blame is crucial and a number of approaches to this have been developed, which are discussed in the manual. Epidemiologically, these reviews do not provide whole-population data as they only cover deaths in hospital but making a start by improving clinical care for those women who have managed to access facility-based care is already a positive step even when more mothers are dying at home.

Confidential enquiries into maternal deaths

The methodology with the potential to have the most sustained impact is that of a CEMD. These enquiries consider all maternal deaths, or a statistically representative sample of deaths, in a particular area or country and draw up clinical, service and public health recommendations suitable for widespread implementation. The deaths covered include both the women who die at home and the women who die in the facilities, and a standardised system of case identification is essential. These enquiries also need to be supported by stakeholders working at a level where they can influence policy and guideline development. Enquiries that have the most impact have either been commissioned by the national or regional ministry of health or implemented with the ministry as a key stakeholder. Their ownership by other healthcare groups and professional associations leads to the development or revision, dissemination and implementation of professional clinical guidelines. They also provide data for healthcare planners and politicians to use to change or develop policies and raise investment levels in health care where practicable.[2]

The longest running example of a CEMD is that of the UK, where an enquiry process is now in its sixth decade and which has made a considerable impact on maternity care. Over time, other countries have adopted or adapted the methodology and have introduced their own versions. Among the earliest of these were in Egypt,[18] Sri Lanka[19] and Malaysia,[20,21] where the maternal mortality rates have substantially declined. More recently, CEMDs have commenced in a number of more developed countries, and the state of Kerala in southern India published its first report in 2009.[22] The powerful South African Enquiry, 'Saving Mothers', first published in 1998, has started to have a major impact on the development of maternal health policies in that country as well as being held up as a leading example in other parts of Africa and beyond.[23]

The major beneficial difference with this approach is that, being owned at a national or regional level at which policies can be made and guidelines developed, the results and recommendations can have a far wider impact on maternal health than is the case for enquiries carried out only within local facilities or communities. Such wider enquiries provide data for health planners and ministers to change or develop policies and to raise investment levels in health care when practical.

Confidential enquiries take time and coordination to set up and require the support of the ministry of health and of healthcare professionals and their organisations. They usually also require a functioning statistical and health system infrastructure in which to identify all maternal deaths. Although they may require more resources or personal commitment than some of the other methodologies discussed in this guideline, they are not necessarily hugely resource-intensive. The methodology can be adapted to suit the available resources. Most of the work is usually undertaken by motivated, unpaid, local staff, thus requiring only a small number of paid personnel. Participation in the process can also be made explicit in job descriptions.

Surveys of severe morbidity (near miss reviews)

Near miss case reviews consider the management of those women who survived an episode of major maternal morbidity. These reviews provide a valuable adjunct to maternal death reviews, especially in settings where deaths are rare. They can be undertaken on a subset of, or all, cases occurring in one or more health facilities in conjunction with facility-based case reviews, and are already incorporated in the CEMD methodologies used in South Africa and Scotland, with the rest of the UK about to follow suit. Because cases are easier to identify within health facilities, such reviews are unlikely to be very helpful in identifying avoidable factors in community-based settings, but they can provide valuable additional information about access to services and socio-cultural barriers, since the mother herself is alive and can report on her own pathway through pregnancy.

The main advantage of using near misses rather than deaths for audits or case reviews is that obstetric complications occur much more frequently than maternal deaths, enabling a more comprehensive quantitative analysis. In hospitals in Benin and South Africa, for example, near misses were between five and ten times more frequent than deaths.[24,25] Depending on the definition used, this ratio can be as high as 117 near miss cases per maternal death in developed countries.[26]

Near miss reviews are also less threatening. Firstly, if the woman survived in the face of great odds, staff may find it easier to discuss her case, as the enquiry may be less likely to assign blame. And, since she survived, positive elements in the care may appear and staff may be congratulated for saving the woman's life. Secondly, as she survived, she rather than her family members can be interviewed about the quality of the care she received. This may reveal important aspects of the quality of care that might otherwise have been overlooked. The interview with the woman may also complement the information from records.[2]

The problems lie with agreeing a local definition of a 'near miss' and also what is evidence-based good clinical practice. Achieving such consensus is by no means straightforward and agreeing a local definition requires a concerted effort and support by all those involved in the review process. A further issue is that near miss events can usually only be identified in health facilities and do not provide community data. Case ascertainment may require reviewing a large number of registers and case notes in each facility. In settings with a high volume of severe morbidity events, a subsample of cases might be required for in-depth case reviews. Selection criteria for this might include, for example, focusing on events that only occurred at night or weekends, or reviewing only a specific type of complication.

Experience to date

Since the initial publication of BTN in 2004, there have been numerous regional and national workshops organised by WHO, UNFPA, UNICEF, the Commonwealth Secretariat and other safe motherhood partners, and one or more methodologies have subsequently been implemented in a significant number of countries around the world. To date, representatives from the ministries of health and professional organisations in over 60 countries have attended BTN planning workshops and have already started one or more of the methodologies, or are aiming to do so soon. These range from parts of Western Europe to countries in Eastern Europe and Central Asia such as Moldova and Kyrgyzstan, many African nation states, several cities in India and its neighbouring countries and the state of Kerala, as well as several countries in the Far East and Central America.

During the workshops, a number of points became clearer. Deciding which method to adopt depends on three overarching considerations:

■ the level of political and professional support

■ where the review is to be conducted

■ which maternal deaths are to be included.

In terms of level, there are some basic options: community, health facility, or district, regional or national levels. In terms of cases, these can be all maternal deaths, a proportion of deaths or deaths occurring in one facility or region, or from one or more, or all causes. Experience has shown that, at country level, even though a confidential enquiry is the 'gold standard' to which many aspire, the easiest methodologies to start with are community- and facility-based reviews as they are generally the easiest to pilot and introduce, especially in resource-poor settings.[12] Box 3.2 summarises the 'Rule of P's' – the key lessons learnt from the BTN workshops held in the WHO European region, covering mainly the Central Asian republics and newly emerging states.

Conclusion

Since its introduction, BTN has proven to be popular and useful in helping to develop national and local strategies to improve access to, and the quality of, maternity services. Five years after its first publication, individuals from over 60 countries have

---

| **Box 3.2** | Lessons learnt from *Beyond the Numbers* (BTN) implementation in the WHO European region: the Rule of P's; reproduced with permission from Bacci *et al.*[12] |

The introduction of any technique for maternal and perinatal death reviews should be:

1. **practical**, using whichever of the five BTN approaches is realistic and feasible for any country's specific circumstances. Country representatives all agree that it is important to 'start small' and to learn and refine programmes based on acquired experience. For the majority of countries, it proved easier to start with facility-based reviews or, in some places, verbal autopsies, before going for national confidential enquiries.

2. **piloted** – as a basis for good practice, whatever approach is chosen should be piloted first so that questionnaires can be refined in the light of experience and so that any other problems or difficulties that may emerge owing to local particularities can be addressed before national implementation.

3. **partnership based** – developing and implementing the clinical audit methodology should be done in partnership with all key stakeholders (ministry of health, leading obstetricians and midwives, public health officials). All stakeholders should be involved from the beginning at the planning phase through to interpreting and assessing results to allow development and implementation of recommendations.

4. **done with political commitment and support** – it was recognised that although there are benefits from undertaking case reviews at facility level these depend on the enthusiasm and commitment of particular individuals. Experience has shown that by working through the ministry of health national ownership is assured and necessary actions, such as development of a national programme of evidence-based management and/or clinical guidelines, can be taken at central level.

5. **supportive and not punitive** – it was agreed that BTN-style case reviews will require a shift in attitude towards a 'no blame, no shame' culture.

attended workshops and more are planned. The BTN methodologies are attractive and achievable. Experience has shown the practical steps that need to be taken to enable easier implementation. It is therefore planned to update the publication and add additional modules covering in-house death and near miss reviews, to provide a CD-ROM with a usable database, a simple analytical package and a list of suitable generic questionnaires, and, finally, to extend these methodologies into a manual for perinatal death and near miss review.

Ideally, every country should have a functioning national maternal and neonatal death review and audit committee supported by the professional associations and the ministry of health. It should have the ability and authority to undertake maternal death reviews and to make the necessary recommendations for improving maternal and newborn health within that country.

A network of regional BTN (or similar) centres throughout the world would be able to lead and coordinate these activities throughout the region and to act both as centres of excellence and as training institutions for the development of sustainable programmes in future.

References

1. Callaghan WM. Epilogue. In: Berg C, Danel I, Atrash H, Zane S, Bartlett L, editors. *Strategies to Reduce Pregnancy-Related Deaths: From Identification and Review to Action.* Atlanta: Centers for Disease Control and Prevention; 2001. p. 53.

2. World Health Organization. *Beyond the Numbers: Reviewing Maternal Deaths and Complications to Make Pregnancy Safer.* WHO: Geneva; 2004 [http://www.who.int/making_pregnancy_safer/documents/9241591838/en/].

3. United Nations. *United Nations Millennium Declaration.* General Assembly resolution 55/2. New York: United Nations; 2000. [www.un.org/millenniumgoals].

4. World Heath Organization. *Maternal Mortality in 2005. Estimates developed by WHO, UNCEF, UNFPA and The World Bank.* Geneva: WHO; 2007 [www.who.int/reproductive-health].

5. Lewis G, editor. *Saving Mothers' Lives: Reviewing Maternal Deaths to Make Motherhood Safer 2003–2005. The Seventh Report on Confidential Enquiries into Maternal Deaths in the United Kingdom.* London: CEMACH; 2007 [www.cmace.org.uk].

6. Lewis G, CEMACH. *Why Mothers Die 2000–2002 – The Sixth Report of Confidential Enquiries into Maternal Deaths in the United Kingdom.* London: RCOG Press; 2004 [www.cmace.org.uk].

7. Department of Health. *Maternity Matters: Choice, Access and Continuity of Care in a Safe Service.* London: Department of Health; 2007 [www.dh.gov.uk/publications].

8. Thaddeus S, Maine D. Too far to walk: maternal mortality in context. *Soc Sci Med* 1994;38:1091–110.

9. Lewis G. Reviewing maternal deaths to make pregnancy safer. *Best Pract Res Clin Obstet Gynaecol* 2008;22:447–63.

10. World Health Organization [www.who.int/reproductive-health].

11. Royal College of Obstetricians and Gynaecologists [www.rcog.org.uk].

12. Bacci A, Lewis G, Baltag V, Betrán AP. The introduction of confidential enquiries into maternal deaths and near-miss case reviews in the WHO European Region. *Reprod Health Matters* 2007;15:145–52.

13. Department of Health. *The Confidential Enquiries into Maternal Deaths in England and Wales 1952–54.* London: Department of Health for England; 1954.

14. Godber G. The origin and inception of the Confidential Enquiries into Maternal Deaths. *BJOG* 1994;101:946–7.

15. Ronsmans C, Campbell O. *Verbal Autopsies for Maternal Deaths.* Report of a WHO workshop. WHO/FHE/MSM/95.15. Geneva: WHO; 1995.

16. Langer A, Hernandez B, Garcia-Barrios C, Saldana-Uranga GL; National Safe Motherhood Committee of Mexico. Identifying interventions to prevent maternal mortality in Mexico: a

verbal autopsy study. In: Berer M, Ravindran TKS, editors. *Safe Motherhood Initiatives: Critical Issues.* London: Blackwell Science; 1999.

17. G Lewis, personal communication.

18. Ministry of Health. *National Maternal Mortality Study: Egypt 1992–1993.* Cairo: Ministry of Health, 1994.

19. Sri Lanka College of Obstetricians and Gynaecologists. *Maternal Deaths in Sri Lanka: a Review of Estimates and Causes 1996.* Colombo: Sri Lanka College of Obstetricians and Gynaecologists; 1996.

20. Pathmanathan I, Liljestrand J, Martins JM, Rajapaksa LC, Lissner C, de Silva A, *et al. Investing in Maternal Health: Learning from Malaysia and Sri Lanka.* Washington, DC: The World Bank; 2003.

21. Ministry of Health. *Evaluation and Implementation of the Confidential Enquiries Into Maternal Deaths in the Improvement of Maternal Health Services.* Kuala Lumpur: Ministry of Health; 1998.

22. Paily V, editor. *Why Mothers Die, Kerala 2004–05. The First Report of the Confidential Enquiries into Maternal Deaths, Kerala 2004 and 2005.* Cochin: Kerala Federation of Obstetrics and Gynaecology; 2009.

23. Department of Health. *First Interim Report on Confidential Enquiries into Maternal Deaths in South Africa.* Pretoria: National Committee on Confidential Enquiries into Maternal Deaths; 1998.

24. Filippi V, Alihonou E, Mukantaganda S, Graham WJ, Ronsmans C. Near misses: maternal morbidity and mortality. *Lancet* 1998;351:145–6.

25. Mantel GD, Buchmann E, Rees H, Pattinson RC. Severe acute maternal morbidity: a pilot study of a definition for a near-miss. *Br J Obstet Gynaecol* 1998;105:985–90.

26. Waterstone M, Bewley S, Wolfe C. Incidence and predictors of severe obstetric morbidity: case–control study. *BMJ* 2001;322:1089–93.

Chapter 4
Human resource challenges

Soo Downe

Introduction

It has become increasingly clear that one of the key solutions to the problem of maternal and infant mortality is the provision of sufficient skilled, up-to-date and empathic birth attendants when and where women need them, in the context of a system that permits rapid escalation of care and emergency treatment where this is necessary. There is almost universal agreement on this principle, even if there is intense debate on the implications for the nature and location of maternity services provision. Despite the rhetorical consensus, in 2006 the World Health Organization (WHO) noted that 57 countries had a severe lack of healthcare workers in general, including maternity care workers.[1] In 2008, the Kampala Declaration[2] on 'health workers for all and all for health workers' announced that:

> Everyone committed to this agenda shares the vision that 'all people, everywhere, shall have access to a skilled, motivated and facilitated health worker within a robust health system'.

At the 2006 World Health Assembly, WHO issued Resolution WHA59.23,[3] which called for rapid scaling up of health workforce production, and WHA59.27,[4] which called for the strengthening of nursing and midwifery globally.[5] In 2009, the WHO *Making Pregnancy Safer* report[6] estimated that there was a 50% shortfall on the 700 000 midwives that were needed worldwide and that 47 000 doctors with obstetric skills were still required, particularly in rural areas. This chapter deals with some of the issues to be addressed if the Resolutions are to be met.

There is a clear relationship between countries and socio-economic groups without good access to skilled birth attendants and rates of maternal and infant mortality (Figure 4.1).

For example, in Cuba there are 170 people to each doctor but in Malawi and Tanzania this is 50 000 to 1. Cuba has a reported perinatal mortality of 15.5 per 1000 live births,[7] against 34 per 1000 pregnancies in Malawi[8] and 42 per 1000 pregnancies in Tanzania.[9] In terms of nurses and midwives per 10 000 population, this varies from 1 in Haiti (neonatal mortality 25 per 1000 live births)[10] to 195 in Ireland (perinatal mortality 2.37/1000).[11] However, countries with the highest resource allocation to health (such as the USA) do not necessarily experience the lowest rates of mortality, possibly because the health funding system restricts access to appropriately skilled and

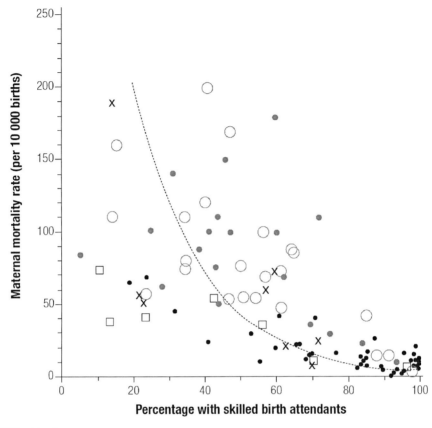

Figure 4.1 Rates of maternal mortality and skilled birth attendant by region; reproduced with permission from Woods[55]

trained health professionals for those who do not have sufficient insurance. Given these data, it could be argued that there is no need to debate the issue of the skilled birth attendant any further. The solution to the persisting failure to progress towards achieving Millennium Development Goals (MDGs) 4 and 5 is for all countries to train, upskill or task shift more individuals to be appropriately trained skilled birth attendants as soon as possible and to ensure all women have access to them.

The fact that this has not happened to date indicates that the human resource issue is rather more complex than this solution suggests. The barriers to effective human resource solutions appear to relate to the following key areas:

▨ disagreement about the nature of the skilled birth attendant

▨ debate about the optimum location of practice

▨ the response of local communities to imposed solutions

- issues around education, training and updating (including upskilling and task shifting)
- problems with sufficient employment and sustainable retention, particularly in rural and remote areas
- the lack of an effective supervision, management and policy infrastructure.

This chapter explores each of these areas in turn and then summarises the key issues in each case. The final section presents some examples of countries and settings where coverage of maternity care has been increased and where maternal and infant mortality rates have fallen. The key lessons from these sites are summarised at the end of the paper.

Barriers to effective human resource solutions

Nature of the skilled birth attendant

There appear to be two paradigmatic designs of formal professional maternity care across the world. In the first, obstetricians are the lead professionals, assisted by nurses, nurse-midwives, auxiliary staff and/or medical assistants who have a greater or lesser degree of formal training and a greater or lesser degree of autonomy. In the second model, midwives are the lead professionals for normal birth and obstetricians are the lead professionals for problematic pregnancy and birth, and there is a greater or lesser degree of control by obstetricians over the work of midwives; nurses and auxiliary staff may be assistants to midwives and/or doctors. The former model is most prevalent in North America and other countries under its sphere of influence, whereas the latter is the prevalent model in Europe and other countries with a legacy of European influence.

However, in many countries of the world, an informal non-professional service design is the norm. In this context, local care is given by family members, by dayas/traditional birth attendants (TBAs) or by traditional midwives, and health-centre care may be given by nonmedical clinicians. Some of these carers see their work as a calling, either secular or divine, and many are highly skilled by virtue of many years of experience.

WHO uses four summary categories to characterise the range of groups providing formal health care across the world:[12]

- medical doctors
- non-physician clinicians
- nurses
- community health workers.

This list does not include the informal traditional caring sector. The diversity of provision raises many questions about the nature of the skilled birth attendant. One of the most widely quoted definitions is:[13]

> an accredited health professional – such as a midwife, doctor or nurse – who has been educated and trained to proficiency in the skills needed to manage normal (uncomplicated) pregnancies, childbirth and the immediate postnatal period, and in the identification, management and referral of complications in women and newborns.

It is of interest that this definition is skills based. It does not cover attitudes and behaviours, or knowledge of techniques to integrate effectively into and across local contexts. There is reasonable anecdotal evidence that systems of care that deliver the best outcomes most economically include well-respected, well-trained, genuinely caring and adequately rewarded and deployed professional midwives working locally and effectively with local respected and experienced traditional community workers and with local service users, with rapid access to effective referral and transfer systems and well-resourced, efficient and empathic emergency professional medical treatment at central locations.

However, in some counties, midwifery is illegal and, in others, the cost of full midwifery and medical training to ensure sufficient numbers of both midwives and obstetricians for all childbearing women to access is beyond local or even governmental budgets. In some locations, the introduction of midwifery and other new cadres is seen as a competitive challenge to existing professional groups, thus creating resistance. In other settings, cultural elements, such as caste and gender bias and low education levels for women, preclude the majority from contemplating midwifery as a respected and suitable professional. In some communities, allegiance to the local traditional midwife or experienced TBA is strong and there is resistance to the imposition of a new cadre of worker with a biomedical perspective (midwife or obstetrician), especially where this is seen as counter-cultural or in contravention of religious teaching. These factors all need to be considered as an element in the decision making about the appropriate cadre of skilled birth attendant for a specific local context.

Location of practice

In 2008, WHO stated that, in countries of all levels of available resource, a primary care based health system has the greatest chance of producing better outcomes, improving equity and meeting social expectations.[14] Worldwide, it has been estimated that around one in three births are not attended by a skilled birth attendant.[15] Although half the world's population lives in rural areas, only about one-third of nurses and about one-quarter of all physicians work there (Table 4.1).[16]

The vast majority of the world's medical and nursing training centres are in cities and most graduates of these programmes want to work where they trained, or in locations that provide at least equivalent work and lifestyle opportunities. As a result, and in situations of constrained human resources, remote and rural communities consistently lose out. These are also the communities that are least likely to have access to means of transport and to effective transportation infrastructures, so any countrywide human resource deficits are amplified in rural and remote settings. In terms of pregnancy and childbirth, the impact of this deficit is severe, as the acute nature of emergency events demands a local response. This situation is a long way from the primary care focused health system envisaged by WHO.

Table 4.1 Rural versus urban worldwide distribution of populations, nurses and physicians; data from WHO[16]

	Rural	Urban
World population	50%	50%
Nurses worldwide	38%	62%
Physicians worldwide	24%	76%

This is not just a problem in the Southern countries of the world. In the USA, the frontier nurse-midwives were set up in the 1950s to serve remote, disadvantaged communities where other cadres did not want to work.[17] They were effective in improving outcomes, specifically in terms of stillbirths and maternal and infant mortality. In Australia, remote aboriginal populations are the least well served in terms of health care in general and maternity care in particular, and they have the worst outcomes.[18] In Canada, the centralising solution of flying pregnant Inuit women to hospitals hundreds of miles away from their local community to await the birth of their baby was a relative failure in terms of maternal wellbeing and this has led to a range of initiatives to improve local access to skilled and culturally appropriate care.[19,20]

As an early attempt to address the maternity skills shortage in community settings, UNFPA supported the training of TBAs in hygienic practices and basic emergency skills in the early 1970s. Some of the intentions of training TBAs were to ensure capacity at the community/village level, to prevent harm in childbirth, to detect and refer in cases of pathology, and to treat some acute emergencies, such as postpartum haemorrhage. The evidence on the effectiveness of the TBA programme is mixed.[21] Some possible reasons for this are explored later in this chapter. The lack of the expected level of success has led to a rethink and a call to institute local area health centres where skilled birth attendants can be based.[22] This proposal is a pragmatic solution to the fact that training sufficient qualified nurses and/or midwives to attend all women in their communities is not a realistic proposition in the short term for many countries. However, making this new approach work may depend on learning the lessons from previous attempts to centralise maternity care away from communities. These include the problems inherent in the need for women to travel in late pregnancy and labour, the financial burden of accessing such centres in communities where cash is scarce, and the emerging routinisation (and even dehumanisation) of care in centralised locations. Ultimately, these are all factors that will affect the desire of skilled birth attendants to work in such centres and the willingness of local women and communities to access them.

Community acceptability

Although provision of skilled maternity care providers in district level health buildings/locations might be a pragmatic solution to the skills shortage that exists in many countries today, there is evidence that, where they are provided, women do not always use these facilities.[23] This is partly to do with the 'three delays':[24]

1. seeking help
2. getting to help
3. receiving adequate help.

It is also, however, partly to do with the dehumanised care women receive in some of these centralised locations,[25] and with disarticulation between the local and the central care systems.[26] Disarticulation can arise as a result of dysfunctional relationships between staff in the central unit and those referring or bringing women in from the community, and also as a consequence of the clash between cash and subsistence economies.[27] The negative atmosphere set up in this situation prevents women from attending for future visits and demotivates staff, causing a vicious circle to develop. Junior staff, or staff groups lower in the hierarchy, feel overworked, undervalued and victimised, and they have no positive feedback from those they care for. Classic vertical bullying can develop, with childbearing women at the bottom of the heap. It may be increasingly hard to persuade skilled birth attendants to work in such settings, which then creates understaffing, burn-out in remaining staff and delay in treatment. This makes the central setting even more unacceptable to women, even if they are in dire need. The experience of those who do use the service feeds back to others in the community and to the local TBA or traditional midwife, who is not welcomed at the central location. This vicious circle is self-perpetuating and persistent.

There is evidence that systems that consciously build mutual trust and respect can overcome this barrier.[28] The consequence can be improved use of central services, increased willingness of local workers to refer appropriately and the development of mutual regard so that traditional and professional carers can effectively learn together and from each other.[19] Participatory approaches to solving the problems of maternal mortality can make the local health centre and community more attractive places for women to use and for skilled birth attendants to live and work. Absolutely crucially, they appear to have a significant impact on maternal and infant mortality.[29] Improving community acceptability has the potential to change a vicious circle into a virtuous cycle.

Education, training and updating (including upskilling and task shifting)

There is arguably a moral duty for local and governmental political entities to educate and train enough healthcare staff to provide skilled birth attendance to all childbearing women within their jurisdiction. Given even basic data on populations and demographics, it should be possible for government agencies to have an understanding of how many skilled birth attendants are needed, even if the type of cadre required is subject to local debate and to available resources. The content of the basic training is fairly uncontroversial. WHO and UNICEF have tools and resources to underpin care for normal pregnancy and birth, as well as for a wide range of chronic and acute pathologies. Emergency obstetric care courses are well established. The standards for professional midwifery and obstetric courses have been determined by the respective international organisations – the International Confederation of Midwives (ICM) and the International Federation of Gynecology and Obstetrics (FIGO) – and a wide range of standard-setting authorities across the world. The debate seems to be around how local beliefs, cultures and norms are integrated into the authoritative knowledge that is represented by the standard psychosocial biomedical model of midwifery and obstetric training taught in most university settings. There is a growing recognition that it is important to base at least some professional maternity care training in rural and remote areas and to incorporate education in the issues, cultures and diseases that are important to marginalised groups in any specific country. This is seen as one way of ensuring that at least some trained professionals will choose to work in these areas.[30]

Where there is not enough time or resource to train professional staff from the outset, upskilling and task shifting have been proposed. The process has also been termed 'substitution'. Following a formal systematic review of studies undertaken in African countries, Dovlo[31] characterised four levels of practice in this area:

- ■ indirect substitution (such as enhanced midwife roles and nurse anaesthetists)
- ■ direct substitution (new cadres of staff such as medical assistants)
- ■ intra-cadre skills assignment (delegating specific specialist tasks to other groups with less formal training)
- ■ delegation of nonprofessional tasks (for example, task shifting to health aides or TBAs).

Dovlo noted that 'the cost-effectiveness of using substitutes and their relative retention within countries and in rural communities underlies their advantages to African health systems. Some studies comparing clinical officers and doctors show minimal differences in outcomes to patients.'

These findings raise a series of questions. As Dovlo[31] observed, the blurring of professional and cadre boundaries can lead to intergroup hostility, with poor-quality services as a consequence. Taking a reductionist task-led approach may antagonise both those groups who see their professional projects being eroded and those groups to whom the tasks are substituted, or shifted, who may see their workload expand beyond their control. In a Global Health Workforce Alliance Community of Practice (CoP) debate on task shifting in 2009, it was suggested that the better approach is 'task-sharing'.[32] In this case, the shift in tasks and the upskilling process are both discussed and mutually agreed, with a clear back-up plan if escalation of care is required. This approach also pays attention to skills built up over years of experiential learning, and recognises and values these capacities. The process of task and/or skill sharing in this way can in itself provide an opportunity to create effective teams who like each other. Building effective relationships at this stage may bear fruit in future, in terms of shared decision making, appropriate referral and willingness to learn from each other.

In the same Global Health Workforce Alliance debate, it was suggested that natural crises can provide unexpected opportunities to identify individuals who may be capable of taking on healthcare tasks and, eventually, formal training. Local people who respond rapidly and who demonstrate leadership and generate respect may be the ideal catalysts around whom effective local community provision can be built. Part of the development of sustainable local health provision might include deliberate attention to this kind of emergence.

However task sharing or upskilling opportunities are developed, it is essential to ensure that sustainability is enhanced with formal support systems. These include clear roles and job descriptions, or role scopes, allowing for flexibility around the tasks that can be done by a range of groups at role boundaries. Systems of updating knowledge and skills are essential to ensure that practitioners remain skilled and aware of new developments, drugs and techniques that will improve the health of the local population. The Healthcare Information For All by 2015 (HIFA2015) campaign was set up to promote and fulfil the aim that 'by 2015, every person worldwide will have access to an informed healthcare provider'.[33] The HIFA2015 *Foundation Document* illustrates the chronic lack of information among health providers for even basic treatments in pregnancy and childbirth and in general healthcare situations. A few countries have systems of supervision and of mandatory updating but these often require expensive attendance at study days and more junior staff may find it hard to be released to attend. Books are often out of date, especially where they are exported to resource-poor centres when new editions are published in resource-rich countries.

The electronic revolution might be seen as a solution to this problem, and, for some, it has made a dramatic difference. One of the partnership priorities for donor countries is to build up systems of open access and data transfer that can revolutionise knowledge locally, assuming that this can be contextualised culturally and philosophically.

Where internet access is available, initiatives such as the launch of free online access to the *African Journal of Primary Care and Family Medicine*, launched by Open Journals Publishing in 2009, can help. The journal contains a facility to help aspiring authors to improve their papers before publication, which, in turn, can contribute to a virtuous cycle of building capacity and self-esteem. However, this depends on access to reliable power sources, then hardware, then the internet, then sufficient bandwidth, then the resources to pay to access journals, educational sites and downloads, and then on access to a printer with enough ink and paper to keep printing. The revolutions in communication and education that are offered by Skype and virtual worlds such as Second Life are not available to many rural and remote communities. Organisations such as TALC (Teaching Aids at Low Cost) are addressing some of these issues with CD-ROMs, and the provision of a high-speed internet link to South Africa will help some countries in that area, but the real revolution seems to be in mobile phone technology. Given the phenomenal spread of mobile phones, the minimal resources needed to run them and the almost universal access to satellite technology, this may be where educational resources are best sited for most.

The local community is also a valuable resource. Training staff in community action and participatory action research techniques, and in self-reflection and reflexivity, possibly in combination with virtual (e- or m-media based) CoP,[34] might in itself create learning through grounded feedback loops. The growing interest in narrative medicine[35] and in learning from 'N-of-1' studies[36] provides a background for this kind of education and training for remote workers. *Cases Journal* (casesjournal.com), which was launched in 2008, is an example of a forum where experiential learning is contextualised by research and theory. This clinically embedded approach may be particularly valuable for maternity care workers who work with small numbers of women in rural and remote areas.

Sufficient employment and sustainable retention, particularly in rural and remote areas

Even if enough of the right kinds of maternity care provider are educated, prepared and updated, the human resource solution depends on adequate levels of employment and retention. In some countries, enough staff are prepared but they are lost before they even start clinical work, or soon after they have done so. The problem includes:

- lack of employment opportunities
- lack of attractiveness of rural locations
- lack of career progression
- loss of staff through external brain drain to developed countries where the pay and rewards are greater and where the opportunities for self-development are improved
- internal brain drain to non-governmental organisations (NGOs), topic-specific global health initiatives and government health agencies
- in some countries, loss of healthcare workers to HIV/AIDS and to endemic diseases such as malaria and tuberculosis.

All of these conditions further extend the numbers of years that would be necessary to train an adequate healthcare cohort for all women, including those in the most remote areas. A number of strategies to overcome this issue have been proposed and tested.

As noted above, in 2006 WHO produced a Resolution[3] for rapid scaling up of human resources and for establishing productive partnerships between resource-rich and resource-poor counties in this area. Intergovernmental or interagency partnership arrangements can seem to be an answer, potentially including basic education, skills development, postgraduate training and research. However, they carry risks, specifically in terms of staff that leave for a short-term educational visits and then do not return. One of the key strategies in the 2008 Kampala Declaration[2] is to manage the pressures of the international health workforce market and its impact on migration (Strategy 6).

The High-Level Forum on Health MDGs has set up best practice principles for global partnerships, with an emphasis on in-country funding, including in-country education and training.[37] WHO is also currently finalising a voluntary code on the international recruitment of health personnel.[38] This requires recruiting countries to ensure they train enough staff locally, that they are not denuding countries of their essential workforce and that any concerted recruitment drive is agreed with and managed at government level.

All of these agreements and policies have been made and endorsed at the governmental level. However, the main driver for most healthcare practitioners to leave their country of origin is personal: the promise of better financial rewards and of professional and personal advancement. Free movement of individuals is an important right but this needs to be balanced with local need. In seeking to make this balance, some strategies are focused on the retention of a service, if not of specific individuals, particularly in rural areas. These include the requirement for healthcare staff who have been publicly funded in their training to work in less well-served areas for a set amount of time (usually 2–5 years). This strategy has had mixed results.[39] Retention schemes based on compulsion can come at a cost to day-to-day commitment, which can result in poor service provision. Those forced to serve their time in difficult and unsanitary conditions are unlikely to perform at their best, either technically or in terms of interpersonal skills. This might again generate a negative cycle of poor-quality care leading to rejection by women, non-attendance, increased morbidity and mortality and decreased staff morale.

Incentive-based retention schemes seem to be more successful. In Zambia, a health worker retention scheme was set up in 2003 to encourage the retention of medical staff in rural areas.[40] The plan was to offer a flexible package of incentives that paid attention to the range of issues that were of concern to staff. The package included improving the basic working infrastructure and the availability of essential equipment, offering good-quality staff accommodation, providing access to guaranteed sources of power and water, and offering monetary and non-monetary salary top-ups. Eighty-eight percent of the original staff were retained until the end of the 3-year contract period and 65% renewed for a second 3-year term. This scheme is now being extended to nurses and to enrolled midwives, among others.

Another effective strategy seems to be a deliberate effort to train members of local communities as skilled health practitioners at all levels.[39] It appears that a higher percentage of these individuals return to work for long stretches, or even permanently, in their community of origin. For example, in Afghanistan, the Community Midwifery Education Programme enrols students from districts with a significant deficit in provision.[41] The candidates must also be endorsed by their local community and they are expected to return there. Since the programme was introduced in 2002, the number of midwives available in Afghanistan increased from 467 to 2167 (mid-2008) and the number of births attended by skilled workers rose from roughly 6% in 2003 to 19.9% in 2006. Longombe[42] reported in 2009 on a small-scale comparative study in the Congo that assessed the retention of doctors trained in a medical school based in a rural setting and one based in an urban setting. Of the 97.7% of the rural graduates who were employed in the province where they trained, the majority (81.4%) stayed in rural areas. Of the 40.0% of urban graduates who stayed in their local province, only 23.7% worked in a rural area.

Offering locally based pre-registration education for health workers may also bring added value, in that personnel known to the local community might be more likely to understand local issues and values, to trust and respect local people, and to be trusted and respected in their turn. Programmes that explicitly build in modules on local community issues and diseases are also more likely to retain qualified staff locally.[39]

The issue of the internal brain drain is less well recognised than that of intercountry recruitment. This is the phenomenon of the movement away from practice and into management and administration positions in NGOs. The NGO Code of Conduct for Health Systems Strengthening is designed to counteract this movement.[43] This code is intended to alert NGOs to the problem and to encourage them to build sustainability into their planning and recruitment strategies so that sufficient healthcare workers are reseeded into clinical practice.

It appears that sustainable recruitment and retention of skilled birth attendants, both medical and midwifery/nursing, is dependent on a complex and interconnected set of factors. The systematic narrative review undertaken by Lehmann and colleagues[39] synthesises 55 papers in this area and concluded that bundles of interventions are the best solution to what is a complex and multifactorial issue. These bundles included:

- elements relating to living conditions, including access to clean water, good housing and education for children
- working environments, including reducing overwork and increasing access to equipment and resources that are appropriate for local need and fully functioning
- development opportunities, including continuing education and involvement in research
- changing the locus of decision-making power so that it is devolved to the most local level possible.

In summary, they concluded that incentives can be divided into three core groups:
- education and regulatory interventions
- monetary compensation (direct and indirect financial incentives)
- management, environment and social support.

Dieleman and colleagues[44] reached a similar conclusion in 2009 relating to the factors that improve health workers' performance, using realist review techniques. They concluded that change for the better happens in the context of increased knowledge and skills, and of feeling a need or obligation to change. Motivation is increased by a sense of local problems, being empowered, having and accepting new information, having a sense of belonging and being respected, experiencing clear improvements in the quality of care that can be delivered and having an increase in remuneration.

In summary, the problem of recruitment and retention of skilled maternity care workers is not simple. The new and more nuanced designs used by researchers in this area offer the potential to be the basis of whole-system complexity-based solutions at governmental and organisational level that might succeed where simple solutions have previously failed. Places where such strategies have been implemented can provide powerful learning opportunities. The examples given at the end of this chapter indicate the possibilities for this approach.

Supervision, management and policy infrastructure

Once staff are in place and their skills up to date, it is essential to ensure that they practise effectively, that they are linked into working management structures and that the policy infrastructure continues to support sustainable systems. This is true of the skilled maternity care practitioner as well as for those who are taking up task sharing, delegation and upskilling roles. A degree of command and control is necessary to ensure good quality but there is a risk that completely top-down systems of supervision and management can create rigid hierarchies that limit innovation and repress individualised care that might violate strict role definitions and tasks. Whole-system approaches, such as the one that has been instituted in Sri Lanka (see below), allow for local knowledge to inform the staffing needs at the community level. Such intelligence is essential to enable management systems to ensure that there are enough of the most appropriate staff available.

Clear job descriptions and regular assessment of updating needs and skill deficits are essential elements in ensuring good-quality clinical care. This needs to be based on self-assessment and on simple, locally relevant forms of measurement, ideally with the input of women using the local service. Systems that build in flexible learning from novel situations are more likely to be responsive to the needs of childbearing women and their communities. The creation of face-to-face, or virtual (e- or m-technology) CoPs, where the contributions of all members are equally valued, can provide mutual, reflexive learning opportunities for staff at all levels who are based across the range of settings used by local women. The theoretical basis for the effectiveness of CoPs is mutuality of interest and willingness to learn from each other.[34] Over time, effective CoPs can contribute to and catalyse a spontaneous desire in individuals to be up to date and to learn. They can also be catalytic in building mutual trust and respect between staff that work in different parts of the system. As a consequence, movement of pregnant and labouring women between systems and locations may become easier. In some settings, gender and caste hierarchies may interact with professional role boundaries, making it difficult to create a forum in which honest debate can take place. In this case, CoPs may need to be tailored for homogeneous groups in the first instance. As these groups gain confidence, it may become possible to support mergers between CoPs of different interest groups, all of which have a mutual interest in reaching MDGs 4 and 5.

Effective management and policy systems depend on local intelligence, open channels so that information can flow freely upwards and downwards, the capacity and willingness of management cadres to address identified needs, and the capacity and willingness of policy makers to learn from the information they receive and to plan for the future. The integrated approach used in Sri Lanka, discussed below, provides an example. Such examples suggest that whole-system approaches will usually need to take a realist view in the first instance. This involves identifying what needs to change at all levels and then working with those elements that can be manipulated with a minimum of resistance first, with a longer-term plan to tackle the more resistant elements as the innovation evolves and becomes embedded. Figure 4.2 illustrates some of the complexities that can influence the recruitment and retention of staff.

A successful whole-system approach to the human resource issues relating to MDGs 4 and 5 requires attention to the continuing sustainability of new innovations in maternity staffing. Strategies for doing this include both formal top-down systems of management and supervision and more informal self-supervision and interprofessional development through approaches such as CoPs. To ensure effective policy and planning for the future, the knowledge generated by these systems must be transmitted freely between local and regional levels, to central government, and back again.

Stories of success in whole-system approaches

The Mobile Obstetric Maternal Health Worker and the Midwives and Others with Midwifery Skills initiatives

The Mobile Obstetric Maternal Health Worker (MOM) initiative was initially developed in response to the problems with maternity care in Burma.[45] Before the project began, the maternal mortality ratio was 1000–1200 per 100 000 live births

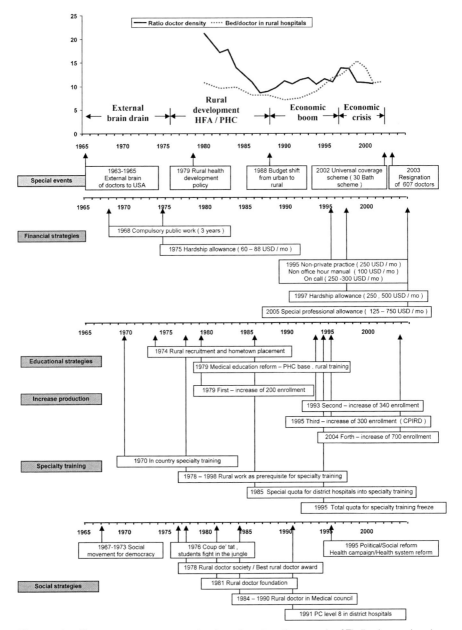

Figure 4.2 Human resources as a complex dynamic system: the example of Thailand; reproduced with permission from Noree *et al*.[56]

and the infant mortality rate was 218 per 1000 live births. Apart from deficits in the maternity services infrastructure and endemic socio-economic problems, the country was experiencing civil war and regular attacks on health workers and healthcare facilities. Recognising the complex issues in the Burmese situation, a multi-ethnic collaborative developed the MOM project, which was designed to bring maternal and child services to local women using a community-based approach. It was decided that, for this particular setting, maternal health workers should be trained to bring maternity care, including emergency care, to the home. This entailed a 6-month training programme that included clinical elements, strategies for community mobilisation, counselling skills, and training and supervision. The package included skills updating, protocol standardisation and ensuring adequate supplies of equipment, and information exchange. It was designed to address all three key delays, as well as building community resilience. As the programme only commenced in 2006, it is too early to see an effect on maternal and infant mortality rates. However, the case studies presented by Teela and colleagues[45] indicate high levels of commitment and of functioning in the maternal health workers, and effects on the wider community. As one maternal health worker respondent said, her role 'brings together families and communities'. In an extreme context of war and poverty, this is an important effect.

The Midwives and Others with Midwifery Skills (MOMS) is a UNFPA/UNICEF and ICM initiative launched in 2006.[46] The project report cites a range of instances in which this approach is used, from all regions of the world. Many of the projects cited in the report have the following operational approaches in common with the Burmese initiative:

1. identify local health workers (such as traditional midwives) who intend to remain local, who are respected and who have years of experiential learning

2. undertake a local needs assessment, paying attention to local cultural norms, beliefs and skills, and identifying issues such as out-of-date materials, in languages that do not make sense to locals, and that are solely based on biomedical constructions of physiology and reality

3. ensure that essential skills (for example, the physiology of the pelvis) are taught but also include knowledge of relevance to the local community, such as building community capacity in general

4. identify local learning styles and prepare materials that take this into account

5. ensure continuous and continuing support

6. link up local healthcare systems with referral locations, through joint training and education sessions, and use this to recognise unique local knowledge, to share relevant biomedical knowledge and to build mutual trust and respect

7. continue to educate and retain increasing numbers of skilled birth attendants alongside and in partnership with these local systems.

Medical officer of health units in Sri Lanka

In Sri Lanka, primary healthcare services are channelled via medical officer of health units (MOHUs).[47,48] Every household is linked to one of the MOHUs. Each MOHU has a medical officer of health, around 20 public health midwives, each with a designated subpopulation to cover, and about six public health inspectors, also with designated subpopulations. The midwife does her work in home visits, or visits to local clinics. The public health inspector is concerned with notifiable infections and water and food hygiene. This role is carried out via community visits. The staff are generally held in high regard by the local community. They have strong allegiances to their local areas and to the other staff members in the MOHU. The motto in each MOHU is 'to know your people, know your area'. This work runs in parallel with the provision of free education to girls, in recognition of the societal complexities of good maternal, family and societal health. However, some of these benefits are being undermined by bribery and corruption at local and regional government levels. This is the next component of the system to be addressed. Despite this problem, the introduction of the system has been associated with reductions in maternal and child mortality and increased coverage of vaccination.

Community voluntary health workers in Nepal and Bangladesh

In Nepal, the female community voluntary health workers scheme was established in 1988.[49] Of all women who see a female community voluntary health worker, 85% attend for antenatal care. Ninety-seven percent of all rural wards are covered. The scheme includes the set-up of local mothers' groups and facilitation of mutual community support networks that encourage health awareness.

In Bangladesh, the community voluntary support system has been in place since 2005.[50] Trained volunteers make household visits to advise on health issues and to check up on the wellbeing of pregnant women. They communicate regularly with health workers, refer women with complications, and accompany women who transfer. The volunteers are rewarded in terms of microfinance. They are permitted to sell ionised salt to those they visit and they receive commission for selling health micro-insurance.

In both Nepal and Bangladesh, the schemes are underpinned with clearly defined roles and regular supervision, updating and support. Maternal mortality ratios in Nepal are falling and there have been no maternal deaths in the 30 pilot communities in Bangladesh since the scheme began there.

Linking up systems in South America

In Otavalo, Ecuador, a project was set up in 2008 that sought to integrate cultural practices and beliefs into the hospital setting.[51] This included the use of upright position for labour, traditional herbs and remedies, and companionship from the woman's chosen birth partners. Crucially, the scheme was developed in partnership between local traditional midwives and registered medical, nursing and midwifery hospital staff. Compared with eight maternal deaths in the hospital in the year before the change, there was only one in the year after the change (and that was deemed to be unavoidable). The infant mortality rate was 7.8 per 1000 live births, less than half the national average. Intriguingly, caesarean sections reduced from 18% to 8%. Significantly, the project also increased hospital births by 8%, as women who were previously afraid of the hospital become more convinced of the possible benefits of attending. The centre is now at the hub of a roll-out project, as these collaborative and culturally sensitive practices begin to spread to other local provinces.

The 104 Advice hotline in India

The 104 Advice telemedicine project was set up in the Andhra Pradesh state in India in 2007 with two aims:[52]

- to offer health advice, information on health care and counselling to callers
- to provide primary screening to rural pregnant women, growing children and people with chronic diseases to reduce maternal and infant mortality rates.

The service offers a toll-free telephone service where callers can get basic health advice and counselling for mental health problems. It depends on health personnel who volunteer to staff the hotline for 2 hours a week. It has been scaled up across the state, and, in 2009, 400 staff at any one time offer advice 24 hours a day to an average 1 500 000 callers per month. It also has a wider systems-based remit. This includes the hosting of a complaints service relating to the services in government hospitals so that a feedback loop can be developed to improve overall quality. The service now also funds outreach vehicles that visit local villages and provide cold-chain facilities for drugs, facilities to store blood and urine, medicines, and a television for public education. Each unit covers 56 villages a month. The project is now developing public health-based street plays and sound-and-light shows.

Discussion

Despite some notable successes, maternity care systems are not working for many childbearing women and their babies across the world. Project- and task-orientated solutions that are based on population-level evidence and simple linear thinking have been very successful in specific circumstances, such as magnesium sulphate for pre-eclampsia and emergency obstetric care training. However, they may not be enough to resolve the more complex system-wide problems that underpin the general lack of progress, towards MDG 5 in particular. It may be time to integrate specific project-based solutions based on theoretical population-based evidence with those based on whole-system thinking, and on what works, for whom and in what circumstances,[53] in real contexts, where implementation has been successful.

The need for whole-system thinking

Simple one-size-fits-all solutions are unlikely to be effective in the context of the global human resource crisis in health care in general, and in maternity care in particular. The six interconnected strategies in the 2008 Kampala Declaration on Health Workers for All are:[2]

1. building coherent national and global leadership for health workforce solutions
2. ensuring capacity for an informed response based on evidence and joint learning
3. scaling up health worker education and training
4. retaining an effective, responsive and equitably distributed health workforce
5. managing the pressures of the international health workforce market and its impact on migration
6. securing additional and more productive investment in the health workforce.

As this chapter has illustrated, these are all essential elements in a human resources strategy for maternity care. However, even with all six elements in place, problems can arise when top-down solutions are imposed without regard for local experiential expertise, cultures, beliefs and solutions. This may be one reason why TBA training did not bring the benefits that were intended. A whole-system approach would have paid attention to whether the training was locally appropriate (in context and in teaching techniques), whether those trained had a prior history as trusted and experienced local traditional midwives, how local beliefs and cultures could be integrated into the training, how regular updating could be provided, and how mutually respectful bridges could be built between the community and referral units. This would have ensured that transfer was straightforward, accepted by the woman and her community, and welcomed by the central unit when it became necessary. It is not clear whether the TBA training programme did this.

Whole-system solutions can also provide a more coherent basis for deciding on the overall shape and design of the optimum maternity care system to be provided, the kind of education needed for all grades and cadres of medical and other staff, and on methods of recruiting, employing and sustaining human resource provision. This would integrate the formal and the informal care provision systems.

Figures 4.3 and 4.4 give an example of such a whole-system solution, from the point of view of Scotland.[54]

It is of interest that, although it is a resource-rich country, Scotland has been reported to have among the highest rates of maternal mortality in Europe[11] and it has particular issues with the provision of services to very rural and remote communities. All the resources indicated in Figures 4.3 and 4.4 would not be available in all settings. However, the closely integrated mix of team members and of service provision is probably relevant to various degrees everywhere. The Scottish *Delivering for Remote and Rural Healthcare* report[54] notes that:

> Services must be well planned and co-ordinated with a greater focus on more collective and collaborative responses within and across communities. This will include the formalisation of networks to ensure that larger centres are obligated to support and sustain healthcare services in remote and rural areas. … Future models for healthcare delivery are based on integrated teams, demonstrating a range of competencies, defined by patient need. These competencies can overlap, between traditional professional roles, to the benefit of holistic care and utilises resources to better effect. Most of the team will be based within the remote and rural community, in primary or community care, within the hospital service or in combination, some team members will be based in the larger centre, with responsibility for supporting local delivery and providing a visiting service, where appropriate. … In order to sustain the competent workforce, appropriate training and education is required. This workforce must be supported in a variety of ways including formal networks and mentoring arrangements with larger centres, up to date equipment, modern Information Technology (IT) and technological links and robust transport systems.

This would seem to be relevant for maternity care across the world.

Beyond the health system, the examples above indicate that, in many countries, whole-system thinking will need to pay attention to wider social and cultural issues, such as culturally appropriate education of women and microfinance opportunities. Systems that catalyse the interrelationships between health and social wellbeing and that use this opportunity to build authentically respectful and caring relationships seem to be the most effective in reducing maternal and infant mortality. We dismiss the power of this effect at our peril.

Conclusion: learning from what works well

Skilled birth attendants are more likely to be attracted to the job, to learn and work effectively, to stay in post, to pass on their skills to others and to treat women well if they come from the local community, are educated locally, are able to live in good conditions, are equipped to deliver a good service, have opportunities to participate in updating and further training and are able to work in mutual respect with others in the maternity care system, including traditional midwives. Whole-system approaches that

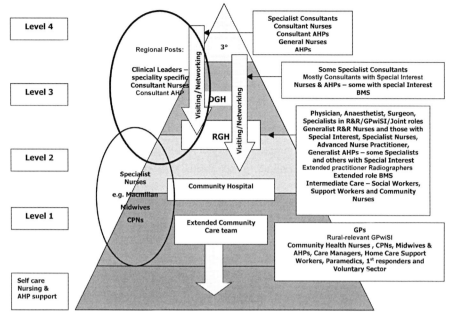

Figure 4.3   Remote and rural staffing model, Scotland: levels of staffing; reproduced from The Scottish Goverment;[54] Crown Copyright

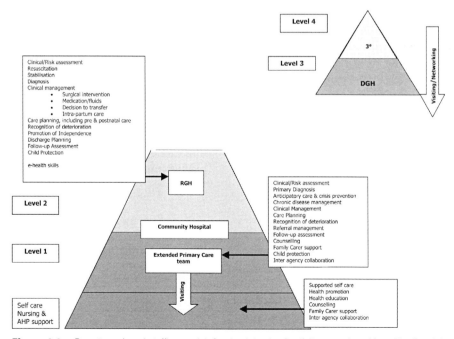

Figure 4.4   Remote and rural staffing model, Scotland: levels of activity; reproduced from The Scottish Government;[54] Crown Copyright

recognise these drivers and that provide the infrastructure to support them are most likely to deliver on a range of targets, including MDGs 4 and 5. These solutions do not just deal with health care but recognise the need to engage with societal issues such as free education for young girls and microfinancing. In their turn, the benefits generated by these societal changes create better living conditions locally and more attractive environments in which to recruit and retain staff. In summary, effective approaches to human resource provision for maternity care require a cyclical process, based on the following steps at the policy, educational, management and local delivery level:

- assess the context:
  - the degree of buy-in at national, regional and local government levels
  - the available resources, including educational opportunities and trained staff who are not practising
  - local cultural norms, particularly in relation to women and girls
  - local health beliefs
  - local health needs
  - existing traditional provision and gaps in provision
- prepare for the change process:
  - find out what works, for who, locally and in similar contexts elsewhere
  - identify local stakeholders with influence in this area (who may or may not be in senior positions)
  - establish the drivers for these stakeholders
  - engage the stakeholders in identifying gaps and finding solutions, based on what works
  - ensure educational and supervisory systems are in place
- take action:
  - tailor solutions to the context as identified in the first two steps
  - evaluate the impacts, both positive and negative
  - disseminate success stories locally, regionally, nationally and internationally
- continue the cycle.

Albert Einstein apparently believed that problems cannot be solved at the same level of awareness that created them. Cutting-edge thinkers in this area are beginning to respond to the need for whole-system solutions to the complex issue of effective staffing for optimum maternity care worldwide. This chapter suggests a way forward.

Acknowledgement

Some of the observations in this chapter are based on continuing debate within the Global Alliance for Nursing and Midwifery (GANM), the MDG Annual Ministerial Review (AMR) and HIFA2015 on online communities.

References

1. World Health Organization. *The Global Shortage of Health Workers and Its Impact.* Fact sheet no 302. Geneva: WHO; 2006 [www.who.int/mediacentre/factsheets/fs302/en/index.html].

2. World Health Organization, Global Health Workforce Alliance. *The Kampala Declaration and Agenda for Global Action.* Geneva: WHO; 2008 [www.who.int/workforcealliance/knowledge/publications/alliance/en/].

3. World Health Organization. *Resolution WHA59.23: Rapid Scaling Up of Health Workforce Production.* Geneva: WHO; 2006 [apps.who.int/gb/or/e/e_wha59r1.html].

4. World Health Organization. *Resolution WHA59.27: Strengthening Nursing and Midwifery.* Geneva: WHO; 2006 [apps.who.int/gb/or/e/e_wha59r1.html].

5. Task Force for Scaling Up Education and Training for Health Workers, Global Health Workforce Alliance. *Scaling Up, Saving Lives.* Geneva: World Health Organization; 2008 [www.who.int/workforcealliance/about/taskforces/education_training/en/].

6. World Health Organization. *Making Pregnancy Safer.* Geneva: WHO; 2009 [www.who.int/making_pregnancy_safer/topics/skilled_birth/en/index.html].

7. MINSAP. Cuba: Health Profile. Annual Health Statistics, 2006 [www.medicc.org/publications/cuba_health_reports/cuba-health-data.php].

8. World Health Organization. *Malawi Country Profile.* Geneva: WHO; 2009 [www.who.int/making_pregnancy_safer/countries/mai.pdf].

9. World Health Organization. *Tanzania Country Profile.* Geneva: WHO; 2009 [www.who.int/entity/making_pregnancy_safer/events/2008/mdg5/countries/final_cp_tanzania_19_09_08.pdf].

10. World Health Organization. *Haiti Country Profile.* Geneva: WHO; 2009 [www.who.int/entity/making_pregnancy_safer/countries/hai.pdf].

11. EURO-PERISTAT. *European Perinatal Health Report.* 2008 [www.europeristat.com/publications/european-perinatal-health-report.shtml].

12. World Health Organization. *Task Shifting: Rational Redistribution of Tasks Among Health Workforce Teams: Global Recommendations and Guidelines.* Geneva: WHO; 2008.

13. World Health Organization. *Making Pregnancy Safer: the Critical Role of the Skilled Attendant.* A joint statement by WHO, ICM and FIGO. Geneva: WHO; 2004 [www.who.int/making_pregnancy_safer/topics/skilled_birth/en/index.html].

14. World Health Organization. *The World Health Report 2008 – Primary Health Care (Now More Than Ever).* Geneva: WHO; 2008 [www.who.int/whr/2008/en/index.html].

15. World Health Organization. *Proportion of Births Attended by a Skilled Health Worker: 2008 Updates.* Geneva: WHO; 2008 [www.who.int/reproductivehealth/publications/maternal_perinatal_health/2008_skilled_attendants/en/index.html].

16. World Health Organization. *Increasing Access to Health Workers in Remote and Rural Areas through Improved Retention.* Geneva: WHO; 2009 [www.who.int/hrh/migration/background_paper.pdf].

17. Isaacs G. The frontier nursing service. Family nursing in rural areas. *Clin Obstet Gynecol* 1972;15:394–407.

18. Sullivan EA, Ford JB, Chambers G, Slaytor EK. Maternal mortality in Australia, 1973–1996. *Aust N Z J Obstet Gynaecol* 2004;44:452–7.

19. Van Wagner V, Epoo B, Nastapoka J, Harney E. Reclaiming birth, health, and community: midwifery in the Inuit villages of Nunavik, Canada. *J Midwifery Womens Health* 2007;52:384–91.

20. Couchie C, Sanderson S, Society of Obstetricians and Gynaecologists of Canada. A report on best practices for returning birth to rural and remote aboriginal communities. *J Obstet Gynaecol Can* 2007;29:250–60.

21. Sibley LM, Sipe TA, Brown CM, Diallo MM, McNatt K, Habarta N. Traditional birth attendant training for improving health behaviours and pregnancy outcomes. *Cochrane Database Syst Rev* 2007;(3):CD005460.

22. Campbell OM, Graham WJ, Lancet Maternal Survival Series steering group. Strategies for reducing maternal mortality: getting on with what works. *Lancet* 2006;368:1284–99.

23. Gabrysch S, Campbell OM. Still too far to walk: literature review of the determinants of delivery service use. *BMC Pregnancy Childbirth* 2009;9:34.

24. Thaddeus S, Maine D. Too far to walk: maternal mortality in context. *Soc Sci Med* 1994;38:1091–110.

25. el-Nemer A, Downe S, Small N. 'She would help me from the heart': an ethnography of Egyptian women in labour. *Soc Sci Med* 2006;62:81–92.

26. Davis-Floyd R. Home-birth emergencies in the US and Mexico: the trouble with transport. *Soc Sci Med* 2003;56:1911–31.

27. Jenkins GL. Burning bridges: policy, practice, and the destruction of midwifery in rural Costa Rica. *Soc Sci Med* 2003;56:1893–909.

28. Misago C, Kendall C, Freitas P, Haneda K, Silveira D, Onuki D, *et al.* From 'culture of dehumanization of childbirth' to 'childbirth as a transformative experience': changes in five municipalities in north-east Brazil. *Int J Gynaecol Obstet* 2001;75 Suppl 1:S67–72.

29. Manandhar DS, Osrin D, Shrestha BP, Mesko N, Morrison J, Tumbahangphe KM, *et al.* Effect of a participatory intervention with women's groups on birth outcomes in Nepal: cluster-randomised controlled trial. *Lancet* 2004;364:970–9.

30. Bärnighausen T, Bloom DE. Designing financial-incentive programmes for return of medical service in underserved areas: seven management functions. *Hum Resour Health* 2009;26;7:52.

31. Dovlo D. Using mid-level cadres as substitutes for internationally mobile health professionals in Africa. A desk review. *Hum Resour Health* 2004;18;2:7.

32. Global Health Workforce Alliance. '*Task Shifting*', *1st Topic of the Exchange*. Geneva: WHO; 2009 [www.who.int/workforcealliance/knowledge/e_solutions/TaskShifting/en/index.html].

33. Healthcare Information for All by 2015. *Foundation Document*. Oxford: HIFA2015; 2009 [www.hifa2015.org/publications].

34. Li LC, Grimshaw JM, Nielsen C, Judd M, Coyte PC, Graham ID. Evolution of Wenger's concept of community of practice. *Implement Sci* 2009;1;4:11.

35. Greenhalgh T, Hurwitz B. *Narrative Based Medicine*. London: BMJ Books; 1998.

36. Madhok V, Fahey T. N-of-1 trials: an opportunity to tailor treatment in individual patients. *Br J Gen Pract* 2005; 55:171–2.

37. High-Level Forum on the Health MDGs. *Best Practice Principles for Global Health Partnership Activities at Country Level*. Paris: High-Level Forum on the Health MDGs; 2005.

38. Dayrit M, Taylor A, Yan J, Braichet JM, Zurn P, Shainblum E. WHO code of practice on the international recruitment of health personnel. *Bull World Health Organ* 2008;86:737–816.

39. Lehmann U, Dieleman M, Martineau T. Staffing remote rural areas in middle- and low-income countries: a literature review of attraction and retention. *BMC Health Serv Res* 2008;8:19.

40. Koot J, Martineau T. *Mid Term Review: Zambian Health Workers Retention Scheme (ZHWRS) 2003–2004.* 2005 [www.hrhresourcecenter.org/hosted_docs/Zambian_Health_Workers_Retention_Scheme.pdf].

41. UNICEF Devpro Resource Centre. *Afghanistan's Community Midwives*. 2008 [www.unicef.org/devpro/46000_46782.html].

42. Longombe AO. Medical schools in rural areas – necessity or aberration? *Rural Remote Health* 2009;9:1131 [www.rrh.org.au/articles/subviewnew.asp?ArticleID=1131].

43. Health Alliance International. *The NGO Code of Conduct for Health Systems Strengthening*. Seattle: Health Alliance International; 2009 [ngocodeofconduct.org/pdf/ngocodeofconduct.pdf].

44. Dieleman M, Gerretsen B, van der Wilt GJ. Human resource management interventions to improve health workers' performance in low and middle income countries: a realist review. *Health Res Policy Syst* 2009;17;7:7.

45. Teela KC, Mullany LC, Lee CI, Poh E, Paw P, Masenior N, *et al.* Community-based delivery of maternal care in conflict-affected areas of eastern Burma: perspectives from lay maternal health workers. *Soc Sci Med* 2009;68:1332–40.

46. UNFPA-ICM. *Investing in Midwives and Others with Midwifery Skills to Save the Lives of Mothers and Newborns and Improve Their Health*. 2008 [www.unfpa.org/public/publications/pid/909].

47. Alailama P, Sanderatne N. Social policy in a slowly growing economy: Sri Lanka. In: Mehrotra S, Jolly R, editors. *Development with a Human Face: Experiences in Social Achievement and Economic Growth*. Oxford: Oxford University Press; 2000. p. 248–9.

48. Personal communication via MDG-AMR CoP e-exchange (strengthening health systems), 29 January to 11 February, volume 7.

49. USAID. *Female Community Health Volunteers.* Nepal Family Health Programme Technical Brief #1. 2007 [www.jsi.com/NFHP/Docs/TechnicalBriefs/01_female_community_health_volunteers.pdf].

50. UNICEF Devpro Resource Centre. *Bangladesh's Community Support Systems for Maternal and Newborn Health.* 2009 [www.unicef.org/devpro/46000_47709.html].

51. Soguel D. 'Gravity birth' pulls women into Ecuador hospital. *Women's e-News.* 15 February 2009 [www.womensenews.org/article.cfm/dyn/aid/3920].

52. Health Management and Research Institute. *104 – Advice* [www.supporthmri.com/104-Advice.aspx].

53. Pawson R, Greenhalgh T, Harvey G, Walshe K. Realist review – a new method of systematic review designed for complex policy interventions. *J Health Serv Res Policy* 2005;10 Suppl 1:21–34.

54. The Scottish Government. *Delivering for Remote and Rural Healthcare: The Final Report of the Remote and Rural Workstream.* Edinburgh: The Scottish Government; 2008 [www.scotland.gov.uk/Publications/2008/05/06084423/0].

55. Woods R. Long-term trends in fetal mortality: implications for developing countries. *Bull World Health Organ* 2008;86:417–96 [www.who.int/bulletin/volumes/86/6/07-043471/en/index.html].

56. Noree T, Chokchaichan H, Mongkolporn V. *Abundant for the Few, Shortage for the Majority: the Inequitable Distribution of Doctors in Thailand.* Thailand: International Health Policy Program; 2005 [www.aaahrh.org/reviewal/1166639104_Thailand%20-%20Revised.pdf].

Section 2

Clinical problems and solutions – maternal

Chapter 5
Postpartum haemorrhage

Andrew Weeks

Introduction

Postpartum haemorrhage (PPH) is the most common cause of maternal deaths worldwide, responsible for 30% of all maternal deaths.[1] This is equivalent to 150 000 deaths annually or a death every 4 minutes. The danger of PPH comes not only from its rapid onset post delivery but also from the speed with which it causes maternal death. To prevent and treat PPH, therefore, a skilled birth attendant capable of managing PPH needs to be available at the birth. In the UK, despite universal access to heath care, around five women per year still die from PPH.[2] The scale of the medical care needed to prevent death from PPH in the UK is reflected in the fact that 315 women undergo peripartum hysterectomy annually for massive haemorrhage, half of whom have an atonic uterus.[3]

PPH is traditionally defined as the loss of over 500 ml blood in the first 24 hours after delivery. In reality, however, blood loss appears to be frequently higher than this in settings without prophylaxis. Measured median blood loss varies from 200 to 496 ml and the percentage of women with losses of over 500 ml varies from 12% to 51%.[4,5] In clinical practice, therefore, birth attendants often use their clinical judgement to assess 'abnormal loss'. In 2009, the RCOG amended its definition of PPH so that 500 ml is used as a point of 'alert' while treatment is only given once the women has lost 1000 ml.[6] Useful practical ways of assessing blood volume are making comparisons with the volume of a hand (300 ml), a soaked large swab (350 ml), or a soaked kanga (a traditional African piece of printed cotton fabric; 250 ml).[7] Charts are available that provide aids to estimating blood loss.[8] As many women cope well with blood loss of up to 1000 ml, researchers generally use a blood loss of over 1 litre ('severe PPH') as a cut-off.[6]

Aetiology

The most common reason for a PPH is an atonic uterus where the loss of myometrial tone allows the maternal blood flow to the placental bed (500 ml per minute during pregnancy) to continue unchecked. Other causes include retained placental tissue, tears of the uterus, cervix or vagina, and clotting disorders. These have been summarised into the '4T' mnemonic – tone, tissue, trauma and thrombin. Major risk factors for PPH include placental abruption, placenta praevia, multiple pregnancy, retained placenta, previous PPH and delivery by emergency caesarean section. Other risk factors include obesity, anaemia, Asian ethnicity, induction of labour, prolonged labour, large baby, delivery by elective caesarean section, episiotomy, operative vaginal delivery, age over 40 years and intrapartum pyrexia.[6]

There has been a long-standing debate over the association between prolonged labour and PPH. It is unclear whether this is due to a primary myometrial problem causing the uterus to contract inefficiently both before and after delivery, myometrial acidaemia[9] or the association of both with increased fetal size. There is also an association with the use of oxytocin infusions in labour but randomised controlled trials (RCTs) of intrapartum oxytocin show no effect on PPH rates.[10]

Strategies for preventing postpartum haemorrhage deaths

All women have some blood loss at the time of delivery. For most, it is mild and will have no ill effect on their health. For a small number, however, the blood loss becomes excessive and intervention is required if they are not to die.

The natural history of PPH is not fully known. In settings where there is no or little access to health care, the maternal mortality ratio is around 2000 per 100 000 live births.[11,12] If 30% of these deaths are from PPH,[1] then untreated PPH can be estimated to cause death in about 0.7% (one in 150) of pregnant women.

Healthy women can tolerate blood loss of up to 40% of their blood volume – approximately 2.8 litres in women with a blood volume of 7 litres.[6] Malnourished or anaemic women will be able to tolerate much less. Women who lose more than 2.8 litres of blood therefore enter a 'death zone' where they are at risk of death without rescue therapies. A histogram of measured blood loss is available from a study in which 330 women were given placebo for PPH prophylaxis (Figure 5.1).[5] In this study, 1%

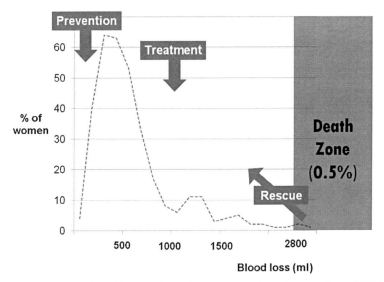

Figure 5.1 Histogram of blood loss at delivery, showing the 'death zone' at loss of over 40% blood volume and the three strategies for intervention; the rise at 1200 ml reflects the response to treatment, with an increase in women stopping bleeding shortly after medical therapy is given; data adapted from Hoj *et al.* (2005)[5] with corrections from Hoj[59]

of women had blood loss of over 2800 ml. It was not reported how many women had additional uterotonics but the figure was 1% in a similar study.[4] There were no deaths in any of the women in these studies, which reflects the ability of the medical community to adequately rescue women despite severe blood loss.

There are three main areas of intervention that need to be addressed if the mortality from PPH is to be reduced: prevention, treatment and rescue (Figure 5.1). PPH prevention covers antenatal strategies together with appropriate management of the third stage of labour and interventions for retained placenta. PPH treatment covers both medical treatment (oxytocin, prostaglandins and tranexamic acid) and surgical treatment (balloon tamponade, compression sutures and hysterectomy). PPH rescue therapies include intravenous fluids and blood transfusion, coagulation correction and supportive care such as compression garments. These areas for intervention are not mutually exclusive and need to be considered together. Each will be considered in turn in this chapter.

Preventing postpartum haemorrhage

Reducing risk antenatally

Prevention of PPH starts in the antenatal clinic. A review of the list of associated factors above shows an association with anaemia as well as an association with surgical intervention, irrespective of whether this is induction, episiotomy, operative vaginal delivery or caesarean section. Anaemia increases risk both through reducing the woman's tolerance to blood loss and through a direct effect on the myometrium. Thus, treatment of anaemia – whether through giving oral iron for iron-deficiency anaemia or deworming with mebendazole – is an important public health strategy.

As well as leading to an increased number of severe tears after delivery, routine episiotomy is associated with a 27% increase in PPH at normal birth and so should be used sparingly for delivery.[13]

Reducing the risk of operative vaginal delivery and caesarean section is not so easy, but it should not be forgotten that PPH is one of the hidden costs of these interventions. Added to the problem of immediate blood loss with caesarean section are the risks for future pregnancies of PPH through placenta praevia and placenta accreta. In the event of placenta praevia or placenta accreta, it is recommended that senior staff be consulted to reduce the associated morbidity. Leaving a morbidly adherent placenta in place in the uterus at the time of caesarean section may reduce morbidity from this condition.[14]

Active management of the third stage of labour

Active management of the third stage of labour was first described when oxytocin became available as a therapeutic agent.[15] Oxytocin was given to contract the uterus and the controlled cord traction prevented retained placenta. Early cord clamping was already part of standard practice and entered the protocol by default.[16] In 1988, the Bristol third stage trial[17] showed that this 'active management' package reduced the risk of PPH and it became incorporated into the modern management of labour. The importance of the problem of PPH worldwide and the simplicity of the intervention meant that the use of active management quickly became a mantra for the safe motherhood movement.

Overall, active management of the third stage reduces blood loss of over a litre (RR 0.33; 95% CI 0.21–0.51), the use of blood transfusion (RR 0.34; 95% CI 0.22–

0.53) and the need for additional uterotonics (RR 0.20; 95% CI 0.17–0.25).[18] The speed of placental delivery is increased but there is no overall increase in need for manual delivery of placenta.

The components of active management are still under investigation. The debates around the choice of oxytocic are considered below and there is a large continuing randomised trial to assess the benefit of controlled cord traction.[19] The place of early cord clamping has attracted intense debate and it has now been removed from the active management protocol by the World Health Organization (WHO)[20] and the International Federation of Gynecology and Obstetrics (FIGO)[21] as it reduces neonatal iron stores without reducing PPH rates.

Medical prophylaxis

Oxytocin and carbetocin

Throughout Europe, by far the most common prophylactic in use is oxytocin, given after delivery of the baby or placenta.[22] Oxytocin is also the drug recommended by WHO,[20] FIGO[21] and the National Institute for Health and Clinical Excellence (NICE)[23] and is given as 10 iu intramuscularly at the time of the delivery of the baby. It can also be given as an intravenous bolus but this causes a large, transient decrease in blood pressure and so should be administered slowly and with care (Figure 5.2).

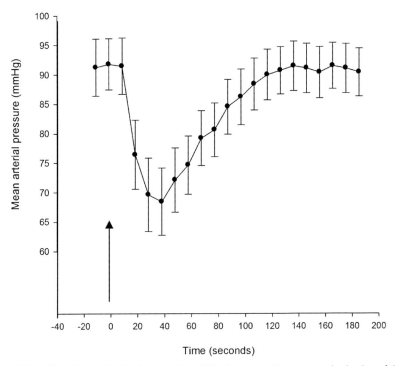

Figure 5.2   Effect of an oxytocin bolus on maternal blood pressure; the arrow marks the time of the oxytocin bolus; adapted from Carlin[60]

Oxytocin is now also packaged in a simple, single-use syringe (Uniject®; BD, Franklin Lakes, New Jersey), a move that should facilitate its use outside of hospitals. Widespread community trials of the device are currently under way.

Although oxytocin acts rapidly on the uterus (within 1 minute when given intravenously and 2 minutes when given intramuscularly), the half-life of oxytocin is only 10 minutes. A number of strategies have therefore been developed to prolong the oxytocic effect. These include the giving of oxytocin as an intravenous infusion, combining oxytocin with the long-acting ergometrine, or the use of carbetocin, an oxytocin agonist. The clinical and pharmacological properties of carbetocin are similar to those of naturally occurring oxytocin, resulting in rhythmic contractions of the uterus within 2 minutes that last for 1–2 hours. There is evidence from randomised studies that carbetocin may be more effective than oxytocin[24] and some countries have already adopted it as their first-line recommended oxytocic for PPH prevention at the time of caesarean section.[25]

Ergometrine and oxytocin/ergometrine (Syntometrine®)

Ergometrine is a plant-derived medicine and was the first treatment described for PPH. Administration causes an intense and sustained uterine contraction (in contrast to the intermittent contractions caused by oxytocin). Clinical trials of its use for prophylaxis show it to reduce the PPH rate (when used as part of the active management of the third stage of labour) compared with physiological management.[26] However, there are increases in hypertension, vomiting and pain associated with its use, as well as an increase in retained placenta when it is administered intravenously.[27]

Oxytocin may be given with ergometrine as a way of providing a sustained contraction after the oxytocin has worn off. The drug Syntometrine® (Alliance, Chippenham, Wilts) is commonly used in the UK (as compared with the rest of Europe)[22] and contains 5 iu oxytocin and 500 µg ergometrine. A systematic review has shown Syntometrine to be slightly more effective than oxytocin alone in preventing blood loss.[28] For blood loss over 500 ml, the odds ratio (OR) was 0.82 (95% CI 0.71–0.95) and for loss over 1000 ml the OR was 0.78 (95% CI 0.58–1.03). However, adverse effects are more common in groups receiving ergometrine-based active management, with increased levels of hypertension (OR 2.81; 95% CI 1.17–6.73), nausea (RR 1.83; 95% CI 1.51–2.23) and vomiting (RR 2.19; 95% CI 1.68–2.86). The adverse-effect profile has led to ergometrine being reserved for treatment rather than universal prophylaxis.

Carboprost and sulprostone

Intramuscular carboprost (15-methyl prostaglandin $F_{2\alpha}$; Hemabate®; Pfizer, Walton-on-the-Hill, Surrey) and sulprostone (prostaglandin E_2) have been used for the prevention of PPH but their use is restricted by their cost and adverse-effect profile. A number of small trials have been conducted that show no major differences between intramuscular prostaglandins and conventional uterotonics (oxytocin or ergometrine) in reducing the blood loss.[29]

Misoprostol

Misoprostol is a synthetic prostaglandin E_1 analogue licensed for the prevention of peptic ulcers caused by nonsteroidal anti-inflammatory drugs.[30] Its cost is similar to that of oxytocin with syringe and needle but its long shelf life and oral administration make it especially attractive for use in low-resource areas. Furthermore, it has no effect on blood pressure and can be safely used in asthma sufferers (in contrast to many of the prostaglandins that cause bronchoconstriction). It does, however, commonly cause hyperthermia, a symptom preceded by shivering. This appears to be related to route, gestation and patient population, with the rates being higher in the third trimester, with sublingual administration and with higher doses. Although the high fevers caused alarm when they were first seen and resulted in admission to the intensive care unit,[31] experience has shown that the fevers are self-limiting and respond rapidly to tepid sponging and paracetamol.

Misoprostol has been introduced for PPH management in a number of low-resource countries. In some settings, misoprostol has been given to women for self-administration immediately following home birth. However, in 2009 WHO issued a communiqué that specifically advised against doing this, owing to a lack of evidence of its benefit and the potential for harm.[32]

Initial small randomised trials comparing oral misoprostol with standard oxytocic regimens suggested that misoprostol might be as effective as oxytocic drugs for PPH prevention. However, a large multicentre trial[33] of nearly 20 000 women comparing 600 μg of oral misoprostol with 10 iu of oxytocin showed that the rate of severe PPH (blood loss more than 1000 ml) was higher in the misoprostol group (4% versus 3%). Oxytocin is therefore now recommended over misoprostol as first-line treatment for PPH prophylaxis as part of the active management of the third stage of labour by WHO and FIGO.[20,21]

The evidence as to whether misoprostol is better than placebo is more complex. The Cochrane review of all RCTs[29] shows there to be no overall difference in efficacy. There is, however, evidence that misoprostol is beneficial in community settings.[34] The reason for this is unclear but may relate to the differing management of placental delivery. In hospital settings, there is often a tradition of enthusiastic early controlled cord traction timed to coincide with the peak level of oxytocin. However, if early controlled cord traction is used with misoprostol, the placental detachment (and haemorrhage) may occur before the misoprostol reaches effective serum levels. In community settings, however, the timing of controlled cord traction is usually later and is likely to coincide with the peak serum levels of misoprostol at 20 minutes. This may explain why misoprostol is relatively ineffective in hospital settings.

Based on the above evidence, WHO currently recommends the use of oxytocin rather than misoprostol for the prevention of PPH.[20] However, they recommend the use of either oxytocin or misoprostol in settings where active management is not being practised or where no skilled birth attendants are available. Specifically, they warn that, when misoprostol is used, no other components of the active third stage should be used.[32]

The optimal dosage and route is not known and studies have used mainly oral or sublingual doses of 600 or 800 μg. Concerns about hyperthermia and an excess of deaths in the misoprostol arms of RCTs led Hofmeyr et al.[35] to recommend a reduction in dosage to 400 μg. However, an expert group that was convened to recommend optimal misoprostol doses suggested a single dose of 600 μg of oral or sublingual misoprostol.[34] They advised that the dose should not be repeated for 2 hours to prevent the hyperthermia associated with high dosages.

Tranexamic acid

Tranexamic acid is a powerful antifibrinolytic agent that is used for the treatment of menorrhagia and the reduction of operative blood loss in general surgery. There is, however, little research into its use for the prevention of PPH. A systematic review of three small RCTs (a total of 460 women were recruited) found a 56% reduction in PPH but the authors concluded that there is insufficient evidence from RCTs to confirm or refute a clinically important treatment effect.[36] A large RCT is currently under way into its use for PPH treatment.

Other third-stage components

Controlled cord traction

There are no randomised trials that assess the effect of controlled cord traction on labour outcomes. There are, however, concerns that controlled cord traction can lead to premature placental separation, cord tearing and uterine inversion without compensatory benefit, and a large WHO trial is now in progress.[19]

Early cord clamping

Early cord clamping was introduced as part of the active management of the third stage of labour package. A systematic review[37] of 11 trials (3000 women), however, suggests that the timing of cord clamping has no effect on PPH rates or timing of placental delivery. The placental transfusion that results from deferred cord clamping shifts the normal curve for neonatal haemoglobin to the right. This results in less neonatal anaemia but more hyperbilirubinaemia in the newborn. Early cord clamping is thus not recommended in settings where iron-deficiency anaemia is common.[20,21]

Cord drainage

There are very few trials that consider the issue of cord drainage (two trials with 600 women) but a systematic review found some evidence that it reduces the length of the third stage.[38] Deferred cord clamping should have a comparable effect (that is, of draining blood from the placenta) but the meta-analysis[37] of trials comparing early and deferred cord clamping showed no effect on the length of the third stage.

Treating retained placenta

Women in whom the placenta is retained have an increased risk of PPH from 20–30 minutes onwards[39,40] and it is therefore suggested that a diagnosis of retained placenta is made at 30 minutes.[14,41] The usual management has been manual removal of the placenta in theatre but several alternative medical strategies have been investigated to encourage expulsion.[42]

Umbilical cord injection with oxytocin or prostaglandin

There has been some evidence that the intra-umbilical injection of oxytocin may be effective in encouraging spontaneous expulsion of the placenta.[43] However, a large RCT[44] of 50 iu umbilical oxytocin in nearly 600 women with retained placenta that was published in 2010 found no benefit over placebo. Despite this, the meta-analysis[43] of all trials still shows a borderline statistical effect on the need for manual removal and, therefore, WHO's guideline[45] still states that umbilical oxytocin injection 'may be offered'.

Two small randomised trials have assessed the benefits of an intra-umbilical prostaglandin injection and have reported conflicting results. Bider *et al.*[46] randomised 17 women to receive prostaglandin F$_{2\alpha}$ or saline and found that the technique was successful in all those who received prostaglandin, while Rogers *et al.*[47] compared misoprostol solution with placebo and found little benefit.

Glyceryl trinitrate

The use of systemic glyceryl trinitrate (GTN) may be of some benefit for women with retained placenta.[42] Uterine relaxation occurs about 60 seconds after injection and lasts for 2 minutes. Numerous observational studies (mainly using intravenous boluses of 50–200 µg) had suggested some benefit and a randomised trial has now supported this. Bullarbo *et al.*[48] randomised 24 women to receive 1 mg of GTN or placebo sublingually 20 minutes after an intravenous bolus of 10 iu oxytocin. The efficacy was 100% in those given GTN, but only 8% (one of 12) in those treated with placebo ($P < 0.0001$). GTN treatment also reduced the mean blood loss by nearly 300 ml.

Treatment of postpartum haemorrhage

Medical treatment

Oxytocin

Despite being the first-choice oxytocic for the management of atonic PPH, there are no randomised trials to demonstrate the efficacy of oxytocin compared with placebo. Evidence for its efficacy for PPH comes from the trials on its prophylactic use, outlined above. On the basis of this, WHO[45] recommends 10 iu oxytocin as a slow intravenous infusion as first-line treatment, followed by ergometrine (with or without oxytocin) as second-line treatment and intramuscular prostaglandin F$_{2\alpha}$ (carboprost) as third-line treatment.

Misoprostol

A number of studies have generated encouraging evidence on the use of misoprostol as an emergency treatment for PPH. The vast majority of these have been small observational studies showing dramatic effects.[34] However, three large RCTs recently conducted by Gynuity Health Projects have provided important new evidence regarding the efficacy of misoprostol. The first examined the role of misoprostol as an adjunct treatment for women who had already been given oxytocin to treat PPH. Although currently unpublished, the results were made available to WHO for their guideline on PPH treatment.[45] The study recruited 1400 women with PPH and compared the use of combined oxytocin and 600 µg misoprostol with oxytocin alone. The results showed no difference between the groups in additional blood loss of 500 ml (RR 1.01; 95% CI 0.78–1.30) or 1000 ml (RR 0.76; 95% CI 0.43–1.34).[45] The conclusion is that, in settings where oxytocin is available for the treatment of PPH, there is no role for additional misoprostol.

The other two Gynuity studies[49,50] compared the efficacy of misoprostol and oxytocin as first-line treatments for PPH. In these two studies, a total of 40 000 women were recruited in early labour and had their blood loss measured by blood collection in conical plastic drapes. The studies were conducted in a range of units throughout the world – some which routinely gave oxytocin for prophylaxis (who were in study 1)[49] and some which gave no prophylaxis (study 2).[50] Those women who developed PPH (defined as a measured blood loss of 700 ml) were randomly assigned to either a high-dose oxytocin infusion (40 iu over 15 minutes) or misoprostol 800 µg sublingually, each with placebos so as to ensure double-blinding. As expected, the PPH rate was much higher in the units where no oxytocin prophylaxis was used, where 10.5% developed a PPH. In this study there was less additional blood loss in those given oxytocin than for those given misoprostol. The difference was statistically significant for an extra loss of 300 ml (30.1% versus 16.7%; RR 1.78; 95% CI 1.40–2.26) but not for a loss of over 1000 ml (1.0% versus 0.6%; RR 1.67; 95% CI 0.40–6.96). In the units where women were given routine prophylaxis, only 2.6% developed a PPH. There was no difference in additional blood loss of 300 ml (34.4% versus 30.7%; RR 1.12; 95% CI 0.92–1.37) but more women in the misoprostol group had an additional loss of over 1000 ml (2.7% versus 0.7%; RR 3.61; 95% CI 1.02–12.85). The percentage of women recruited (as opposed to those with a PPH) with severe PPH in each of the four arms of the two trials was similar.

These three studies have produced some fascinating results and three conclusions can be drawn from them:

- Oxytocin is more effective than misoprostol for the treatment of PPH if it has not been previously given as prophylaxis. This is no great surprise and is in agreement with the results of the previous WHO prophylaxis study.[33]

- This advantage is reduced if oxytocin has already been given as prophylaxis although it may still be marginally more effective.

- Perhaps most interestingly, comparison of the results from the two studies[49,50] suggests that women can safely undergo physiological management as long as they are rapidly given an oxytocic in the event of haemorrhage.

It is clear from previous prophylaxis studies that active management reduces both the median blood loss and losses of over 500 ml and 1000 ml. However, as long as women have prompt access to oxytocics, there appears to be little difference in the higher levels of blood loss. The main benefit of universal PPH prophylaxis (as compared with targeted PPH treatment) may therefore be to reduce the levels of postpartum anaemia. Both strategies may be equally effective at preventing maternal mortality, although there is no adequately powered study that compares the two strategies. These data will be reassuring for those settings where the limited supply of oxytocin is reserved for PPH treatment alone.

There are no placebo-controlled trials of PPH treatment conducted in very rural low-resource settings where there is no access to oxytocin and misoprostol may still have a role there. In rural African settings, some women are given misoprostol antenatally so that they can self-administer at the time of delivery, although in 2009 WHO[32] recommended against doing this until more evidence is available. For places where it is used, the Bellagio expert group recommended 600 µg of oral or sublingual misoprostol for PPH treatment.[51] As with the prophylactic doses, they recommended that a second dose should not be repeated before 2 hours. This dosage remains controversial, however, and many African countries now have approved a dosage of 1000 µg rectally despite pharmacokinetic evidence that serum levels are low following rectal administration.[52] The large doses used in the Gynuity studies (800 µg sublingually) resulted in relatively high rates of adverse effects and it has been argued that 400 µg will be as effective but with fewer adverse effects.[35] There is currently no consensus.

Tranexamic acid

The antifibrinolytic agent tranexamic acid is potentially attractive for PPH management as it would provide an alternative way of achieving haemostasis and reducing bleeding irrespective of whether it came from uterine atony or lacerations. However, there are theoretical concerns regarding its use:[53]

▓ pregnant women are already at risk of peripartum thromboembolism and tranexamic acid might increase this risk

▓ women with severe PPH can develop disseminated intravascular coagulation and tranexamic acid would theoretically increase the damaging microvascular thrombosis that occurs in this process

▓ rapid intravenous administration of tranexamic acid can cause hypotension, thus exacerbating the hypotensive effects of PPH.

Published reports of its use for PPH treatment are very limited and amount to three case reports only.[53] However, randomised trials of its use for PPH prophylaxis and in those undergoing surgery show promise. An continuing large randomised study should clarify its role in PPH management (www.womantrial.lshtm.ac.uk).

Ergometrine

There is minimal evidence regarding the use of ergometrine for the treatment of PPH, although it is included in all the major PPH guidelines.[23,45] Its inclusion has been justified on the basis of its demonstrated efficacy in the prophylaxis trials.

Physical treatment

There are several physical treatments for PPH available. However, there are no randomised trials to evaluate their efficacy and observational trials are highly prone to bias, especially given the natural history of PPH to improve spontaneously ('natural' death rates without intervention are only around 0.05%,[11] despite a physiological 700 ml PPH rate of around 10%).[49]

The simplest options are those of uterine compression. This can be achieved through bimanual compression (classically using a fist in the vagina and hand on the abdominal wall) but compression sutures are now commonly used. The most popular is the B–Lynch suture but inserting this suture requires a lower segment caesarean section uterine incision, which is often absent. It was therefore modified by Hayman *et al.*[54] so as to enable the brace suture to be used without a caesarean section incision. In this alternative, two front-to-back sutures are inserted the whole way through the uterine lower segment on the left and right side of the midline, brought up over the uterus and tied either side of the fundus. Drainage of blood can occur between the sutures. This achieves the same compression as the B–Lynch but without the need to open the lower segment. Initial observational studies suggest that it is as effective as the B–Lynch suture.[55] The simplicity of these procedures and their use of widely available surgical materials make these ideal for low-resource settings.

The alternative to external compression is internal tamponade. This was traditionally achieved through the use of uterine packing with gauze. However, balloon catheters are now recommended instead because of their simplicity, ease of insertion and removal, and lack of trauma to the endometrium on removal. A range of options are available but the purpose-made Bakri balloon provides a central drainage channel and a 500 ml balloon capacity. A low-cost alternative using a condom tied to the end of a large Foley catheter and held in place with a vaginal pack also appears to be effective.[56]

The final alternatives – mass ligation, internal iliac artery ligation and hysterectomy – are surgical operations that require far greater skill. Mass ligation is the simplest and involves placing bilateral sutures into the uterus just above the level of the uterine artery. These horizontally positioned sutures pass from front to back through the lateral part of the myometrium and return anteriorly through the broad ligament, thus enclosing the ascending uterine artery on both sides. This is often used as a low-risk first option before moving on to the more surgically complex internal iliac ligation or hysterectomy.

Rescue of women with severe postpartum haemorrhage

Blood transfusion

The lack of donated blood for emergency transfusion is a major problem in the developing world. In women who die from PPH, at least 26% of the deaths are estimated to be directly attributable to an inability to obtain a blood transfusion.[57] Blood transfusion services are frequently haphazard, with blood acquired from family members at the time of need. Although often adequate for chronic anaemia, this is rarely in time to prevent deaths in women with an acute obstetric haemorrhage. Bates *et al.*[57] call for national blood transfusion policies to be produced and to be enforced by local committees. Policies should promote local voluntary donations, the rationalising of donor screening and use of transfusion, and an effective distribution system. Obtaining a blood transfusion is expensive and Bates *et al.* also call for novel financing systems such as microfinance to be developed to provide a financial buffer for the poorest families.

Compression anti-shock garments for transfer

There has been a lot of interest in this novel technique, which provides haemodynamic support to a woman with PPH. The technique was developed by the military as a way of maintaining a soldier's blood pressure during transfer from the battlefield to hospital. It works on the principle that compression of the legs and abdomen squeezes blood out of them and into the central vessels. In animal studies, the translocation of blood is up to 30% of the total blood volume.[58] The garment also reduces the available intravascular space, which in turn raises the blood pressure.

The modern garment is typically made of neoprene and wraps around the limbs and trunk, using Velcro® to hold it in place. It is available in both a pneumatic form (where, like a giant blood pressure cuff, air is pumped into the compression suit to provide the pressure) and a non-pneumatic form (where a compression of 30 mmHg is provided by the elasticity and tightness of the suit alone). Large quasi-randomised trials in trauma patients have, however, found no reduction in morbidity or mortality and its use in trauma settings is therefore sporadic.[58]

The non-pneumatic anti-shock garment offers considerable potential for use in low-resource settings as it is simple to apply, reusable and relatively inexpensive (US$160 per garment). Large observational studies have shown it to have potential[58] and the results of much larger continuing studies are awaited.

Conclusion

PPH is a major cause of maternal death worldwide. The rapid onset and progression of PPH means that high-quality community services are required if PPH-related mortality is to be prevented. The strategies for overcoming this problem can be divided into prevention, treatment and rescue. While universal access to prophylaxis with oxytocics will prevent PPH in some women, around 3% of low-risk women will still lose over 1000 ml of blood. These women require rapid access to life-saving PPH treatment and rescue therapies. Other women, with placental abruption, placenta praevia, obstructed labour or multiple pregnancy, are at much higher risk and almost all of these will need PPH therapies or rescue treatment to prevent morbidity.

To date, the focus of the world health community has been on the provision of the active management of third stage to all women. This is important and the availability of misoprostol and Uniject® will help to reach those women who do not otherwise access health services. However, recent studies of women with PPH suggest that the main benefit of prophylaxis over treatment is only a small reduction in rates of postpartum anaemia. In isolation, therefore, universal prophylaxis will prevent relatively few PPH deaths. Achieving significant improvements in PPH-related mortality requires a scaling up of rural obstetric services, including the provision of surgical services to prevent PPH (caesarean section and manual removal of placenta), PPH medical treatments (oxytocin and possibly tranexamic acid), physical treatments (balloon tamponade and surgery) and rescue packages (blood transfusion and the non-pneumatic anti-shock garment). More research is now required to determine the most cost-effective way of providing these services.

References

1. Khan KS, Wojdyla D, Say L, Gülmezoglu AM, Van Look PFA. WHO analysis of causes of maternal death: a systematic review. *Lancet* 2006;367:1066–74.
2. Lewis G, editor. *Saving Mothers' Lives: Reviewing Maternal Deaths to Make Motherhood Safer 2003–2005. The Seventh Report on Confidential Enquiries into Maternal Deaths in the United Kingdom.* London: CEMACH; 2007.
3. Knight M, UKOSS. Peripartum hysterectomy in the UK: management and outcomes of the associated haemorrhage. *BJOG* 2007;114:1380–7.
4. Derman RJ, Kodkany BS, Goudar SS, Geller SE, Naik VA, Bellad MB, *et al.* Oral misoprostol in preventing postpartum haemorrhage in resource-poor communities: a randomised controlled trial. *Lancet* 2006;368:1248–53.
5. Hoj L, Cardoso P, Nielsen BB, Hvidman L, Nielsen J, Aaby P. Effect of sublingual misoprostol on severe postpartum haemorrhage in a primary health centre in Guinea-Bissau: randomised double blind clinical trial. *BMJ* 2005;331:723.
6. Royal College of Obstetricians and Gynaecologists. *Prevention and Management of Postpartum Haemorrhage.* Green-top Guideline no. 52. London: RCOG Press; 2009.
7. Prata N, Mbaruku G, Campbell M. Using the kanga to measure postpartum blood loss. *Int J Gynaecol Obstet* 2005;89:49–50.
8. Bose P, Regan F, Paterson-Brown S. Improving the accuracy of estimated blood loss at obstetric haemorrhage using clinical reconstructions. *BJOG* 2006;113:919–24.
9. Quenby S, Pierce SJ, Brigham S, Wray S. Dysfunctional labor and myometrial lactic acidosis. *Obstet Gynecol* 2004;103:718–23.
10. Saunders NJ, Spiby H, Gilbert L, Fraser RB, Hall JM, Mutton PM, *et al.* Oxytocin infusion during second stage of labour in primiparous women using epidural analgesia: a randomised double blind placebo controlled trial. *BMJ* 1989;299:1423–6.
11. Kaunitz AM, Spence C, Danielson TS, Rochat RW, Grimes DA. Perinatal and maternal mortality in a religious group avoiding obstetric care. *Am J Obstet Gynecol* 1984;150:826–31.

12. World Health Organization. *Maternal Mortality in 2005: Estimates Developed by WHO, UNICEF, UNFPA, and the World Bank.* Geneva: WHO; 2007.

13. Carroli G, Mignini L. Episiotomy for vaginal birth. *Cochrane Database Syst Rev* 2009;(1):CD000081.

14. Palacios-Jaraquemada JM. Diagnosis and management of placenta accreta. *Best Pract Res Clin Obstet Gynaecol* 2008;22:1133–48.

15. Spencer PM. Controlled cord traction in management of the third stage of labour. *Br Med J* 1962;1:1728–32.

16. Weeks AD. Umbilical cord clamping after birth. *BMJ* 2007;335:312–13.

17. Prendiville WJ, Harding JE, Elbourne DR, Stirrat GM. The Bristol third stage trial: active versus physiological management of third stage of labour. *BMJ* 1988;297:1295–300.

18. Prendiville WJ, Elbourne D, McDonald S. Active versus expectant management in the third stage of labour. *Cochrane Database Syst Rev* 2000(3):CD000007.

19. Gülmezoglu AM, Widmer M, Merialdi M, Qureshi Z, Piaggio G, Elbourne D, *et al.* Active management of the third stage of labour without controlled cord traction: a randomized non-inferiority controlled trial. *Reprod Health* 2009;6:2.

20. World Health Organization. *WHO Recommendations for the Prevention of Postpartum Haemorrhage.* Geneva: WHO; 2006.

21. International Confederation of Midwives, International Federation of Gynaecology and Obstetrics. *Prevention and Treatment of Post-partum Haemorrhage: New Advances for Low Resource Settings.* Joint Statement. London: FIGO; 2006 [www.figo.org/files/figo-corp/docs/PPH%20Joint%20Statement%202%20English.pdf].

22. Winter C, Macfarlane A, Deneux-Tharaux C, Zhang WH, Alexander S, Brocklehurst P, *et al.* Variations in policies for management of the third stage of labour and the immediate management of postpartum haemorrhage in Europe. *BJOG* 2007;114:845–54.

23. National Collaborating Centre for Women's and Children's Health. *Intrapartum Care.* London: RCOG Press; 2007.

24. Su LL, Chong YS, Samuel M. Oxytocin agonists for preventing postpartum haemorrhage. *Cochrane Database Syst Rev* 2007;(3):CD005457.

25. Leduc D, Senikas V, Lalonde AB, Ballerman C, Biringer A, Delaney M, *et al;* Clinical Practice Obstetrics Committee; Society of Obstetricians and Gynaecologists of Canada. Active management of the third stage of labour: prevention and treatment of postpartum hemorrhage. *J Obstet Gynaecol Can* 2009;31:980–93.

26. Liabsuetrakul T, Choobun T, Peeyananjarassri K, Islam QM. Prophylactic use of ergot alkaloids in the third stage of labour. *Cochrane Database Syst Rev* 2007;(2):CD005456.

27. Begley CM. A comparison of 'active' and 'physiological' management of the third stage of labour. *Midwifery* 1990;6:3–17.

28. McDonald SJ, Abbott JM, Higgins SP. Prophylactic ergometrine-oxytocin versus oxytocin for the third stage of labour. *Cochrane Database Syst Rev* 2004;(1):CD000201.

29. Gülmezoglu AM, Forna F, Villar J, Hofmeyr GJ. Prostaglandins for preventing postpartum haemorrhage. *Cochrane Database Syst Rev* 2007;(3):CD000494.

30. Elati A, Weeks AD. The use of misoprostol in obstetrics and gynaecology. *BJOG* 2009;116 Suppl 1:61–9.

31. Chong YS, Chua S, Arulkumaran S. Severe hyperthermia following oral misoprostol in the immediate postpartum period. *Obstet Gynecol* 1997;90(4 Pt 2):703–4.

32. World Health Organization. *WHO Statement Regarding the Use of Misoprostol for Postpartum Haemorrhage Prevention and Treatment.* WHO/RHR/09.22. Geneva: WHO; 2009.

33. Gülmezoglu AM, Villar J, Ngoc NT, Piaggio G, Carroli G, Adetoro L, *et al;* WHO Collaborative Group To Evaluate Misoprostol in the Management of the Third Stage of Labour. WHO multicentre randomised trial of misoprostol in the management of the third stage of labour. *Lancet* 2001;358:689–95.

34. Alfirevic Z, Blum J, Walraven G, Weeks A, Winikoff B. Prevention of postpartum hemorrhage with misoprostol. *Int J Gynaecol Obstet* 2007;99 Suppl 2:S198–201.

35. Hofmeyr GJ, Gülmezoglu AM, Novikova N, Linder V, Ferreira S, Piaggio G. Misoprostol to prevent and treat postpartum haemorrhage: a systematic review and meta-analysis of maternal deaths and dose-related effects. *Bull World Health Organ* 2009;87:645–732.

36. Ferrer P, Roberts I, Sydenham E, Blackhall K, Shakur H. Anti-fibrinolytic agents in post partum haemorrhage: a systematic review. *BMC Pregnancy Childbirth* 2009;9:29.

37. McDonald SJ, Middleton P. Effect of timing of umbilical cord clamping of term infants on maternal and neonatal outcomes. *Cochrane Database Syst Rev* 2008;(2):CD004074.

38. Soltani H, Dickinson F, Symonds IM. Placental cord drainage after spontaneous vaginal delivery as part of the management of the third stage of labour. *Cochrane Database Syst Rev* 2005;(4):CD004665.

39. Combs CA, Laros RK. Prolonged third stage of labour: morbidity and risk factors. *Obstet Gynecol* 1991;77:863–7.

40. Magann EF, Evans S, Chauhan SP, Lanneau G, Fisk AD, Morrison JC. The length of the third stage of labor and the risk of postpartum hemorrhage. *Obstet Gynecol* 2005;105:290–3.

41. World Health Organization. *Managing Complications in Pregnancy and Childbirth: A Guide for Midwives and Doctors.* Geneva: WHO; 2007.

42. Weeks AD. The retained placenta. *Best Pract Res Clin Obstet Gynaecol* 2008;22:1103–17.

43. Carroli G, Bergel E. Umbilical vein injection for management of retained placenta. *Cochrane Database Syst Rev* 2001;(4):CD001337.

44. Weeks AD, Alia G, Vernon G, Namayanja A, Gosakan R, Majeed T, *et al.* Umbilical vein oxytocin for the treatment of retained placenta (Release Study): a double-blind, randomised controlled trial. *Lancet* 2010;375:141–7.

45. World Health Organization. *WHO Guidelines for the Management of Postpartum Haemorrhage and Retained Placenta.* Geneva: WHO; 2009.

46. Bider D, Dulitzky M, Goldenberg M, Lipitz S, Mashiach S. Intraumbilical vein injection of prostaglandin F2 alpha in retained placenta. *Eur J Obstet Gynecol Reprod Biol* 1996;64:59–61.

47. Rogers MS, Yuen PM, Wong S. Avoiding manual removal of placenta: evaluation of intra-umbilical injection of uterotonics using the Pipingas technique for management of adherent placenta. *Acta Obstet Gynecol Scand* 2007;86:48–54.

48. Bullarbo M, Tjugum J, Ekerhovd E. Sublingual nitroglycerin for management of retained placenta. *Int J Gynaecol Obstet* 2005;91:228–32. Erratum in: *Int J Gynaecol Obstet* 2006;92:337.

49. Blum J, Winikoff B, Raghavan S, Dabash R, Ramadan MC, Dilbaz B, Dao B, *et al.* Treatment of post-partum haemorrhage with sublingual misoprostol versus oxytocin in women receiving prophylactic oxytocin: a double-blind, randomised, non-inferiority trial. *Lancet* 2010;375:217–23.

50. Winikoff B, Dabash R, Durocher J, Darwish E, Nguyen TN, León W, *et al.* Treatment of post-partum haemorrhage with sublingual misoprostol versus oxytocin in women not exposed to oxytocin during labour: a double-blind, randomised, non-inferiority trial. *Lancet* 2010;375:210–16.

51. Blum J, Alfirevic Z, Walraven G, Weeks A, Winikoff B. Treatment of postpartum hemorrhage with misoprostol. *Int J Gynaecol Obstet* 2007;99 Suppl 2:S202–5.

52. Tang OS, Gemzell-Danielsson K, Ho PC. Misoprostol: pharmacokinetic profiles, effects on the uterus and side-effects. *Int J Gynaecol Obstet* 2007;99 Suppl 2:S160–7.

53. Searle E, Pavord S, Alfirevic Z. Recombinant factor VIIa and other pro-haemostatic therapies in primary postpartum haemorrhage. *Best Pract Res Clin Obstet Gynaecol* 2008;22:1075–88.

54. Hayman R, Arulkumaran S, Steer P. Uterine compression sutures: surgical management of postpartum hemorrhage. *Obstet Gynecol* 2002;99:502–6.

55. Ghezzi F, Cromi A, Uccella S, Raio L, Bolis P, Surbek D. The Hayman technique: a simple method to treat postpartum haemorrhage. *BJOG* 2007;114:362–5.

56. Akhter S, Begum MR, Kabir J. Condom hydrostatic tamponade for massive postpartum hemorrhage. *Int J Gynaecol Obstet* 2005;90:134–5.

57. Bates I, Chapotera GK, McKew S, van den Broek N. Maternal mortality in sub-Saharan Africa: the contribution of ineffective blood transfusion services. *BJOG* 2008;115:1331–9.

58. Millar S, Martin HB, Morris JL. Anti-shock garment in postpartum haemorrhage. *Best Pract Res Clin Obstet Gynaecol* 2008;22:1057–74.

59. L Hoj, personal communication.

60. A Carlin, personal communication.

Chapter 6

Reducing deaths from hypertensive disorders of pregnancy

Robert Pattinson, G Justus Hofmeyr and Carine Ronsmans

Introduction

Hypertensive disorders of pregnancy (HDP) are among the most important causes of maternal death worldwide. HDP are responsible for 16.1% of maternal deaths in high-income countries, for 9.1% of maternal deaths in Africa and Asia and for 25.7% of maternal deaths in Latin America.[1]

As examples of high-income countries, in the UK there were 18 maternal deaths due to HDP of a total of 132 direct deaths (13.6%) during 2003–05. Ten mothers died because of intracranial haemorrhage, two because of cerebral infarct and six had liver complications.[2]

In South Africa, as an example of a middle-income country, the fourth confidential enquiry into maternal deaths from 2005–07[3] reported 622 maternal deaths due to HDP, which was 15.7% of the total of 3959 maternal deaths, and 34.2% of direct maternal deaths. The deaths were subclassified as being due to eclampsia (55.3%), pre-eclampsia (27.8%), HELLP syndrome (haemolysis, elevated liver enzymes, low platelets) (8.7%), chronic hypertension (6.1%) and other causes (2.1%). The commonly reported final causes of death were cerebral haemorrhage (45.5%), respiratory failure including adult respiratory distress syndrome (ARDS) (25.4%), cardiac failure including pulmonary oedema (22.8%), multiple organ failure (14.1%), disseminated intravascular coagulopathy (DIC) (14.1%), renal failure (10.3%) and liver failure (4.8%).

In Kerala, India, as an example of a low-income country, HDP, with 41 deaths (13.4%), were the second most common cause of maternal death after obstetric haemorrhage (19.8%).[4] In an analysis of 29 deaths reported to the enquiry, 16 women had eclampsia, ten had severe pre-eclampsia, three had HELLP syndrome, and there were four women for whom there was no information. The final causes of death were intracranial haemorrhage in ten women, multiple organ disease in seven, DIC in five, ARDS in two, pulmonary embolus following HDP in two and three deaths were just recorded as 'eclampsia'.[4] Table 6.1 summarises the data from the three geographic areas.

HDP not only contribute to maternal deaths but also have an impact on perinatal deaths. The relationship between HDP and perinatal deaths is complex. Certain conditions that place the baby at risk also increase the risk of HDP, such as

Table 6.1   Maternal deaths recorded in confidential enquiries in three geographic areas

	UK (2003–05)[2]	Kerala (2004–05)[4]	South Africa (2005–07)[3]
Total deaths	295	307	3959
Total direct deaths	132	182	1819
Hypertension related (% of direct deaths)	18 (14%)	41 (22.5%)[a]	622 (34.2%)
Eclampsia (% of HDP)		16 (55%)	344 (55.3%)
Severe pre-eclampsia (% of HDP)		10 (34%)	176 (28.3%)
HELLP syndrome (% of HDP)		3 (10%)	54 (8.7%)
Chronic hypertension (% of HDP)			38 (6.1%)
Liver rupture, acute fatty liver (% of HDP)			10 (1.6%)
Causes (% of HDP)			
Intracranial haemorrhage	10 (56%)	10 (34%)	283 (45.5%)
Cerebral infarct	2 (11%)		
Liver complications	6 (33%)		30 (4.8%)
Multiple organ disease		7 (24%)	88 (14.1%)
DIC		5 (17%)	70 (11.3%)
ARDS/respiratory failure		2 (7%)	158 (25.4%)
Pulmonary embolus		2 (7%)	
Eclampsia		3 (10%)	
Cardiac failure			142 (22.8%)
Renal failure			64 (10.3%)

ARDS = adult respiratory distress syndrome; DIC = disseminated intravascular coagulopathy; HDP = hypertensive disorders of pregnancy; HELLP = haemolysis, elevated liver enzymes low platelets

[a] There were 41 deaths reported to the Demographic and Health Surveys (DHS) and confidential enquiry. In only 29 deaths (the confidential enquiry cases) were the subcategories of disease recorded. The percentages for the subcategories are of the known 29 deaths.

impaired uteroplacental blood flow and conditions that increase placental volume (diabetes, multiple pregnancy, syphilis, red cell immunisation and partial molar pregnancy). HDP increase the risk of placental abruption. Catastrophic maternal complications such as persistent eclampsia, intracranial haemorrhage, pulmonary oedema and cardiac arrest, as well as maternal death, may be a direct cause of fetal death. Pregnancy termination in the mother's interest may lead to iatrogenic preterm birth, and labour induction may lead to fetal distress. There may also be an inflammatory fetal syndrome similar to that seen in the mother: a large observational study[5] found that pre-eclampsia was associated with neonatal encephalopathy (odds ratio [OR] 25.5; 95% confidence interval [CI] 8.4–74.7), which was independent of obstetric intervention and could not be explained by either acidaemia or maternal fever. The authors concluded that a systemic inflammatory response in the fetus could explain the link between maternal pre-eclampsia and neonatal encephalopathy, and that this may occur through cerebral vasoconstriction.

In South Africa, HDP was classified as the primary cause of perinatal deaths in 13% of cases, representing approximately 3894 perinatal deaths per year. The majority of these were stillbirths (75%) and the remaining 25% were neonatal deaths.[6]

In the UK perinatal mortality report for 2006,[7] the data do not allow a calculation of the total impact of HDP on perinatal deaths; however, about 3% of stillbirths were classified as being due to pre-eclampsia. The biggest cause of neonatal deaths was immaturity (47%) but the proportion of these neonates that died resulting from early delivery due to HDP was not reported. However, HDP is the most common cause of iatrogenic preterm birth and the impact of HDP on perinatal mortality in the UK will be substantial. The data from the West Midlands collected by the Perinatal Institute from 1997 to 2007 indicate that HDP were recorded in 7.1% of stillbirths, in 4.8% of early neonatal deaths and in 5.2% of late neonatal deaths.[8] In neonatal deaths due to preterm birth, 4.8% of the mothers had hypertension recorded. Data from low-income countries are scant but in Matlab, Bangladesh, 2.3% and 3.1% of perinatal deaths were attributed to pre-eclampsia and eclampsia, respectively.[9]

Health system causes of maternal and perinatal death due to HDP

Identifying where women, healthcare providers or health managers fail to respond, or respond inappropriately, are important areas where, if targeted, reductions in maternal and perinatal deaths can be made. In the UK report of 2003–05,[2] 'the single major failing in clinical care in pre-eclampsia in the current triennium was inadequate treatment of systolic hypertension. The sequel, intracranial haemorrhage, occurred in several cases.' In Kerala, the major health system problems were delays in transport, using inappropriate management protocols such as the lytic cocktail to manage eclampsia and not reducing the blood pressure effectively.[4]

In South Africa, 49% of deaths due to HDP were thought to be clearly avoidable within the health system. The major problems occurred at the primary level, with 65% of these women having suboptimal care. The major patient-related problems were lack of attending antenatal care (19.4%) and poor attendance at clinics (7.3%). A transport problem was reported as playing a significant role, with 19.4% of women who died having delay in getting to any health institution and a delay in transport between institutions was a contributing factor in the deaths of 10.9% of the women transferred. The most common healthcare provider errors were not following the standard protocol, poor assessment, and delays in transferring or managing the woman at an inappropriate level.[3]

In perinatal deaths related to HDP in South Africa, 14% were thought to be clearly avoidable within the health system. The major areas of suboptimal care reported were failure to respond to hypertension in antenatal care (7.2%), no or poor attendance at antenatal care (8.8%) and delay in referral to the appropriate level of care (3.0%).[6]

Drug availability and use of magnesium sulphate for the management of HDP varies between countries. A comprehensive audit of medical records of women giving birth in nine hospitals in Indonesia, Malaysia, the Philippines and Thailand found that magnesium sulphate was universally used for the management of eclampsia in all hospitals.[10] In countries such as Mozambique and Zimbabwe, on the other hand, the availability and use of magnesium sulphate remains poor. Magnesium sulphate is cheap and has appeared on the essential medicines list of the World Health Organization (WHO) since 1996. The main reasons for its low availability are the complex mechanisms of approval, acquisition and distribution of drugs in some countries.[11] In addition, the low cost of magnesium sulphate means that market forces cannot be relied on to ensure its availability.

Summary of the impact of HDP on maternal and perinatal deaths

■ HDP are a major contributor to maternal deaths throughout the world but are most significant, proportionally, in middle- and low-income countries. To accelerate progress to reach the Millennium Development Goals (MDGs), low- and middle-income countries will need to be targeted.

▓ Eclampsia is by far the most common complication of HDP associated with maternal death.

▓ Intracranial haemorrhage is the most common cause of death, followed by cardiac and respiratory problems, including pulmonary oedema and DIC.

▓ Major avoidable factors are lack of attendance at antenatal care, referral to the appropriate level, transport between institutions, and following an appropriate protocol that includes magnesium sulphate and aggressive control of the blood pressure.

This chapter will examine the interventions and strategies available to reduce both maternal and perinatal deaths related to HDP.

What interventions are known to be effective?

The effective interventions related to HDP with respect to reducing maternal and perinatal deaths are shown in Tables 6.2 and 6.3, respectively.

Reduction in unplanned pregnancies at the extremes of reproductive age

Unplanned pregnancies are common in middle- and low-income countries. At the East London Hospital Complex, South Africa, one-quarter of all pregnancies are terminated and of the remainder two-thirds are unplanned.[12]

Pregnancy at the extremes of reproductive age is dangerous to mother and baby. Data from the South African confidential enquiries into maternal deaths illustrate that women who die as a result of complications of HDP are more often in the extremes of reproductive life (younger than 20 years 17.4% compared with 11.3% of the general pregnant population, and older than 34 years 19.4% versus 14.9% of the general pregnant population).[13] In relation to perinatal deaths, the South African data indicate that women over the age of 34 years had a significantly higher perinatal mortality rate due to HDP of 5.82 per 1000 births compared with women with HDP between the ages of 20 and 34 years (2.62 per 1000 births).[6] In the UK, eclampsia is more common among teenagers.[14] The greatest proportions of unplanned pregnancies are among teenagers and women over the age of 34 years, and reduction in unplanned pregnancies is likely to reduce the proportions of these age groups in the obstetric population and, hence, HDP-related deaths.

The maternal mortality ratio does not capture reductions in risk due to declining fertility very well but such progress could be monitored by tracking trends in the absolute number of maternal deaths or the maternal mortality ratio. In 2000–05, the global total fertility rate was 2.65 children, about half the rate in 1950–55.[15] As a result, the total number of births has fallen in some countries. In South Asia, total births are projected to remain stationary at about 37 million between 1990 and 2015 but, in sub-Saharan Africa, births will continue to increase by a projected 43% over the same period. Not only will this high fertility add an extra burden to overstretched maternity services, thus potentially increasing obstetric risk, it will also automatically result in increases in the number of maternal deaths from all causes, including HDP.

Prevention of pre-eclampsia

Calcium supplementation

Calcium supplementation during pregnancy in communities with low dietary calcium has been shown to reduce the composite outcome maternal death or serious morbidity:[16]

- ▓ maternal death or serious morbidity is reduced by 20% (four trials, 9732 women: relative risk [RR] 0.80; 95% CI 0.65–0.97)
- ▓ maternal death is possibly reduced (one trial, one death in the calcium supplementation group [$n = 4151$] versus six deaths in the placebo group [$n = 4161$]: RR 0.17; 95% CI 0.02–1.39).

Calcium supplementation has also resulted in a reduction in hypertension in pregnancy (11 trials, 14946 women: RR 0.70; 95% CI 0.57–0.86). There was also a reduction in the risk of pre-eclampsia associated with calcium supplementation (12 trials, 15206 women: RR 0.48, 95% CI 0.33–0.69), with the effect of calcium supplementation was greatest for high-risk women (five trials, 587 women: RR 0.22; 95% CI 0.12–0.42) and for those with low baseline calcium intake (seven trials, 10154 women: RR 0.36; 95% CI 0.18–0.70). There was heterogeneity between trials, with greater effects in the smaller trials.[16]

Calcium supplementation did not impact on perinatal outcomes. There was no overall effect on the risk of preterm birth (ten trials, 14751 women: RR 0.81; 95% CI 0.64–1.03) or stillbirth or death before discharge from hospital (ten trials, 15141 babies: RR 0.89; 95% CI 0.73–1.09).[16]

To date, trials have investigated the effectiveness of calcium supplementation in the second half of pregnancy. Research is needed to assess whether effectiveness is enhanced by prepregnancy supplementation, in which case food fortification programmes would hold the greatest promise for reduction of deaths from HDP on a large scale.[17]

Role of low-dose aspirin

Low-dose aspirin has not been shown to reduce maternal mortality but its use is associated with a reduction in perinatal deaths in pregnancies at high risk of developing pre-eclampsia. However, the number needed to treat is high (NNT 243; 95% CI 131–1666), making it an intervention not useful for widespread use.[18] Low-dose aspirin is associated with a reduction in the risk of pre-eclampsia. There is a 17% reduction in the risk of pre-eclampsia associated with the use of antiplatelet agents (46 trials, 32891 women: RR 0.83; 95% CI 0.77–0.89, NNT 72; 95% CI 52–119). In women at high risk of pre-eclampsia, the risk of developing pre-eclampsia can be reduced and the NNT is acceptable (NNT 19; 95% CI 13–34).

Rest at home

The only other intervention associated with a reduction in relative risk of pre-eclampsia was rest of between 30 minutes and 6 hours at home, with or without a nutritional supplement, for women with normal blood pressure.[19] However, this review included just two small trials with a total of 106 women and its results should be interpreted with caution.

Table 6.2 Efficacy of treatment and prevention of hypertensive disorders of pregnancy (HDP), based on Cochrane reviews

HDP-related maternal outcome	No. of studies	Limitations	No. of events in each group		Relative risk (95% CI)
			Intervention	Control	
Magnesium sulphate versus diazepam for treatment of eclampsia[30]					
Death	6	Three trials are of high quality; for three blinding of treatment allocation was uncertain	26	42	0.59 (0.37–0.94)
Recurring convulsions	6		71	162	0.44 (0.34–0.57)
Blood loss at delivery >500 ml	2		76	78	1.15 (0.82–1.60)
Magnesium sulphate versus phenytoin for treatment of eclampsia[63]					
Death	2	One very large high-quality study; smaller studies did not blind treatment allocation	10	20	0.50 (0.24–1.05)
Recurring convulsions	5		25	83	0.31 (0.20–0.47)
Blood loss at delivery >500 ml	1		71	75	0.98 (0.74–1.30)
Magnesium sulphate versus lytic cocktail for treatment of eclampsia[64]					
Death	2	Trials are small and of average quality	1	6	0.25 (0.04–1.43)
Recurring convulsions	2		4	49	0.09 (0.03–0.24)
Placental abruption	1		3	4	0.84 (0.20–3.57)
Magnesium sulphate versus placebo for treatment of pre-eclampsia[31]					
Death	3	One very large high-quality study; smaller studies did not blind treatment allocation	11	21	0.54 (0.26–1.10)
Eclampsia	7		43	107	0.41 (0.29–0.58)
Serious maternal morbidity	3		196	183	1.08 (0.89–1.32)
Placental abruption	2		92	141	0.64 (0.50–0.83)
Postpartum bleeding	2		754	775	0.96 (0.88–1.05)
Any antihypertensive drug versus placebo/no treatment for treatment of mild to moderate hypertension in pregnancy[23]					
Death	4	All trials are small and their quality is moderate to poor	2	0	2.85 (0.30–27.0)
Eclampsia	5		0	1	0.34 (0.01–8.15)
Proteinuria/pre-eclampsia	22		239	241	0.97 (0.83–1.13)
Severe hypertension	19		115	228	0.50 (0.41–0.61)
Routine calcium supplementation versus placebo during pregnancy[16]					
Death/serious morbidity	4	Results dominated by one large trial; all trials are of good quality	167	210	0.80 (0.65–0.97)
Pre-eclampsia	12		368	480	0.48 (0.33–0.69)
High blood pressure	11		1249	1442	0.70 (0.57–0.86)
Placental abruption	5		36	42	0.86 (0.55–1.34)
Antiplatelet agents versus placebo during pregnancy in women at risk of pre-eclampsia[18]					
Death	3	There is wide variation in study quality	3	1	2.57 (0.39–17.06)
Eclampsia	9		33	36	0.94 (0.59–1.48)
Pre-eclampsia	43		1081	1291	0.83 (0.77–0.89)
Placental abruption	16		172	150	1.10 (0.89–1.37)
Gestational hypertension	34		1077	1103	0.95 (0.88–1.03)

CI = confidence interval; HDP = hypertensive disorders of pregnancy; RR = relative risk

Table 6.3   Effect of interventions for reducing perinatal deaths due to hypertensive disorders of pregnancy (HDP), based on Cochrane reviews

HDP-related perinatal outcome	No. of studies	Limitations	No. of events in each group		Relative risk (95% CI)
			Intervention	Control	
Magnesium sulphate versus diazepam for treatment of eclampsia[30]					
Stillbirth	4	Three trials are of high quality;	51	55	0.89 (0.63–1.26)
Neonatal death		for three blinding of treatment	38	27	1.34 (0.84–2.14)
Perinatal death		allocation was uncertain	87	80	1.04 (0.80–1.36)
Magnesium sulphate versus phenytoin for treatment of eclampsia[63]					
Stillbirth	2	One very large high-quality	57	72	0.83 (0.61–1.13)
Neonatal death	2	study; smaller studies did not	29	32	0.95 (0.59–1.53)
Perinatal death	2	blind treatment allocation	84	103	0.85 (0.67–1.09)
Magnesium sulphate versus lytic cocktail for treatment of eclampsia[64]					
Stillbirth	2	Trials are small and of average	9	16	0.55 (0.26–1.16)
Neonatal death	2	quality	5	13	0.39 (0.14–1.06)
Magnesium sulphate versus placebo for treatment of pre-eclampsia[31]					
Stillbirth	3	One very large high-quality	424	426	0.99 (0.87–1.12)
Neonatal death	1	study; smaller studies did not	187	159	1.16 (0.94, 1.42)
Perinatal death	2	blind treatment allocation	538	541	1.04 (0.93–1.15)
Any antihypertensive drug versus placebo/no treatment for treatment of mild to moderate hypertension in pregnancy[33]					
Miscarriage	7	All trials are small and their	6	17	0.39 (0.17–0.93)
Stillbirth	18	quality is moderate to poor	18	16	1.14 (0.60–2.17)
Neonatal death	4		1	2	0.79 (0.14–4.34)
Perinatal death	20		30	31	0.96 (0.60–1.54)
Routine calcium supplementation versus placebo during pregnancy[16]					
Stillbirth or death before discharge:					
• adequate calcium diet	4		29	26	1.12 (0.66–1.90
• inadequate calcium diet	6		148	174	0.86 (0.69–1.06)
• overall	10		177	200	0.89 (0.73–1.09)
Antiplatelet agents versus placebo during pregnancy in women at risk of pre-eclampsia[18]					
Fetal loss (miscarriage and stillbirth)	28		169	172	0.96 (0.78–1.18)
Neonatal death	19		67	74	0.89 (0.64–1.22)
Perinatal death	15		190	212	0.86 (0.76–0.98)

CI = confidence interval; HDP = hypertensive disorders of pregnancy; RR = relative risk

Other interventions aimed at preventing HDP

Other potential methods of preventing pre-eclampsia have been investigated but there is insufficient evidence for their use (garlic,[20] nitric oxide,[21] progesterone,[22] exercise or other physical activity[23] and altered dietary salt intake[24]) or they are potentially harmful (antioxidants[25] and diuretics[26]). For the use of antioxidants, there was no difference between antioxidant and control in preventing pre-eclampsia or adverse effects, except that women were more likely to experience abdominal pain and require antihypertensive therapy and that women required more antenatal admissions due to hypertension in pregnancy.[25] For the use of diuretics, there were no differences between the diuretic and the control group with respect to HDP and their outcomes, but women on thiazide diuretics had more adverse effects of nausea and vomiting and women taking diuretics were more likely to stop their treatment because of adverse effects than the women in the placebo control group.[26]

Screening for HDP

In an exhaustive review of 27 tests to screen for pre-eclampsia, Meads *et al.*[27] reported that the quality of included studies was generally poor. Some tests appeared to have high specificity but at the expense of compromised sensitivity. The only tests that reached specificities above 90% were a body mass index greater than 34 kg/m^2, high alpha-fetoprotein and bilateral notching of the uterine artery found at Doppler examination. A few tests not commonly performed in routine practice, such as kallikreinuria and sodium dodecyl sulphate polyacrylamide gel electrophoresis (SDS-PAGE) proteinuria, seemed to offer the promise of high sensitivity without compromising specificity but these require further investigation. The reviewers concluded that the tests evaluated are not sufficiently accurate to suggest their routine use in clinical practice. Doppler of the uterine artery would also not be practical to introduce as screening in middle- and low-income countries. The authors speculated that the most cost-effective approach to reducing pre-eclampsia is likely to be the provision of an effective, affordable and safe intervention applied to all mothers without prior testing to assess levels of risk.[27]

The main role of screening for hypertension in pregnancy in developing countries is to identify women whose pregnancy or delivery is likely to raise problems and to refer women at the appropriate time to facilities where the appropriate treatment can be provided. Screening here is related to early detection of hypertension or proteinuria. The risk approach will function properly only if women agree to be referred and effective treatment is available at the place of referral. Compliance with referral may be low, however, particularly where geographical access to hospitals represents a significant barrier.[28] Active collaboration between referral levels may be poor, communication and transport arrangements may not have been formalised, and setting-specific protocols for referrer and receiver may not have been agreed.[29]

Prevention of morbidity and mortality

Magnesium sulphate

Magnesium sulphate is a proven effective intervention for preventing recurrent convulsions and mortality in women with eclampsia and for preventing eclampsia in women with pre-eclampsia. A systematic review comparing magnesium sulphate with diazepam for treatment of eclampsia[30] found a 56% reduction in recurring convulsions (seven trials, 1441 women: RR 0.44; 95% CI 0.34–0.57) and a reduction in maternal death (six trials, 1336 women: RR 0.59; 95% CI 0.37–0.94). Another review comparing magnesium sulphate with other anticonvulsants for women with pre-eclampsia[31] found that magnesium sulphate more than halved the risk of eclampsia (RR 0.41; 95% CI 0.29–0.58, NNT 100; 95% CI 50–100) and non-significantly reduced the risk of dying by 46% (RR 0.54; 95% CI 0.26–1.10).

Magnesium sulphate was not found to alter the risk of stillbirth or neonatal death (RR 1.04; 95% CI 0.93–1.15) or other outcomes for the fetus or neonate. There was a small reduction in risk of placental abruption (RR 0.64; 95% CI 0.50–0.83, NNT 100; 95% CI 50–1000).[31] However, magnesium sulphate has been shown to reduce the incidence of cerebral palsy in preterm infants when given to mothers with preterm labour for neuroprotective purposes. In women with pre-eclampsia with preterm infants, the trend was also for a reduction in cerebral palsy but it was not significant.[32]

However, magnesium sulphate has its drawbacks. Adverse effects were found to be more common with magnesium sulphate (24% versus 5%, RR 5.26; 95% CI 4.59–6.03, NNT for harm 6; 95% CI 6–5). The main adverse effect was flushing. A small increase (5%) in the risk of caesarean section was also reported.[31]

Antihypertensive therapy

The use of antihypertensive therapy is associated with a halving in the risk of developing severe hypertension (19 trials, 2409 women: RR 0.50; 95% CI 0.41–0.61, NNT 10; 95% CI 8–13) but there is little evidence of a difference in the risk of developing pre-eclampsia (22 trials, 2702 women: RR 0.97; 95% CI 0.83–1.13).[33] No clear effect on the risk of the baby dying (26 trials, 3081 women: RR 0.73; 95% CI 0.50–1.08), preterm birth (14 trials, 1992 women: RR 1.02; 95% CI 0.89–1.16) or small-for-gestational-age babies (19 trials, 2437 women: RR 1.04; 95% CI 0.84–1.27) were reported.[33]

In evaluating various drug regimens, Duley et al.[34] concluded that, until better evidence is available, the choice of antihypertensive should depend on the clinician's experience and familiarity with a particular drug, and on what is known about adverse effects. However, diazoxide, ketanserin, nimodipine and magnesium sulphate (as an antihypertensive) are probably best avoided.

The use of antihypertensive therapy has not been reported to reduce maternal deaths. Intracranial haemorrhage or infarct as an endpoint has not been reported in the trials of antihypertensive therapy in pregnancy. In maternal deaths due to HDP, intracranial haemorrhage is by far the most common final cause of death. The most common cause of intracranial haemorrhage is severe hypertension and thus lowering the blood pressure has been regarded as the most important method of preventing intracranial haemorrhage.

Early induction of labour

The only way to 'cure' pre-eclampsia or eclampsia is to remove the placenta. This simple fact is in danger of being forgotten as attempts are made to prolong the pregnancy for the benefit of the infant. It is important to note that both England and Wales and Sweden achieved very low levels of mortality from HDP in the 1970s, long before magnesium sulphate was introduced. In England and Wales, mortality from HDP was 80 per 100 000 live births in 1920, falling to 26 and two deaths per 100 000 live births in 1950 and 1970, respectively.[35] Similarly, dramatic falls in mortality from

HDP were seen in Sweden.[36] These falls were largely due to the introduction of early induction of labour in women with severe pre-eclampsia.[35,36]

Delaying the delivery of an infant whose mother has pre-eclampsia remote from term has also been considered as a management option to improve the outcome for the infant.[37] However, the only two trials included in this review were too small from which to to draw any conclusion. The intervention group had more hyaline membrane disease (RR 2.30; 95% CI 1.39–3.81), more necrotising enterocolitis (RR 5.54; 95% CI 1.04–29.56) and more admission to neonatal intensive care (RR 1.32; 95% CI 1.13–1.55) than those allocated an expectant policy. Nevertheless, babies allocated to the intervention group were less likely to be small for gestational age (RR 0.36; 95% CI 0.14–0.90). Expectant management has its risks and in a prospective case series of 5 years in a tertiary hospital, Hall *et al*.[38] described that 27% of women experienced a major complication, although in their hands few mothers had poor outcomes. These results are very unlikely to be repeated in regional or district hospitals as expectant care can only be practised in situations where the mother can be closely monitored. The safest option for the mother is referral to a tertiary institution or, if that is not available, delivery of the women.

Induction of labour in women with gestational hypertension or mild pre-eclampsia from 36 weeks of gestation was found to result in less poor maternal outcome (mainly progression to severe disease) than women managed expectantly (RR 0.71; 95% CI 0.59–0.86, NNT 8). Surprisingly, fewer caesarean sections were needed in the induction group than in the expectantly managed group (RR 0.75; 95% CI 0.55–1.04). This adds further evidence for the early delivery of women with HDP.[39]

Improvement of knowledge and skills

There is clear evidence that outreach visits,[40] continuing medical education and workshops,[41] influencing opinion leaders[42] and audit and feedback[43] are all associated with small but significant improvements in the quality of care. After reviewing maternal near misses and deaths due to hypertension, a strict protocol was developed in the Pretoria Academic Complex and this resulted in a significant reduction in the mortality index for cases due to hypertension.[44] There are skills-training packages available that have been proven to have an effect.[45–50] The introduction of fire drills (simulation training) also has the added advantage of improving interprofessional cooperation.[51–53]

Summary of effective interventions

The key effective interventions for HDP are:

- calcium supplementation in calcium-depleted populations for preventing pre-eclampsia
- magnesium sulphate to manage eclampsia and to prevent eclampsia in women with pre-eclampsia
- antihypertensive therapy to prevent severe hypertension and to prevent intracranial haemorrhage
- early induction of labour
- improve knowledge and skills by using effective training methods and audit and feedback.

Framework for strategies to reduce deaths from HDP

Prevention

Calcium supplementation reduces HDP and reduces pre-eclampsia by 52%; it is especially effective in women with a low baseline intake, where the reduction is 64%. The biggest effect of calcium supplementation during pregnancy is in women who access prenatal care early. Thus, early attendance for antenatal care to receive calcium supplementation is essential, or alternative methods of supplementing calcium developed for the whole population need to be developed. The scaling up of calcium supplementation to all pregnant women in areas with a low calcium intake must be a high priority.

Early detection strategies

To prevent maternal and perinatal deaths, HDP need to be detected early and women for whom pregnancy or delivery is likely to raise problems need referral at the appropriate time and to the appropriate level of care. Thus, early attendance for antenatal care is again essential. Once hypertension or proteinuria is detected, mechanisms must be in place to refer the woman to the appropriate level of care. Lack of this referral mechanism is a common health system failure and needs to be urgently addressed. In the absence of a better option, screening according to the WHO antenatal care guidelines is probably the best to follow, namely to measure the blood pressure and test the urine for protein at each visit.[54,55] The optimal number of antenatal visits is not known and guideline recommendations have varied from four to nine goal-oriented visits.

Management strategies for pre-eclampsia

Prevention of eclampsia

Administering magnesium sulphate to women with eclampsia or with severe pre-eclampsia is an effective mechanism to reduce severe morbidity and deaths due to HDP.

Prevention of cerebrovascular accidents

Controlling the blood pressure is essential to prevent intracranial haemorrhage. To achieve this, there must a choice of antihypertensive agents available. The drug of choice is unclear but nifedipine is readily available and inexpensive. No adverse events were recorded with the combination of magnesium sulphate and nifedipine in the Magpie Trial and this was the most commonly used antihypertensive.[56]

Prevention of pulmonary oedema

Strict control of fluid intake is necessary to prevent pulmonary oedema.

Treatment (delivery)

Rapid labour induction with low-dose titrated oral misoprostol solution[57] or vaginal misoprostol 25 µg 4-hourly[58] are workable strategies. Misoprostol is inexpensive and thus a feasible induction agent for low- and middle-income countries. It appears that a titrated dose of oral misoprostol is as effective and safe as vaginal misoprostol.

The dosages of misoprostol should not exceed 25 µg vaginally or 50 µg orally as the risk of hyperstimulation increases above these dosages. These low dosages are still as effective in ensuring delivery within 24 hours as other conventional methods and they do not have as many adverse effects. There appears to be no advantage but possible harm from using misoprostol sublingually and this should not be used until there is further evidence available.[59] The WHO Expert Committee on the Selection and Use of Essential Medicines has included misoprostol on its list. It it hoped that this will encourage countries to put it on their own essential drug lists and thus make it available for use in induction of labour.

Previous caesarean section

On the basis of evidence of lower risk of uterine hyperstimulation than with dinoprostone or misoprostol, mechanical methods of labour induction have a theoretical advantage for women with previous caesarean section and unfavourable cervix,[60] although direct evidence of the safety of this strategy is lacking.

Impact of introducing interventions

The magnitude of the impact of various interventions on reductions in HDP mortality is not known, although some rough calculations can be made. The 98% fall in HDP-related mortality in the UK and Sweden over 50 years suggests that HDP-related deaths are highly avoidable. This fall has been largely attributed to a reduction in the number of women with eclampsia, while the incidence of pre-eclampsia has been more resistant to change.[14,35] The package of interventions that has caused this drop has not been documented in detail but antenatal screening for high blood pressure and proteinuria in the second half of pregnancy, with early delivery through induction of labour or caesarean delivery in women diagnosed with pre-eclampsia, is thought to be the main reason.[35]

Today, new effective interventions exist and dramatic reductions in HDP mortality should be possible in middle- and low-income countries if all women have access to a skilled health professional in an enabling environment. In South Africa, for example, where most women have a reduced intake of dietary calcium, the introduction of calcium supplementation in pregnancy should be associated with approximately a halving in the incidence of pre-eclampsia. Further reductions in HDP mortality should also be possible if all women with pre-eclampsia and eclampsia are treated with magnesium sulphate.

It is estimated that a package of interventions including 100% coverage with calcium supplementation in pregnancy and magnesium sulphate for all women with pre-eclampsia and eclampsia could reduce the annual number of HDP-related deaths in South Africa from an estimated 360–480 to 97–129. This would represent a 73% fall in HDP mortality. This is based on the assumption that about 1 million births occur in South Africa per year, an incidence of pre-eclampsia of 6–8%, a current coverage of magnesium sulphate for pre-eclampsia and eclampsia of 50%, a case fatality rate for severe pre-eclampsia and eclampsia of 20%,[61,62] and an efficacy of magnesium sulphate of 59% for the reduction of eclampsia in women with pre-eclampsia and thus a 41% mortality reduction in women with eclampsia.

Conclusion

There are clearly effective interventions available now for HDP that will significantly reduce both maternal and perinatal mortality and accelerate progress to achieve the MDGs. The key interventions are:

- calcium supplementation to all pregnant women
- use of magnesium sulphate to prevent and manage eclampsia
- blood pressure control to prevent intracranial haemorrhage
- early delivery of women with HDP.

The major problem that needs solving is how to get these interventions to those women that need it.

References

1. Khan KS, Wojdyla D, Say L, Gülmezoglu AM, Van Look PFA. WHO analysis of causes of maternal death: a systematic review. *Lancet* 2006;367:1066–74.
2. Neilson J. Pre-eclampsia and eclampsia. In: Lewis G, editor. *Saving Mothers' Lives: Reviewing Maternal Deaths to Make Motherhood Safer 2003–2005. The Seventh Report on Confidential Enquiries into Maternal Deaths in the United Kingdom*. London: CEMACH; 2007. p. 72–7.
3. Moodley J, Molefe N. Hypertensive disorders in pregnancy. In: National Committee for the Confidential Enquiry on Maternal Deaths, Pattinson RC, editor. *Saving Mothers 2005–2007. Fourth Report on Confidential Enquiries into Maternal Deaths in South Africa*. Pretoria: Department of Health; 2009. p. 47–66.
4. Paily VP. Overview of Confidential Review of Maternal Deaths for 2004 and 2005. In: Paily VP, editor. *Why Mothers Die, Kerala 2004–05. First Confidential Review of Maternal Deaths, Kerala*. Thiruvananthapuram: KFOG Press; 2009. p. 39–52.
5. Impey L, Greenwood C, Sheil O, MacQuillan K, Reynolds M, Redman C. The relation between pre-eclampsia at term and neonatal encephalopathy. *Arch Dis Child Fetal Neonatal Ed* 2001;85:F170–2.
6. Pattinson RC, Velaphi S, Moran N, Hardy B, Steyn W. Overview. In: Pattinson RC, editor. *Saving Babies 2006–2007: Sixth Perinatal Care Survey of South Africa*. Pretoria: Tshepesa Press; 2009. p. 1–63.
7. Acolet D, Springett A, Golightly S. *Perinatal Mortality 2006*. London: CEMACH; 2008.
8. J Gardosi, personal communication.
9. Kusiako T, Ronsmans C, Van der Paal L. The contribution of complications of childbirth to perinatal mortality in Matlab, Bangladesh. *Bull World Health Organ* 2000;78:621–7.
10. SEA-ORCHID Study Group, Laopaiboon M, Lumbiganon P, McDonald SJ, Henderson-Smart DJ, Green S, Crowther CA. Use of evidence-based practices in pregnancy and childbirth: South East Asia Optimising Reproductive and Child Health in Developing Countries project. *PLoS One* 2008;3:e2646.
11. Sevene S, Lewin S, Mariano A, Woelk G, Oxman AD, Matinhure S, *et al*. System and market failures: the unavailability of magnesium sulphate for the treatment of eclampsia and pre-eclampsia in Mozambique and Zimbabwe. *BMJ* 2005;331:765–9.
12. Mshweshwe TN, Mgoli A, Hofmeyr GJ, Mangesi L. Assessing the prevalence of unwanted pregnancies and barriers to use of preventive measures in East London. 27th Conference on Priorities in Perinatal Care in Southern Africa, 11–14 March 2008, Gauteng, South Africa.
13. Pattinson RC, Moodley J. Overview and 10 key recommendations. In: National Committee for the Confidential Enquiry on Maternal Deaths, Pattinson RC, editor. *Saving Mothers: Fourth Report on Confidential Enquiries into Maternal Deaths in South Africa 2005–2007*. Pretoria: Department of Health; 2009. p. 1–36.
14. Douglas KA, Redman CWG. Eclampsia in the United Kingdom. *BMJ* 1994;309:1395–400.
15. Ronsmans C, Graham WJ, Lancet Maternal Survival Series steering group. Maternal mortality: who, when, where, and why. *Lancet* 2006;368:1189–200.

16. Hofmeyr GJ, Atallah AN, Duley L. Calcium supplementation during pregnancy for preventing hypertensive disorders and related problems. *Cochrane Database Syst Rev* 2006;(3):CD001059.

17. Hofmeyr G, Duley L, Atallah A. Dietary calcium supplementation for prevention of pre-eclampsia and related problems: a systematic review and commentary. *BJOG* 2007;114:933–43.

18. Duley L, Henderson-Smart DJ, Meher S, King JF. Antiplatelet agents for preventing pre-eclampsia and its complications. *Cochrane Database Syst Rev* 2007;(2):CD004659.

19. Meher S, Duley L. Rest during pregnancy for preventing pre-eclampsia and its complications in women with normal blood pressure. *Cochrane Database Syst Rev* 2006;(2):CD005939.

20. Meher S, Duley L. Garlic for preventing pre-eclampsia and its complications. *Cochrane Database Syst Rev* 2006;(3):CD006065.

21. Meher S, Duley L. Nitric oxide for preventing pre-eclampsia and its complications. *Cochrane Database Syst Rev* 2007;(2):CD006490.

22. Meher S, Duley L. Progesterone for preventing pre-eclampsia and its complications. *Cochrane Database Syst Rev* 2006;(4):CD006175.

23. Meher S, Duley L. Exercise or other physical activity for preventing pre-eclampsia and its complications. *Cochrane Database Syst Rev* 2006;(2):CD005942.

24. Duley L, Henderson-Smart DJ, Meher S. Altered dietary salt for preventing pre-eclampsia, and its complications. *Cochrane Database Syst Rev* 2005;(4):CD005548.

25. Rumbold A, Duley L, Crowther CA, Haslam RR. Antioxidants for preventing pre-eclampsia. *Cochrane Database Syst Rev* 2008;(1):CD004227.

26. Churchill D, Beevers GDG, Meher S, Rhodes C. Diuretics for preventing pre-eclampsia. *Cochrane Database Syst Rev* 2007;(1):CD004451.

27. Meads, C A. Cnossen, J S. Meher, S. Juarez-Garcia, A. ter Riet, G. Duley, *et al.* Methods of prediction and prevention of pre-eclampsia: systematic reviews of accuracy and effectiveness literature with economic modelling. *Health Technol Assess* 2008;12:iii-iv:1–270.

28. Dujardin B, Clarysse G, Criel B, De Brouwere V, Wangata N. The strategy of risk approach in antenatal care: evaluation of the referral compliance. *Soc Sci Med* 1995;40:529–35.

29. Murray S, Pearson SC. Maternity referral systems in developing countries: current knowledge and future research needs. *Soc Sci Med* 2006;62:2205–15.

30. Duley L, Henderson-Smart DJ. Magnesium sulphate versus diazepam for eclampsia. *Cochrane Database Syst Rev* 2003;(4):CD000127.

31. Duley L, Gülmezoglu AM, Henderson-Smart DJ. Magnesium sulphate and other anticonvulsants for women with pre-eclampsia. *Cochrane Database Syst Rev* 2003;(2):CD000025.

32. Doyle LW, Crowther CA, Middleton P, Marret S, Rouse D. Magnesium sulphate for women at risk of preterm birth for neuroprotection of the fetus. *Cochrane Database Syst Rev* 2009;(1):CD004661.

33. Abalos E, Duley L, Steyn DW, Henderson-Smart DJ. Antihypertensive drug therapy for mild to moderate hypertension during pregnancy. *Cochrane Database Syst Rev* 2007;(1):CD002252.

34. Duley L, Henderson-Smart DJ, Meher S. Drugs for treatment of very high blood pressure during pregnancy. *Cochrane Database Syst Rev* 2006;(3):CD001449.

35. Loudon I. *Death in Childbirth: An International Study of Maternal Care and Maternal Mortality 1800–1950*. New York: Oxford University Press; 1992.

36. Hogberg U. *Maternal mortality in Sweden*. Umea University Medical Dissertations New Series No 156. Umea: Department of Obstetrics and Gynaecology; 1985. p. 13.

37. Churchill D, Duley L. Interventionist versus expectant care for severe pre-eclampsia before term. *Cochrane Database Syst Rev* 2002;(3):CD003106.

38. Hall DR, Odendaal HJ, Steyn DW, Grove D. Expectant management of early onset severe pre-eclampsia: Maternal outcome. *BJOG* 2000;107:1252–7.

39. Koopmans CM, Bijlenga D, Groen H, Vijgen SM, Aarnoudse JG, Bekedam DJ, *et al.* Induction of labour versus expectant monitoring for gestational hypertension or mild pre-eclampsia after 36 weeks' gestation (HYPITAT): a multicentre, open-label randomised controlled trial. *Lancet* 2009;374:979–88.

40. O'Brien MA, Rogers S, Jamtvedt G, Oxman AD, Odgaard-Jensen J, Kristoffersen DT, *et al.* Educational outreach visits: effects on professional practice and health care outcomes. *Cochrane Database Syst Rev* 2007;(4):CD000409.

41. Forsetlund L, Bjørndal A, Rashidian A, Jamtvedt G, O'Brien MA, Wolf F, et al. Continuing education meetings and workshops: effects on professional practice and health care outcomes. *Cochrane Database Syst Rev* 2009;(2):CD003030.

42. Doumit G, Gattellari M, Grimshaw J, O'Brien MA. Local opinion leaders: effects on professional practice and health care outcomes. *Cochrane Database Syst Rev* 2007;(1):CD000125.

43. Pattinson RC, Say L, Makin JD, Bastos MH. Critical incident audit and feedback to improve perinatal and maternal mortality and morbidity. *Cochrane Database Syst Rev* 2005;(4):CD002961.

44. Lombaard HA, Pattinson RC, Backer F, Macdonald AP. Evaluation of a strict protocol approach in managing women with severe disease due to hypertension in pregnancy: a before and after study. *Reprod Health* 2005;30:1–7.

45. Draycott T, Sibanda T, Owen L, Akande V, Winter C, Reading S, et al. Does training in obstetric emergencies improve neonatal outcome? *BJOG* 2006;113:177–82.

46. Draycott TJ, Crofts JF, Wilson LV, Yard E, Sibanda T, Whitelaw A. Improving neonatal outcome through practical shoulder dystocia training. *Obstet Gynecol* 2008;112:14–20.

47. Johanson RB, Menon V, Burns E, Kargramanya E, Osipov V. Managing Obstetrics Emergencies and Trauma (MOET) structured skills training in Armenia, utilising models and reality based scenarios. *BMC Med Educ* 2002;2:2–5.

48. Johannson H, Ayida G, Sadler C. Faking it? Simulation in the training of obstetricians and gynaecologists. *Curr Opin Obstet Gynecol* 2005;17:557–61.

49. Anderson ER, Black R, Brockelhurst P. Acute obstetric emergency drill in England and Wales: a survey of practice. *BJOG* 2005;112:372–5.

50. Cameron CA, Robberts CL, Bell J, Fisher W. Getting an evidence-based post-partum haemorrhage policy into practice. *Aus N Z J Obstet Gynaecol* 2007;47:169–75.

51. Reeves S, Zwarenstein M, Goldman J, Barr H, Freeth D, Hammick M, et al. Interprofessional education: effects on professional practice and health care outcomes. *Cochrane Database Syst Rev* 2008;(1):CD002213.

52. Siassakos D, Crofts JF, Winter C, Weiner CP, Draycott TJ. The active components of effective training in obstetric emergencies. *BJOG* 2009;116:1028–32.

53. Osman H, Campbell OM, Nassar AH. Using emergency obstetric drills in maternity units as a performance improvement tool. *Birth* 2009;36:43–50.

54. Villar J, Ba'aquel H, Piaggio G, Lumbiganon P, Belzian JM, Farnot U, et al. WHO antenatal care randomised trial for the evaluation of a new model of routine antenatal care. *Lancet* 2001;357:1551–64.

55. Villar J, Carroli G, Khan-Neelofur D, Piaggio GGP, Gülmezoglu AM. Patterns of routine antenatal care for low-risk pregnancy. *Cochrane Database Syst Rev* 2001;(4):CD000934.

56. Altman D, Carroli G, Duley L, Farrell B, Moodley J, Neilson J, et al; Magpie Trial Collaboration Group. Do women with pre-eclampsia, and their babies, benefit from magnesium sulphate? The Magpie Trial: a randomised placebo-controlled trial. *Lancet* 2002;359:1877–90.

57. Alfirevic Z, Weeks A. Oral misoprostol for induction of labour. *Cochrane Database Syst Rev* 2006;(2):CD001338.

58. Hofmeyr GJ, Gülmezoglu AM. Vaginal misoprostol for cervical ripening and induction of labour. *Cochrane Database Syst Rev* 2003;(1):CD000941.

59. Muzonzini G, Hofmeyr GJ. Buccal or sublingual misoprostol for cervical ripening and induction of labour. *Cochrane Database Syst Rev* 2004;(4):CD004221.

60. Boulvain M, Kelly AJ, Lohse C, Stan CM, Irion O. Mechanical methods for induction of labour. *Cochrane Database Syst Rev* 2001;(4):CD001233.

61. Mantel GM, Buchmann E, Rees HJ, Pattinson RC. Severe acute maternal morbidity: a pilot study of a definition for a near miss. *BJOG* 1998;105:985–90.

62. Pattinson RC, Buchmann EJ, Mantel G, Schoon M, Rees H. Can enquiries into maternal morbidity act as a surrogate for maternal death enquiries? *BJOG* 2003;110:889–93.

63. Duley L, Henderson-Smart D. Magnesium sulphate versus phenytoin for women with eclampsia. *Cochrane Database Syst Rev* 2003;(4):CD000128.

64. Duley L, Gülmezoglu AM. Magnesium sulphate versus lytic cocktail for eclampsia. *Cochrane Database Syst Rev* 2000;(3):CD002960.

Chapter 7
Obstructed labour (including partograms)

Stephen Munjanja

Introduction

Obstructed labour is an important cause of maternal and perinatal mortality[1–3] and in the developing world it always features among the top five causes of maternal deaths. Globally, obstructed labour was responsible for 8% of maternal deaths in 2000.[4] The maternal and neonatal morbidity is also significant. In 1990, obstructed labour was ranked 41st in the World Health Organization (WHO) Global Burden of Disease,[5] which represented 0.5% of the burden of all conditions and 22% of all maternal conditions. Using the disability-adjusted life year indicator, it was estimated to be the condition that results in the most morbidity out of all maternal complications. However, it is one of the complications with the most potential for prevention. Unlike haemorrhage or eclampsia, it takes days rather than hours for maternal mortality or morbidity to occur in association with obstructed labour. For achieving Millennium Development Goals (MDGs) 4 and 5, it is important that this eminently preventable complication be addressed. The contribution of a functioning health system in reducing the risk from obstructed labour is shown by the fact that both the immediate and long-term sequelae of this complication are virtually non-existent in developed countries.

Definition

Obstructed labour is defined as the failure of progress in labour due to mechanical factors, in the presence of good contractions of the uterus. There is no difficulty in detecting severe cases of obstructed labour but minor degrees may escape detection. In the latter situation, the woman may deliver vaginally with or without instrumental assistance but with lower genital tract damage. The fetus may also suffer birth trauma and asphyxia. Because of an apparent 'normal' outcome, the birth may not be recognised as one complicated by obstructed labour.

The definition does not depend on the duration of labour but rather on the presence of obstruction, which in women with a ruptured uterus may become apparent after only a few hours of labour. Prolonged labour may be caused by obstructed labour but it is also frequently due to other problems such as inefficient uterine contractions or failure to diagnose the true onset of labour.

Incidence of obstructed labour

The incidence of obstructed labour in developing countries ranges from 1.9% to 18.3%.[6–10] Worldwide, the incidence is estimated to be 3–6%, with the higher figure applying to the less-developed countries.[4] There are biological and epidemiological reasons why there is variation in the incidence between countries and populations. Firstly, maternal and fetal anthropometric features vary between populations, which determines the prevalence of feto-pelvic disproportion in each setting. Secondly, there are differences in the epidemiological methods and diagnostic criteria used in collecting the data. Most reports from developing countries are from referral institutions and are not population based. The outcomes of women who deliver at home, who are the larger proportion in most of sub-Saharan Africa, are not captured in the data sets.

The diagnostic criteria used for case definition is also a major cause of variation between reports. Criteria that have been used include obstructed labour requiring operative or vaginal instrumental delivery, uterine rupture, prolonged labour, caesarean section and obstetric fistulae. Prolonged labour is a particular problem since it is frequently used interchangeably with obstructed labour in clinical reports at facility level. There is also no agreed definition for how long labour should last before it is called 'prolonged'. Some reports use 12 hours and others 18 hours. The difference that case definition can make to incidence is illustrated by two reports from West Africa that used the same population of women. The first paper[8] published on severe maternal morbidity in seven West African cities reported an incidence of obstructed labour of 2.05% (95% confidence interval [CI] 1.86–2.26%). The second paper,[10] which used prolonged labour of more than 12 hours as an additional criterion, reported an incidence of 18.3% (95% CI 17.7–18.9%).

Another epidemiological problem is the use of caesarean section or instrumental delivery for obstructed/prolonged labour as a proxy for obstructed labour. In developing countries, many women who need caesarean section do not get the procedure. In the latest Demographic and Health Surveys (DHS), the caesarean section rates for Zambia and Mozambique were 3% and 1%, respectively,[11,12] which are below the rates needed to deliver women with obstructed labour and other complications. On the other hand, in more-developed countries, the rates may be inflated because of other factors. In the USA in the 1980s, there were six times as many deliveries by caesarean section for cephalo-pelvic disproportion than in Ireland for women who showed the same characteristics and who were delivered in comparable hospitals.[4]

Maternal deaths and other morbidities due to obstructed labour are often classified under other causes. Ruptured uterus may be classified under haemorrhage and infection following obstruction under puerperal sepsis. The mortality burden due to obstructed labour may be more than 8% globally. Despite this, reports on this condition are under-represented in the scientific literature. Only 2.5% of the scientific literature in maternal health has reported on obstructed labour, indicating a gap between its importance and the scientific interest devoted to it.[13]

Causes of obstructed labour

The direct cause of obstructed labour is a mechanical problem that makes vaginal delivery difficult or impossible. Feto-pelvic disproportion is the most common problem and accounts for at least 75% of the cases in sub-Saharan Africa.[7,9] Other causes are malpresentations (especially brow and shoulder) and malpositions (usually occipito-posterior). Rarer causes include fibroids, ovarian tumours, fetal abnormalities, and tumours and congenital malformations of the uterus or vagina. Where ultrasonography is not readily available, these rarer causes still present significant clinical difficulties and can have disastrous consequences.

The primary cause of feto-pelvic disproportion is a small pelvis that does not allow the delivery of an average-sized fetus. Of course, a macrosomic fetus may fail to pass through an adequate pelvis. This is currently less common in developing countries but may change in the future because of the increasing prevalence of diabetes mellitus.

Human beings have a higher risk of obstructed labour than other primates. The assumption of bipedal gait and locomotion reduced human pelvic size. This problem was compounded by the concurrent increase in fetal brain size (encephalisation).[14] There was obviously some adaptation between fetal skull and pelvic dimensions that allowed the human species to survive and prosper. Exactly how is still the subject of speculation.

Adult female pelvic size is the result of the interplay between the genetic potential from the parents and nutritional intake during childhood and adolescence. The relationship between childhood nutrition, adult height and female pelvic size is well established. Childhood undernourishment increases the risk of short stature and small pelvic size, leading to obstructed labour in future pregnancies. Vitamin D deficiency can lead to osteomalacia and this can result in an acquired pelvic deformity. Better nutrition in childhood results in a bigger pelvis but the change to a higher calorie diet can also lead to larger babies.[15,16] There is, therefore, a theoretical increased risk of obstructed labour and this concern has been raised by some authors.[15,17] However, sustained better nutrition will eventually result in the low incidence of obstructed labour observed in developed countries.

Prediction of obstructed labour

Maternal features that had been described previously as risk factors for obstructed labour, such as young age, short stature, small foot size and small size of the pelvis clinically, have been found to be of no predictive value.[10,18–20] Radiological pelvimetry, which is now contraindicated on other grounds, has also been found to be of no benefit.[21] Recent interventions such as ultrasonography for pelvimetry and estimating fetal weight have not yet been subjected to randomised controlled trials but current evidence suggests they are unlikely to prove beneficial.

The only true antenatal predictor that is associated with a reduced risk of obstructed labour is a past history of a vaginal delivery of a good-sized infant.[19] The WHO manual for antenatal care,[22] based on the best evidence from randomised controlled trials and other studies, does not contain strategies for the prediction of obstructed labour. Apart from obstetric history in multiparous women, observation of the progress of labour in the index pregnancy is the next best predictor. In nulliparae, this means that women who have feto-pelvic disproportion have to undergo an unnecessary trial of labour before having a caesarean section. If a predictor with both a high sensitivity and specificity is eventually found, it will save much unnecessary morbidity.

Reducing the risks of obstructed labour

In developed countries, once obstructed labour is detected, delivery is conducted promptly, usually by caesarean section. However, the situation is not so simple in developing countries, where a host of factors contribute to delay in delivery, leading to the tragic consequences so often seen in association with this condition. Reducing the risks of obstructed labour in developing countries can be more easily conceptualised using the three-delay model,[23] which specifies the three types of delay that can result in an increased risk of maternal mortality or morbidity. These are:

1. delay in deciding to seek care
2. delay in getting to a treatment facility
3. delay in receiving adequate treatment at the facility.

The first delay is caused by failure to recognise the problem and also failure to act on it by seeking care when it has been detected. The women in rural areas of sub-Saharan Africa do not note the time labour has started and have no idea how long it should last. Duration of labour is not measured in hours but in days, or parts of a day. The customary saying in many parts of Africa that 'the sun must not rise twice on a labouring woman' means that labour of a duration of up to 24 hours is considered normal. The diagnosis of obstructed labour is therefore made late for women labouring at home. This is compounded by the fact that, unlike with haemorrhage or eclampsia, the presentation of obstructed labour is not dramatic. It is not immediately obvious in obstructed labour that there is a problem, unless the uterus has ruptured.

Surveys have indicated a poor awareness of maternal health problems by individual women in rural Africa. However, in discussions with participatory women's groups in Malawi,[24] there was awareness of the common maternal health problems. The health problems identified by more than half the groups were anaemia (87%), malaria (80%), retained placenta (77%), obstructed labour (76%), malpresentation (71%), antepartum and postpartum haemorrhage (71%) each, and pre-eclampsia (56%). The five problems prioritised as the most important were, in descending order of importance, anaemia, malpresentation, retained placenta, obstructed labour and postpartum haemorrhage.

Even if the problem of obstructed labour has been recognised, the actions to be taken may be dictated by traditional beliefs and customs. In some rural parts of Zimbabwe, obstructed labour is believed to be caused by infidelity of the woman. The treatment, therefore, is for the woman to confess and seek forgiveness. The delay in seeking care may occur despite the problem having been recognised because a 'cultural diagnosis' has been made that requires the 'correct' treatment. However, even in Zimbabwe, the effects of traditional beliefs and customs are declining. During a maternal and perinatal mortality study performed in 2007,[25] interviews were conducted to determine barriers and facilitators to the access of obstetric care. A total of 328 women, 20 traditional birth attendants, 22 community leaders and 24 nurse-midwives were interviewed. The results showed that cultural beliefs, ritual practices and a woman's inability to decide for herself were no longer barriers causing the first of the three 'delays'. Instead, failure to recognise danger signs, high user fees at district hospitals and membership of some religious sects were the major reasons for the first delay. Table 7.1 summarises the findings of the interview study.

The second delay is caused by failure to reach the health facility on time, because of transport and communication problems. The health facilities are far apart and the roads to them are poor. Neither the villagers themselves nor the health systems have the transport to ferry women from villages, and will not for a long time to come.

The Prevention of Maternal Mortality Network, a non-governmental organisation working in West Africa, investigated the feasibility of involving communities in raising awareness of obstetric complications and arranging transport for women.[26–28] The conclusion was that community-managed loan and transport systems for women with complications can be established and may reduce the delay in obtaining emergency obstetric care. However, there is real doubt that this intervention could be scaled up in the countries that conducted the studies or that it could be replicated in other

Table 7.1   Barriers and facilitators to the access of obstetric care in Zimbabwe; reproduced with permission from the Ministry of Health and Child Welfare[25]

Type of delay	Barriers	Non-barriers	Facilitators
First delay	• Failure to recognise danger signs • High fees at district hospitals • Membership of some religious sects	• Cultural beliefs • Ritual practices • Women's ability to decide	• Most women book for antenatal care • Strong desire to deliver at facility • Some traditional birth attendants refuse high-risk women
Secondary delay	• Lack of communication facilities • Lack of transport • No money for transport • Woman alone at home • No community effort for transport	• Increasing mobile network coverage • Maternity waiting home at some facilities • Increasing availability of scotch carts	
Third delay	• Lack of drugs and supplies • Staff shortage • Inadequate skills • Lack of communication facilities • Lack of transport • Companions not included in care	• Women's ability to decide • Taboos and rituals	• Health workers aware of challenges • Much care still given competently

African countries. This is because the community committees received substantial assistance from the network to start – mobilisation was relatively expensive – and required sustained efforts.

Maternity waiting homes (MWHs) have been recommended for eliminating the first and second delays.[29-31] In southern Africa, they are built next to district hospitals (comprehensive emergency obstetric care units) and are for women at higher risk who live far away from facilities. In Zimbabwe, some lower level facilities also have them. Obstructed labour is the complication most amenable to prevention once the woman has been brought closer to the health facility. However, there are no reports that have studied the effects of MWHs in the prevention of maternal mortality or morbidity due to obstructed labour and there have been no randomised controlled trials of this intervention. Some reports have shown that women staying in MWHs have larger babies[32,33] and that they have a better perinatal outcome.[32-35]

In Zimbabwe, it has been policy that primary care clinics, which do not have facilities to conduct caesarean sections, should not attend to primigravidae in labour. Therefore, women go the nearest district hospital and are admitted into the MWH to await labour. In 2007, 14% of women who delivered in rural areas were already in an MWH when labour started.[25] Thirty percent of primigravidae awaited labour at an MWH, which was the highest percentage among all the parities. Obstructed labour contributed 3.3% to maternal deaths and there were only two women with an obstetric fistula out of 45 240 births. The selective policy for primigravidae, combined with the universal availability of MWHs at district hospitals, does play a role in reducing mortality and morbidity from obstructed labour. However, the condition does allow more time to intervene successfully to prevent maternal morbidity and mortality. Because of challenges in managing other complications with a faster evolution, Zimbabwe continues to experience a high maternal mortality of 725 per 100 000 live births.

Failure to provide appropriate treatment on time is the third delay and it contributes significantly to maternal and perinatal mortality and morbidity in obstructed labour. In most of sub-Saharan Africa, the first point of contact for a woman in labour is a primary health centre, which has to refer women with complications to a district hospital. Failures to communicate with the referral hospital and to transport the woman are important reasons for the third delay. In cases of neglected obstructed labour, the district hospital may feel inadequate in managing the problem and will refer the woman to a tertiary centre, which is usually several hours away from the initial facility of contact. It is not unusual in the tertiary hospitals of Harare, Lusaka or Nairobi to admit a moribund woman who has been referred up through several facilities over 2–3 days of labour. The hierarchical nature of the health systems leads to a pyramidal concentration of skills in a few big centres. Even so, further delays may occur at the tertiary centres. At a large teaching hospital in Nigeria, the mean decision to caesarean delivery time interval was 4.4 hours ± 4.2 (SD) hours (range 0.5–26 hours). The major reasons were bottlenecks within the maternity unit (31.7%), unavailability of paediatrician (19.6%), lack of anaesthetic coverage (13.9%) and non-readiness of operating theatre (11.9%).[36] Thus, a woman may have been referred from a long way away, only for her to join a very long queue at the tertiary hospital.

Quality of routine care of labour in developing countries

The possibility to detect and correctly manage obstructed labour depends on the quality of routine care during the intrapartum period. Evidence-based standards for the management of normal and abnormal labour are now available from several sources.[37–41] WHO also publishes systematic reviews whose applicability is especially relevant to developing countries in its Reproductive Health Library.[42] However, in many developing countries there are no up-to-date published standards, or the existing ones are not evidence based. The quality of care in labour has been reported to be inadequate in several countries in Africa, the Caribbean, South America and South Asia, because of the staff lacking essential knowledge and competencies. In addition, knowledge of and use of the partogram, an instrument recommended in most developing countries for the diagnosis of labour complications, is poor.[43–47]

The quality of intrapartum care is also affected by the shortage of resources. Most sub-Saharan African countries use hand-held maternity records on which details of antenatal care and pregnancy outcome are recorded. There is not enough space to enter the observations of labour and most do not incorporate the partogram. In tertiary institutions, a new and comprehensive maternity record is opened on admission to labour and this usually contains a partogram. At primary facilities and district hospitals, where the majority of women are admitted, a single sheet on which the partogram has been printed may be provided but its availability is inconsistent. This sheet easily becomes separated from the main record on discharge. This means that the details of labour are left out of the main record and are unavailable for the management of the next pregnancy. The value of the record as an epidemiological resource is also weakened. Currently, incorporation of the partogram into the limited space available on the hand-held record is complicated by two problems. Firstly, some countries still use the version of the partogram that includes the latent phase, and, secondly, observations in some women may go beyond the margins of the page. These problems can both be resolved by use of the WHO partogram, which starts when the woman has a cervical dilation of at least 4 cm. However, the value of the partogram itself is still a source of debate[48,49] and this is the subject of the next section.

There have been attempts to improve the introduction and adherence to standards of intrapartum care and evaluation using criterion-based audit.[50,51] These isolated reports indicate that it will be some time before the majority of women, especially in rural areas, have an acceptable quality of intrapartum care in developing countries.

The partogram

Emmanuel Friedman was the first person to provide a graphic description of the progress of labour.[52] Much later, this information was put into clinical use by Philpott,[53,54] who was working in Zimbabwe (then Rhodesia). The labour graph that was developed consisted of a cervicograph, on to which were added essential elements of maternal and fetal monitoring. An alert and an action line were added to improve the detection of abnormal labour. The alert line, which indicates that labour has deviated from normal, was a modification of the mean cervicographic progress of the slowest 10% of normal primigravidae admitted in the active phase of labour. The action line, which indicates that action is required to prevent an adverse outcome, is drawn an arbitrary 4 hours to the right of the alert line to allow primary health centres time to transfer the woman to an institution where definitive treatment, such as caesarean section, could be provided.[55]

The pictorial view of labour that the partogram offered made it an attractive intervention, especially in sub-Saharan Africa. Like many interventions at that time, it was accepted enthusiastically and unquestioningly in some settings without properly controlled trials having been conducted. Many developing countries made it a policy recommendation for labour monitoring even though they did not always ensure that it was used effectively in health facilities. WHO eventually conducted a multicentre trial in South East Asia involving 35 484 women.[56] The use of the partogram was associated with significantly fewer prolonged labours, fewer augmented labours and less postpartum sepsis. WHO claimed that the partogram 'clearly differentiates normal from abnormal progress in labour and identifies those women likely to require intervention'. They recommended its use in all labour wards.

Studies followed in which various aspects of the WHO partogram were assessed. A sub-analysis of the database in the South East Asian study[57] showed that the use of the WHO partogram in the management of breech labour reduced the incidence of prolonged labour and (among multigravidae) caesarean section. Studies in Angola,[58] Indonesia[59] and Kenya[60] showed that educational interventions improved proper documentation of the partogram by midwives. At University College Hospital in Ibadan, Nigeria,[61] its use was universal and associated with positive labour outcome among both low- and high-risk women, and it was recommended as the '*sine qua non* tool for intrapartum monitoring in all health facilities in Nigeria to reduce maternal complications'.

In the meantime, the WHO partogram had undergone some modification. The so-called latent phase part of the partogram had always caused problems for staff. This section was sometimes filled for women who were in 'false' labour. Other women took much longer than the 8 hours allowed for this section of labour and the graph ran out of space. WHO recommended a simplified version that starts at a cervical dilation of 4 cm, cutting out the latent phase entirely. The simplified partogram that is now the recommended version is more user friendly and, in one study,[62] was found to be more likely to be completely filled than the composite partogram.

The promising reports on the partogram belied the fact that very few randomised controlled trials had ever been conducted to test its efficacy. In a review published in 2008,[63] only five studies were of sufficient quality to be included in a meta-analysis of the effect of its use for women in spontaneous labour at term. The five studies of randomised or quasi-randomised design were from Canada,[64] Mexico,[65] South Africa[66] and the UK[67,68] and included 6187 women. The review[63] was conducted to determine the effect of partogram use on perinatal and maternal morbidity and mortality. Two studies assessed partogram versus no partogram and the remainder assessed different partogram designs. There was no evidence of any difference between the partogram and no partogram in rates of caesarean section (risk ratio [RR] 0.64; 95% CI 0.24–1.70) or instrumental delivery (RR 1.00;, 95% CI 0.85–1.17) or in Apgar score less than 7 at 5 minutes (RR 0.77; 95% CI 0.29–2.06) between the groups. When compared with a 4-hour action line, women using the partogram with the 2-hour action line were more likely to require oxytocin augmentation (RR 1.14; 95% CI 1.05–1.22). When the 3-hour and 4-hour action lines were compared, the caesarean section rate was lower in the 4-hour action line group and this difference was statistically significant (one trial, 613 women: RR 1.70; 95% CI 1.07–2.70). The review concluded that routine use of the partogram, or specific types of partogram, cannot be recommended as part of standard labour management and care. It called for further trials to be conducted to establish the efficacy of partograms.

Most countries in sub-Saharan Africa have included the partogram in labour ward protocols and it is expected to be used routinely but actual use varies widely between and within countries.[44,46,60] In settings where the standard of intrapartum care is already high, the use of the partogram is less likely to prove beneficial. On the other hand, if the standard of care is very poor, mere introduction of the partogram is unlikely to make a difference. Attention must be paid to the continuum of care from home to the facility where the woman can be given definitive treatment. Women should arrive at facilities in early labour, there should be provision for transfer if necessary and there should be no delay in treating obstructed labour at the referral facilities. If primary care facilities use the partogram but there is no provision for rapid transfer, the outcome cannot be expected to be different when a partogram is used. If the partogram were proved beneficial in trials and used more widely and effectively in sub-Saharan Africa, the expected outcomes would be fewer women with an obstetric fistula, ruptured uterus, puerperal sepsis, intrapartum stillbirth, intrapartum asphyxia and birth trauma. There would be more caesarean sections, as the intervention would be expected to reduce the late diagnosis and under-diagnosis of obstructed labour. The rates of caesarean section in most of sub-Saharan Africa are between 1% and 4%,[69–74] whereas the incidence of obstructed labour in the region is estimated to be 6%.[4]

Management options for obstructed labour

The options for managing obstructed labour depend on the stage of labour and the condition of both mother and fetus when the diagnosis is made. The list of proven or widely accepted technologies that help to reduce mortality from obstructed labour includes contraception, external cephalic version, use of the partogram, augmentation of labour, selective amniotomy, selective episiotomy, vacuum extraction, caesarean section, symphysiotomy and destructive procedures for non-viable fetuses.[75] Once the diagnosis of obstructed labour has been made, delivery must be effected within 30 minutes if the fetus is alive and within 1 hour if the fetus is dead. When there is borderline obstruction, where the fetus is alive, vacuum extraction with selective episiotomy can successfully deliver the woman. There must be no outlet contraction and early recourse to caesarean section should be available. In many places, the procedure is attempted in theatre.

In confirmed obstruction with a live fetus, symphysiotomy is another option that has been recommended for low-resource settings.[76,77] The procedure is no longer performed in developed countries, and has been discarded perhaps rather too hastily in low-resource settings. It definitely still has a role to play in countries where the caesarean section rates need to be doubled or trebled simply to deal with the incidence of obstructed labour. There are many myths about symphysiotomy, which were refuted in a review published in 2002.[78] The review included 5000 symphysiotomies and 1200 caesarean sections from 28 countries on four continents. The symphysiotomies were performed between 1900 and 1999. The review concluded that the procedure is safe for the mother, confers a permanent enlargement of the pelvis and facilitates vaginal delivery in future pregnancies, and is a life-saving operation for the fetus. It compares favourably with caesarean section in terms of risk to the mother's life, and severe long-term complications are rare. A randomised controlled trial is long overdue in settings where it may take another 30–50 years to eliminate obstetric fistulae. Many women and their babies will have died needlessly in that time or suffered severe morbidity.

When the fetus is dead and it is too risky to perform a caesarean section, a destructive operation is an alternative option to consider.[79,80] The risk of maternal trauma is very high and the decision to perform a destructive operation must be taken carefully to avoid worsening the damage already present. In one uncontrolled series,[81] 45% of women had complications of the procedure: atonic postpartum haemorrhage, vaginal and perineal tears, puerperal sepsis and urinary tract infection. The procedure, therefore, now has only a limited application, for cases where late presentation of obstructed labour is associated with fetal death and puerperal sepsis, and caesarean section is unavailable.

Caesarean section is currently the procedure of choice for obstructed labour, whether the fetus is alive or dead. The techniques for performing the procedure were reviewed in 2008[82] and, in low-resource settings where caesarean sections are often performed by relatively junior staff under difficult circumstances, the most cost-effective practice was found to be use spinal analgesia, Joel-Cohen-based abdominal incision and double layer closure of the uterus. The Joel-Cohen-based technique uses a straight transverse abdominal incision and manual separation of the abdominal wall layers to minimise sharp dissection, and its main advantage is that it is a safer and quicker method of getting into the abdomen. The review found that there was less blood loss, fever and pain and shorter time to recovery compared with the Pfannenstiel method for caesarean section. Much of the morbidity at caesarean section can be caused by the operator tearing the lower segment of the uterus while attempting to deliver the fetal head. A study[83] that investigated this found that it was safer to 'pull' the fetus out of the uterus at the uterine incision than to 'push' the fetus from below. Women in the 'push' group had statistically significant higher rates of maternal morbidity (longer operating time, more blood loss, extension of the uterine incision, endometritis and longer hospital stay) than the 'pull' method. Even if the fetus is dead, the same techniques and care should be exercised in conducting caesarean section.

Multiparous women are more likely to rupture the uterus if obstructed labour has been neglected. It is hypothesised that, unlike in nulliparae, the uterus becomes tolerant to myometrial acidification and does not stop contracting. The continued contractions lead to myometrial oedema and necrosis, contributing to uterine rupture.[48]

The type of operation required to manage uterine rupture will depend on the extent of the tear and the condition at presentation. There are no studies comparing different types of operation for similar degrees of rupture. An uncontrolled study[84] on 96 women with rupture found that subtotal hysterectomy significantly lowered operating time, morbidity, time to discharge and mortality compared with attempts to repair the uterus in women *in extremis* with uterine rupture. Whatever operation is chosen, whether it be repair or hysterectomy, haemostasis must be achieved before the abdomen is closed. Inexperienced operators must be taught that speed in performing the operation is less important than ensuring that haemostasis is achieved.

Maternal morbidity and mortality from obstructed labour

The prevalence of maternal morbidity and mortality due to obstructed labour is difficult to determine because there are few population-based reports. One such study in West African urban areas[8] reported that obstructed labour caused 2% of severe maternal morbidity and uterine rupture 0.1%. As expected, the percentage in tertiary hospitals is higher and two studies in such settings in West Africa[85,86] have reported morbidity rates of 2.7% and 3.6% in Nigeria and Niger, respectively.

In labour, morbidity is due to pain, dehydration and infection, and, if the uterus has ruptured, haemorrhage and shock. If the woman has survived delivery, the major morbidity will be due to caesarean section, instrumental delivery, destructive operations, symphysiotomy and hysterectomy or repair of a ruptured uterus. In survivors, the most serious consequences are obstetric fistulae and loss or damage to the uterus.

Obstructed labour remains the most important cause of genitourinary and rectovaginal fistulae in developing countries. Obstructed labour caused 73% of fistulae in one report from India[87] and 74% in another from Ghana.[88] The incidence of obstetric fistula in sub-Saharan Africa ranges from 0.01% to 0.08% of births but these estimates are based on both hospital- and population-based data.[4] Neglected obstructed labour produces injuries to several organ systems of which vesicovaginal fistula is only the most well known. The injury to surrounding tissues produced by prolonged pressure of the presenting fetal part may also result in total urethral loss, stress incontinence, hydroureteronephrosis, renal failure, rectovaginal fistula, rectal atresia, anal sphincter incompetence, cervical destruction, amenorrhoea, pelvic inflammatory disease, secondary infertility, vaginal stenosis, osteitis pubis and foot drop.[89] The surgical treatment of urinary fistula can be complex and special training is required to give the best results. Conservative management (that is, continuous bladder drainage for 14–21 days) is successful in only 1.9% of vesicovaginal but in 10% of ureterovaginal fistulae.[90] The three approaches to repair are vaginal, abdominal and combined vaginal and abdominal, with or without interposition grafts or flaps. Overall closure rates are high, between 71% and 94% in centres involved in the management of this problem.[87,90,91] Follow-up of the woman after a successful repair is necessary to evaluate the effect of the procedure on urinary continence.[92] The psychosocial consequences of an obstetric fistula can be devastating but the true prevalence and nature of the social implications are unknown.[93] The health services in developing countries are ill equipped to deal with the psychosocial trauma and the women are sometimes forced to find solace in one another.[94] The longevity of women where treatment has failed has not been documented.

The incidence of uterine rupture in tertiary hospitals varies widely, between 0.12% and 3.8% of births in different settings.[95–97] The morbidity from haemorrhage, shock and sepsis is high and so is the mortality. Mortality rates range from 3.3% in India[98] to 13.5% in eastern Nepal[99] and obviously vary with the skills and resources available for resuscitation and surgery. The two major causes of death in cases of ruptured uterus are shock and sepsis. Hysterectomy has significant psychosocial consequences because of subsequent infertility and amenorrhoea. This can cause the break-up of relationships and social ostracism. Where the uterus has been repaired, surgeons in many parts of the world still perform tubal ligation as well because the woman may suffer a repeat rupture in a subsequent pregnancy if she fails to use contraception. This procedure is not required for the woman's recovery from the ruptured uterus and the practice assumes that she would not take the recommended advice to have a tubal ligation subsequently. This paternalism has a dubious ethical standing and is not based on follow-up of pregnancies after conservation of the uterus. One study in Ethiopia[100] followed up 238 women who had had repair of the uterus for intervals ranging from 1 year and 11 months to 6 years and 3 months: 111 mothers gave birth to 117 healthy infants and no mother suffered any complication. The authors concluded that repair is medically safe and culturally acceptable, provided the mothers are willing to spend the latter months of subsequent pregnancies in maternity waiting shelters.

Fetal and neonatal morbidity

Obstructed labour is one of the major causes of perinatal mortality in developing countries.[2,101,102] The incidence of fetal death in neglected obstructed labour is very high and ranges from 30% to 83% when the uterus has ruptured.[85,99] Neonates who have survived intrapartum asphyxia may develop hypoxic ischaemic encephalopathy, with all its possible immediate and long-term consequences. The morbidity from cerebral palsy in sub-Saharan Africa is high mainly because of obstructed labour. The interventions to reduce the burden of stillbirths globally were reviewed in 2009.[103] The interventions of relevance to obstructed labour that were recommended for inclusion and scaling up in programmes because of clear benefit to maternal and/or neonatal health were emergency obstetric care packages, including caesarean section.

Other types of birth trauma, such as nerve palsies, are also much more common in obstructed labour. Brachial plexus and facial nerve injuries are the most common and are seen even when the babies are delivered by caesarean section when it is performed for obstructed labour.[104]

Summary

Obstructed labour is still a significant cause of maternal and perinatal mortality and morbidity in developing countries. It needs to be addressed to improve the chances of reaching MDGs 4 and 5. The causes and associated risk factors are well known but antenatal prediction is unreliable. In sub-Saharan Africa, barriers to access make a significant contribution to the eventual mortality and morbidity. Intrapartum prediction can be assisted by the partogram but the efficacy of this intervention needs to be proven in the settings where it is more likely to be beneficial. There are several evidence-based interventions available for the management of this complication but caesarean section remains the most important. The major maternal and perinatal consequences are maternal death, ruptured uterus, obstetric fistula, stillbirth, neonatal asphyxia and cerebral palsy. The important research issues are to determine whether lower technologies such as MWHs, the partogram and symphysiotomy can reduce the risk and consequences of obstructed labour in developing countries.

References

1. Ronsmans C, Graham WJ, Lancet Maternal Survival Series steering group. Maternal mortality: who, when, where, and why. *Lancet* 2006;368:1189–200.
2. McClure EM, Nalubamba-Phiri M, Goldenberg RL. Stillbirth in developing countries. *Int J Gynaecol Obstet* 2006;94:82–90.
3. Lawn JE, Osrin D, Adler A, Cousens S. Four million neonatal deaths: counting and attribution of cause of death. *Paediatr Perinat Epidemiol* 2008;22:410–16.
4. Dolea C, AbouZhar C. *Global Burden of Obstructed Labour in 2000*. Geneva: World Health Organization; 2003.
5. Murray CJL, Lopez AD, editors. *The Global Burden of Disease. A Comprehensive Assessment of Mortality and Disability from Diseases, Injuries and Risk Factors in 1990 and Projected to 2020*. Geneva: World Health Organization; 1996.
6. Chhabra P, Guleria K, Saini NK, Anjur KT, Vaid NB. Pattern of severe maternal morbidity in a tertiary hospital of Delhi, India: a pilot study. *Trop Doct* 2008;38:201–4.
7. Gaym A. Obstructed labor at a district hospital. *Ethiop Med J* 2002;40:11–18.
8. Prual A, Bouvier-Colle MH, de Bernis L, Breart G. Severe maternal morbidity from direct obstetric causes in West Africa: incidence and case fatality rates. *Bull World Health Organ* 2000;78:593–602.
9. Melah GS, El-Nafaty AU, Massa AA, Audu BM. Obstructed labour: a public health problem in Gombe, Gombe State, Nigeria. *J Obstet Gynaecol* 2003;23:369–73.
10. Ould El Joud D, Bouvier-Colle MH. Dystocia: a study of its frequency and risk factors in seven cities of west Africa. *Int J Gynaecol Obstet* 2001;74:171–8.
11. Central Statistical Office (Zambia), Macro International. *Zambia Demographic and Health Survey 2007*. Report no. FR 211. Calverton, MD: Central Statistical Office and Macro International; 2009.
12. Instituto Nacional de Estatistica, Ministerio da Saude, ORC Macro/DHS Program. *Mozambique Demographic and Health Survey 2003*. Report no. FR 161. Calverton, MD: INE, Ministerio da Saude (Mozambique) and Macro International; 2005.
13. Gil-Gonzalez D, Carrasco-Portino M, Ruiz MT. Knowledge gaps in scientific literature on maternal mortality: a systematic review. *Bull World Health Organ* 2006;84:903–9.
14. Wittman AB, Wall LL. The evolutionary origins of obstructed labor: bipedalism, encephalization, and the human obstetric dilemma. *Obstet Gynecol Surv* 2007;62:739–48.
15. Rush D. Nutrition and maternal mortality in the developing world. *Am J Clin Nutr* 2000;72(1 Suppl):212S–40S.
16. Konje JC, Ladipo OA. Nutrition and obstructed labor. *Am J Clin Nutr* 2000;72(1 Suppl):291S–7S.
17. Garner P, Kramer MS, Chalmers I. Might efforts to increase birthweight in undernourished women do more harm than good? *Lancet* 1992 24;340:1021–3.
18. Moller B, Lindmark G. Short stature: an obstetric risk factor? A comparison of two villages in Tanzania. *Acta Obstet Gynecol Scand* 1997;76:394–7.
19. Villar J, Bergsjo P. Scientific basis for the content of routine antenatal care. I. Philosophy, recent studies, and power to eliminate or alleviate adverse maternal outcomes. *Acta Obstet Gynecol Scand* 1997;76:1–14.
20. Brabin L, Verhoeff F, Brabin BJ. Maternal height, birthweight and cephalo pelvic disproportion in urban Nigeria and rural Malawi. *Acta Obstet Gynecol Scand* 2002;81:502–7.
21. Pattinson RC. Pelvimetry for fetal cephalic presentations at term. *Cochrane Database Syst Rev* 2000;(2):CD000161.
22. World Health Organization. *WHO Antenatal Care Randomised Trial: Manual for the Implementation of the New Model*. Report No. WHO/RHR/01.30. Geneva: WHO; 2001.
23. Thaddeus S, Maine D. Too far to walk: maternal mortality in context. *Newsl Womens Glob Netw Reprod Rights* 1991;Sep(36):22–4.
24. Rosato M, Mwansambo CW, Kazembe PN, Phiri T, Soko QS, Lewycka S, et al. Women's groups' perceptions of maternal health issues in rural Malawi. *Lancet* 2006 30;368:1180–8.
25. Ministry of Health and Child Welfare. *Maternal and Perinatal Mortality Study 2007*. Harare: Government of Zimbabwe; 2009.
26. Chiwuzie J, Okojie O, Okolocha C, Omorogbe S, Oronsaye A, Akpala W, et al. Emergency loan funds to improve access to obstetric care in Ekpoma, Nigeria. The Benin PMM Team. *Int J Gynaecol Obstet* 1997;59 Suppl 2:S231–6.

27. Fofana P, Samai O, Kebbie A, Sengeh P. Promoting the use of obstetric services through community loan funds, Bo, Sierra Leone. The Bo PMM Team. *Int J Gynaecol Obstet* 1997;59 Suppl 2:S225–30.

28. Olaniran N, Offiong S, Ottong J, Asuquo E, Duke F. Mobilizing the community to utilise obstetric services, Cross River State, Nigeria. The Calabar PMM Team. *Int J Gynaecol Obstet* 1997;59 Suppl 2:S181–9.

29. World Health Organization. *Maternity Waiting Homes: A Review of Experiences*. Report no. WHO/RHT/MSM/96:21. Geneva: WHO; 1996.

30. Philpott RH. Obstructed labour. *Clin Obstet Gynaecol* 1982;9:625–40.

31. Poovan P, Kifle F, Kwast BE. A maternity waiting home reduces obstetric catastrophes. *World Health Forum* 1990;11:440–5.

32. Millard P, Bailey J, Hanson J. Antenatal village stay and pregnancy outcome in rural Zimbabwe. *Cent Afr J Med* 1991;37:1–4.

33. Tumwine JK, Dungare PS. Maternity waiting shelters and pregnancy outcome: experience from a rural area in Zimbabwe. *Ann Trop Paediatr* 1996;16:55–9.

34. Chandramohan D, Cutts F, Millard P. The effect of stay in a maternity waiting home on perinatal mortality in rura   l Zimbabwe. *J Trop Med Hyg* 1995;98:261–7.

35. van Lonkhuijzen L, Stegeman M, Nyirongo R, van Roosmalen J. Use of maternity waiting home in rural Zambia. *Afr J Reprod Health* 2003;7:32–6.

36. Onwudiegwu U, Makinde ON, Ezechi OC, Adeyemi A. Decision–caesarean delivery interval in a Nigerian university hospital: implications for maternal morbidity and mortality. *J Obstet Gynaecol* 1999;19:30–3.

37. Enkin M, Keirse MJ, Neilson J, Crowther C, Duley L, Hodnett E, *et al. A Guide to Effective Care in Pregnancy and Childbirth*. New York: Oxford University Press; 2000.

38. World Health Organization, UNFPA, UNICEF, World Bank. *Pregnancy, Childbirth, Postpartum and Newborn Care. A Guide for Essential Practice*. Geneva: WHO; 2006.

39. World Health Organization, UNFPA, UNICEF, World Bank. *Integrated Management of Pregnancy and Childbirth: Managing Complications in Pregnancy. A Guide for Midwives and Doctors*. Geneva: WHO; 2003.

40. World Health Organization. *Managing Prolonged and Obstructed Labour. Midwifery Education Module 3*. Geneva: WHO; 2003.

41. The Cochrane Collaboration. *Cochrane Reviews: Pregnancy and Childbirth* [www2.cochrane.org/reviews/en/topics/87_reviews.html].

42. World Health Organization Reproductive Health Library. 2005 [www.who.int/rhl].

43. Delvaux T, Ake-Tano O, Gohou-Kouassi V, Bosso P, Collin S, Ronsmans C. Quality of normal delivery care in Cote d'Ivoire. *Afr J Reprod Health* 2007;11:22–32.

44. Maimbolwa MC, Ransjo-Arvidson AB, Ng'andu N, Sikazwe N, Diwan VK. Routine care of women experiencing normal deliveries in Zambian maternity wards: a pilot study. *Midwifery* 1997;13:125–31.

45. Harvey SA, Blandon YC, McCaw-Binns A, Sandino I, Urbina L, Rodriguez C, *et al.* Are skilled birth attendants really skilled? A measurement method, some disturbing results and a potential way forward. *Bull World Health Organ* 2007;85:783–90.

46. Oladapo OT, Daniel OJ, Olatunji AO. Knowledge and use of the partograph among healthcare personnel at the peripheral maternity centres in Nigeria. *J Obstet Gynaecol* 2006;26:538–41.

47. Liabsuetrakul T, Promvijit T, Pattanapisalsak C, Silalai S, Ampawa T. A criterion-based obstetric morbidity audit in southern Thailand. *Int J Gynaecol Obstet* 2008;103:166–71.

48. Neilson JP, Lavender T, Quenby S, Wray S. Obstructed labour. *Br Med Bull* 2003;67:191–204.

49. Hofmeyr GJ. Evidence-based intrapartum care. *Best Pract Res Clin Obstet Gynaecol* 2005;19:103–15.

50. Kongnyuy EJ, Mlava G, van den Broek N. Establishing standards for obstructed labour in a low-income country. *Rural Remote Health* 2008;8:1022.

51. Hunyinbo KI, Fawole AO, Sotiloye OS, Otolorin EO. Evaluation of criteria-based clinical audit in improving quality of obstetric care in a developing country hospital. *Afr J Reprod Health* 2008;12:59–70.

52. Friedman E. The graphic analysis of labor. *Am J Obstet Gynecol* 1954;68:1568–75.

53. Philpott RH, Castle WM. Cervicographs in the management of labour in primigravidae. I. The alert line for detecting abnormal labour. *J Obstet Gynaecol Br Commonw* 1972;79:592–8.

54. Philpott RH, Castle WM. Cervicographs in the management of labour in primigravidae. II. The action line and treatment of abnormal labour. *J Obstet Gynaecol Br Commonw* 1972;79:599–602.

55. Philpott RH. Graphic records in labour. *Br Med J* 1972;4:163–5.
56. World Health Organization Maternal Health and Safe Motherhood Programme. World Health Organization partograph in management of labour. *Lancet* 1994;343:1399–404.
57. Lennox CE, Kwast BE, Farley TM. Breech labor on the WHO partograph. *Int J Gynaecol Obstet* 1998;62:117–27.
58. Pettersson KO, Svensson ML, Christensson K. Evaluation of an adapted model of the World Health Organization partograph used by Angolan midwives in a peripheral delivery unit. *Midwifery* 2000;16:82–8.
59. Fahdhy M, Chongsuvivatwong V. Evaluation of World Health Organization partograph implementation by midwives for maternity home birth in Medan, Indonesia. *Midwifery* 2005;21:301–10.
60. Wamwana EB, Ndavi PM, Gichangi PB, Karanja JG, Muia EG, Jaldesa GW. Quality of record keeping in the intrapartum period at the Provincial General Hospital, Kakamega, Kenya. *East Afr Med J* 2007;84:16–23.
61. Fawole AO, Fadare O. Audit of use of the partograph at the University College Hospital, Ibadan. *Afr J Med Med Sci* 2007;36:273–8.
62. Mathews JE, Rajaratnam A, George A, Mathai M. Comparison of two World Health Organization partographs. *Int J Gynaecol Obstet* 2007;96:147–50.
63. Lavender T, Hart A, Smyth RM. Effect of partogram use on outcomes for women in spontaneous labour at term. *Cochrane Database Syst Rev* 2008;(4):CD005461.
64. Windrim R, Seaward PG, Hodnett E, Akoury H, Kingdom J, Salenieks ME, *et al.* A randomized controlled trial of a bedside partogram in the active management of primiparous labour. *J Obstet Gynaecol Can* 2007;29:27–34.
65. Walss Rodriguez RJ, Gudino Ruiz F, Tapia Rodriguez S. [Trial of labor. A comparative study between Friedman's partogram and the conventional descriptive partogram]. *Ginecol Obstet Mex* 1987;55:318–22.
66. Pattinson RC, Howarth GR, Mdluli W, Macdonald AP, Makin JD, Funk M. Aggressive or expectant management of labour: a randomised clinical trial. *BJOG* 2003;110:457–61.
67. Lavender T, Alfirevic Z, Walkinshaw S. Partogram action line study: a randomised trial. *Br J Obstet Gynaecol* 1998;105:976–80.
68. Lavender T, Wallymahmed AH, Walkinshaw SA. Managing labor using partograms with different action lines: a prospective study of women's views. *Birth* 1999;26:89–96.
69. Hussein J, Goodburn EA, Damisoni H, Lema V, Graham W. Monitoring obstetric services: putting the 'UN Guidelines' into practice in Malawi: 3 years on. *Int J Gynaecol Obstet* 2001;75:63–73; discussion 74.
70. Bailey PE, Paxton A. Program note. Using UN process indicators to assess needs in emergency obstetric services. *Int J Gynaecol Obstet* 2002;76:299–305; discussion 306.
71. Lalonde AB, Okong P, Mugasa A, Perron L. The FIGO Save the Mothers Initiative: the Uganda–Canada collaboration. *Int J Gynaecol Obstet* 2003;80:204–12.
72. Mekbib T, Kassaye E, Getachew A, Tadesse T, Debebe A. The FIGO Save the Mothers Initiative: the Ethiopia–Sweden collaboration. *Int J Gynaecol Obstet* 2003;81:93–102.
73. AMDD Working Group on Indicators. Program note. Using UN process indicators to assess needs in emergency obstetric services: Niger, Rwanda and Tanzania. *Int J Gynaecol Obstet* 2003;83:112–20.
74. Pearson L, Shoo R. Availability and use of emergency obstetric services: Kenya, Rwanda, Southern Sudan, and Uganda. *Int J Gynaecol Obstet* 2005;88:208–15.
75. Hofmeyr GJ. Obstructed labor: using better technologies to reduce mortality. *Int J Gynaecol Obstet* 2004;85 Suppl 1:S62–72.
76. Bergstrom S, Lublin H, Molin A. Value of symphysiotomy in obstructed labour management and follow-up of 31 cases. *Gynecol Obstet Invest* 1994;38:31–5.
77. Ersdal HL, Verkuyl DA, Bjorklund K, Bergstrom S. Symphysiotomy in Zimbabwe; postoperative outcome, width of the symphysis joint, and knowledge, attitudes and practice among doctors and midwives. *PLoS One* 2008;3:e3317.
78. Bjorklund K. Minimally invasive surgery for obstructed labour: a review of symphysiotomy during the twentieth century (including 5000 cases). *BJOG* 2002;109:236–48.
79. Gupta U, Chitra R. Destructive operations still have a place in developing countries. *Int J Gynaecol Obstet* 1994;44:15–19.

80. Biswas A, Chakraborty PS, Das HS, Bose A, Kalsar PK. Role of destructive operations in modern day obstetrics. *J Indian Med Assoc* 2001;99:248, 50–1.

81. Singhal SR, Chaudhry P, Sangwan K, Singhal SK. Destructive operations in modern obstetrics. *Arch Gynecol Obstet* 2005;273:107–9.

82. Hofmeyr GJ, Mathai M, Shah A, Novikova N. Techniques for caesarean section. *Cochrane Database Syst Rev* 2008;(1):CD004662.

83. Fasubaa OB, Ezechi OC, Orji EO, Ogunniyi SO, Akindele ST, Loto OM, *et al.* Delivery of the impacted head of the fetus at caesarean section after prolonged obstructed labour: a randomised comparative study of two methods. *J Obstet Gynecol* 2002;22:375–8.

84. Thakur A, Heer MS, Thakur V, Heer GK, Narone JN, Narone RK. Subtotal hysterectomy for uterine rupture. *Int J Gynaecol Obstet* 2001;74:29–33.

85. Nwogu-Ikojo EE, Nweze SO, Ezegwui HU. Obstructed labour in Enugu, Nigeria. *J Obstet Gynecol* 2008;28:596–9.

86. Prual A, Huguet D, Garbin O, Rabe G. Severe obstetric morbidity of the third trimester, delivery and early puerperium in Niamey (Niger). *Afr J Reprod Health* 1998;2:10–9.

87. Rathee S, Nanda S. Vesicovaginal fistulae: a 12-year study. *J Indian Med Assoc* 1995;93:93–4.

88. Danso KA, Martey JO, Wall LL, Elkins TE. The epidemiology of genitourinary fistulae in Kumasi, Ghana, 1977–1992. *Int Urogynecol J Pelvic Floor Dysfunct* 1996;7:117–20.

89. Arrowsmith S, Hamlin EC, Wall LL. Obstructed labor injury complex: obstetric fistula formation and the multifaceted morbidity of maternal birth trauma in the developing world. *Obstet Gynecol Surv* 1996;51:568–74.

90. Kumar A, Goyal NK, Das SK, Trivedi S, Dwivedi US, Singh PB. Our experience with genitourinary fistulae. *Urol Int* 2009;82:404–10.

91. Raassen TJ, Verdaasdonk EG, Vierhout ME. Prospective results after first-time surgery for obstetric fistulas in East African women. *Int Urogynecol J Pelvic Floor Dysfunct* 2008;19:73–9.

92. Creanga AA, Genadry RR. Obstetric fistulas: a clinical review. *Int J Gynaecol Obstet* 2007;99 Suppl 1:S40–6.

93. Roush KM. Social implications of obstetric fistula: an integrative review. *J Midwifery Womens Health* 2009;54:e21–33.

94. Wall LL. Fitsari 'dan Duniya. An African (Hausa) praise song about vesicovaginal fistulas. *Obstet Gynecol* 2002;100:1328–32.

95. Adanu RM, Obed SA. Ruptured uterus: a seven-year review of cases from Accra, Ghana. *J Obstet Gynaecol Can* 2003;25:225–30.

96. Ezegwui HU, Nwogu-Ikojo EE. Trends in uterine rupture in Enugu, Nigeria. *J Obstet Gynaecol* 2005;25:260–2.

97. Zeteroglu S, Ustun Y, Engin-Ustun Y, Sahin HG, Kamaci M. Eight years' experience of uterine rupture cases. *J Obstet Gynaecol* 2005;25:458–61.

98. Rashmi, Radhakrisknan G, Vaid NB, Agarwal N. Rupture uterus – changing Indian scenario. *J Indian Med Assoc* 2001;99:634–7.

99. Chuni N. Analysis of uterine rupture in a tertiary center in Eastern Nepal: lessons for obstetric care. *J Obstet Gynaecol Res* 2006;32:574–9.

100. Kelly J, Fekadu S, Lancashire RJ, Poovan P, Redito A. A follow-up of repair of ruptured uterus in Ethiopia. *J Obstet Gynaecol* 1998;18:50–2.

101. Kusiako T, Ronsmans C, Van der Paal L. Perinatal mortality attributable to complications of childbirth in Matlab, Bangladesh. *Bull World Health Organ* 2000;78:621–7.

102. Chalumeau M, Bouvier-Colle MH, Breart G. Can clinical risk factors for late stillbirth in West Africa be detected during antenatal care or only during labour? *Int J Epidemiol* 2002;31:661–8.

103. Bhutta ZA, Darmstadt GL, Haws RA, Yakoob MY, Lawn JE. Delivering interventions to reduce the global burden of stillbirths: improving service supply and community demand. *BMC Pregnancy Childbirth* 2009;9 Suppl 1:S7.

104. Bhat V, Ravikumara, Oumachigui A. Nerve injuries due to obstetric trauma. *Indian J Pediatr* 1995;62:207–12.

Chapter 8

Puerperal sepsis in low- and middle-income settings: past, present and future

Julia Hussein and Leighton Walker

Introduction

Puerperal sepsis is an infective condition in the mother following childbirth and one of the leading causes of maternal mortality worldwide. It is the third most common cause of maternal death as a result of childbirth, after haemorrhage and abortion, accounting for as much as 15% of the 500 000 maternal lives lost annually. In low- and middle-income countries, infections occurring in the puerperium are reportedly the sixth leading cause of disease burden for women in their reproductive years.[1] Complications in the mother such as secondary postpartum haemorrhage and infertility can result, and there is an association with early-onset neonatal sepsis.

Reducing puerperal sepsis in women will contribute to achieving Millennium Development Goals (MDGs) 4 and 5 on child survival and maternal health. Despite the importance of puerperal sepsis globally, there is surprisingly little current interest in the condition. Even in industralised countries such as the UK, although deaths from puerperal sepsis are now rare, the latest Confidential Enquiry into Maternal Deaths[2] suggests that the incidence of complications is increasing and failure of clinicians to recognise signs and symptoms of puerperal sepsis have contributed to maternal mortality.

In developing countries, puerperal sepsis continues to cause many unnecessary deaths, mainly because of inadequate access to care during childbirth and poor quality of care. Women may not be able to reach health professionals during labour and delivery care provided in the home setting with attendants who lack the necessary skills can increase the risk of infection. The urgency to make progress towards reaching the MDGs by 2015 has led to the fast-tracking of strategies to improve the uptake of delivery care with skilled health professionals. However, any consequent increase in uptake of services can place an added burden on health facilities and health personnel where resources are limited. Such a situation can also result in increased morbidity and mortality from poor infection control, especially from nosocomial routes of transmission. In countries where the incidence of HIV is high, the need for good infection prevention is accentuated because of increased risks of puerperal sepsis in women infected by the virus as well as concerns for the safety of health personnel.

This review summarises current knowledge on puerperal sepsis and draws from lessons from the past to identify strategies for progress in reducing this neglected but important cause of maternal death.

Definition of puerperal sepsis

Puerperal sepsis was known as childbed fever in the past. Its association with a vivid and well-documented history spans over 200 years since its first recognition as a separate disease entity in the 18th century. Difficulties in case identification led to inaccurate recording and reporting of the condition,[3,4] a problem that remains to this day.

Various international definitions of puerperal sepsis have been proposed but none are used universally (Table 8.1). This has contributed to difficulties in estimating the incidence of the condition. To compound the problem, many sources of epidemiological data and information combine puerperal sepsis with other puerperal infections of the genital tract, surgical wounds and urinary tract infections, such as the WHO Global Burden of Disease,[1] which categorises these as cases of 'maternal sepsis'. Genital tract sepsis, maternal sepsis, puerperal infections and puerperal fever are terms used in the literature without clarity on their definition. Such terms may or may not include infections of the breast or urinary tract, localised infections or those acquired after abortion. The tenth revision of the International Classification of Diseases (ICD-10)[5] provides the most specific terminology, indicating conditions included as well as excluded from the definition of puerperal sepsis (Table 8.2).

Identification of puerperal sepsis is primarily based on clinical signs and symptoms, leading to difficulties in case ascertainment. Fever and confirmation of infection of the uterine lining or wall and bloodstream infections are the mainstay of diagnosis. Presence of pyrexia alone is insufficient for diagnosis of puerperal sepsis because not all women with fever in the postpartum period necessarily have a uterine infection. Fevers may not be due to infection, and infection can originate from other sites such as the breast or urinary tract, which are commonly affected in the postpartum period. Localising

Table 8.1   International definitions of puerperal sepsis

Document	Definition of puerperal sepsis
International Statistical Classification of Diseases and Related Health Problems, 10th revision (ICD-10) (World Health Organization)[5]	A complication of the puerperium with endometritis, fever, peritonitis and septicaemia, but excluding obstetric pyaemic and septic embolism, and septicaemia during labour
Mother–Baby Package: Implementing Safe Motherhood in Countries (World Health Organization)[83]	Infection of the genital tract occurring at any time between the onset of the rupture of the membranes or labour and the 42nd day postpartum in which fever and one or more of the following are present: • pelvic pain • abnormal vaginal discharge, e.g. presence of pus • abnormal smell/foul odour of discharge • delay in the rate of reduction of size of the uterus (< 2 cm/day during the first 8 days)
Managing Puerperal Sepsis (World Health Organization and International Confederation of Midwives)[84]	Any bacterial infection of the genital tract that occurs after the birth of a baby. It is usually more than 24 hours after delivery before the symptoms and signs appear

Table 8.2 Puerperal sepsis and related maternal conditions in the International Classification of Diseases (ICD-10)[5]

ICD code	
O85	Puerperal sepsis Puerperal: endometritis, fever, peritonitis, septicaemia Excludes obstetric pyemic and septic embolism, and septicaemia during labour
O86	Other puerperal infections Excludes infection during labour
O86.0	Infection of obstetrical surgical wound (caesarean section wound, perineal repair following delivery)
O86.1	Other infection of genital tract following delivery (cervicitis, vaginitis)
O86.2	Urinary tract infection following delivery
O86.3	Other genitourinary tract infections following delivery
O86.4	Pyrexia of unknown origin following delivery Excludes puerperal fever and pyrexia during labour
O86.8	Other specified puerperal infections

signs can be difficult to identify. Infections originating from within the genital tract but outside the uterus (for example, an episiotomy wound) can be confused with puerperal sepsis but should not in themselves lead to symptoms such as pelvic tenderness or failure of uterine involution. Even if there is a uterine infection present, signs and symptoms are variable: fever may not be pronounced, the uterus not always tender and the lochia not invariably malodorous. Microbiological confirmation is useful to confirm the diagnosis but may not be available in low-resource settings. Even when available, contamination of samples from the uterine cavity by normal flora from the vagina and cervix is difficult to avoid. Blood cultures are usually taken only when the woman is seriously ill.

In addition to the problems of clinical diagnosis, estimation of incidence of the condition, especially in developing countries, poses some challenges. Puerperal sepsis can manifest several days after childbirth or after leaving a health facility, making cases difficult to trace. Women may present to different health facilities or be treated in the community. Women with low-grade infections may not present for care as these infections can eventually resolve themselves without treatment.

Epidemiology

Individual studies from developing countries suggest that the incidence of puerperal sepsis is between 0.1% and 10% of deliveries (Table 8.3). This wide range reflects the problems

Table 8.3 Estimated incidence, case fatality rate and mortality of puerperal sepsis in developing countries

Study	Incidence	Case fatality rate	Maternal deaths due to puerperal sepsis
Dolea and Stein (2003)[6]	0.07–9.3% (live births)	4–50%	–
Seale et al. (2009)[10]	1.4–9% (women)	–	–
Khan et al. (2006)[13]	–	–	0.5–15.1% globally
Loudon (2000)[4]	–	37% (Aberdeen, 1789–1792)	–

of estimating incidence: the diagnostic criteria for puerperal sepsis differ from study to study and data are variously obtained from hospitals, ambulatory records or population-based community surveys. Self-reported morbidity through household surveys can overestimate the incidence of puerperal sepsis,[6] whereas hospital-based studies may underestimate incidence because cases of sepsis can occur outside the hospital setting.

A global review[6] of puerperal sepsis provides data from seven developing country studies. A hospital-based study from South Africa[7] reported an incidence of 0.07 per 100 live births, diagnosed using set criteria for severe obstetric complications in hospitals assessed by a medical panel. Women's self-reports of symptoms or medical diagnosis were used in community surveys to establish the incidences of 9.3 cases of puerperal sepsis per 100 live births in El Salvador[8] and 0.09 per 100 live births in West Africa.[9] Two other reviews of sepsis[10,11] in the postpartum period in sub-Saharan Africa reported incidence rates of 9% in Zambian women attending hospital for any reason postpartum. One study[12] reported incidence rates as high as 19% in HIV-infected women, although other common infections seen in the puerperium were included.

Case fatality rates of between 4% and 50% are recorded in sub-Saharan Africa.[6] It is of interest to compare these case fatality rates with those in the late 18th and 19th centuries at the height of the childbed fever epidemics, before the advent of antisepsis and the discovery of disease transmission modalities. Case fatalities as high as 37% were reported in obstetric units of the time, with as many as 600 maternal deaths per 10 000 deliveries being due to puerperal sepsis. These levels did not fall dramatically until the introduction of sulphonamides in hospitals in the 1930s, after which large declines in maternal mortality were observed.[4]

A systematic review published in 2006[13] provides further information on the contribution of puerperal sepsis in relation to other causes of maternal death. Data from individual studies were used to generate combined estimates of cause of death distribution by region: 11.6% of maternal deaths in Asia were due to puerperal sepsis, 9.7% in Africa, and 7.7% in Latin America and the Caribbean, compared with only 2.1% in developed countries. Of the four most common causes of death (haemorrhage, hypertensive disorders, sepsis and abortion), those due to sepsis showed the highest inequity between developing and developed countries, with odds ratios of 2.71 in Africa, 1.91 in Asia, and 2.16 in Latin America and the Caribbean, compared with developed nations.

Aetiology of infection

Puerperal sepsis may be acquired either outside a health facility or within a facility. Nosocomial infections describe those originating in hospital or other health facilities and that are not detectable when an individual is admitted to the facility. The term can include infections introduced by health workers, so the broader description of 'healthcare-associated infections' is sometimes preferred.[14] In developing countries, rates of puerperal infection in home births have been reported to be twice as high as health facility births. A study in Nigeria showed rates of infection of 15% in home births and 8% in facility births, while another from Senegal showed rates of 9% at home and 2% in facilities.[6,15] Nevertheless, the risk of nosocomial infections when health facility-based deliveries are of poor quality still remains.

A number of risk factors are thought to introduce infection into the uterine cavity (Box 8.1). Multivariate analysis has shown that caesarean section delivery and bacterial vaginosis are predictive of endometritis but other risk factors such as duration of labour and preterm rupture of membranes are likely to facilitate, rather than predict, infection.[16,17] The risk factors serve to emphasise that prevention and early detection

---

Box 8.1   Risk factors associated with puerperal sepsis

Socio-economic:
- low status/education of women
- delays in seeking care

Prepregnancy/antenatal:
- malnutrition
- anaemia
- underlying disease
- bacterial vaginosis
- group B streptococcus
- history of prolonged rupture of membranes
- chorioamnionitis (inflammation of the fetal membranes)

Labour and delivery:
- poor infection control practices
- long labour
- multiple vaginal examinations
- instrumental delivery
- caesarean section
- retained products of conception
- haemorrhage
- lacerations of the genital tract

---

of infections are important ways of reducing the occurrence of puerperal sepsis. Prevention can be considered at various stages before pregnancy, during the antenatal period and during labour.

Uterine infection usually results from ascending infection from the vagina into the uterine cavity. Progressive invasion of the layers of the uterus, the endometrium and the myometrium, causes endometritis and myometritis, respectively.[18] Pathogenic organisms have also been reported within the uterus in 19% of women in spontaneous term labour with intact membranes, so microbial invasion of the amniotic cavity can be a cause as well as a consequence of labour.[19] Bacterial vaginosis describes a condition where various pathogenic bacteria colonise the lower genital tract. It is associated with postpartum endometritis and chorioamnionitis but interest in the condition has mostly been with the aim of preventing preterm birth.[20] The finding of group B streptococcal vaginal colonisation is also associated with puerperal sepsis although the current focus of attention in this condition is primarily on the neonate.[21,22]

The majority of women with puerperal sepsis have a mix of organisms. Studies in developing countries report causative organisms such as *Bacteroides*, enterobacteriaceae, *Escherichia coli*, *Klebsiella*, *Neisseria gonorrhoeae*, *Pseudomonas*, *Proteus*, *Staphylococcus aureus*, streptococci, *Trichomonas vaginalis* and various anaerobes.[11,17,23–27] Most literature describing the microbiology of puerperal sepsis is over a decade old. There seems to be little information on changes in microbiological profile in the literature.

In severe cases of puerperal fever, *Streptococcus pyogenes*, the classic group A streptococcus of childbed fever, is commonly implicated, although reports from developing countries recording *S. pyogenes* as a causative organism are few.[17] Its presentation can be diverse, although it is associated with fulminant infections because it can cause rapid tissue destruction.[18,28,29] Severe endotoxic shock with high mortality rates have also been reported with *E. coli* infections.[26]

The immediate complications of puerperal sepsis are peritonitis, abscess formation, pelvic thrombophlebitis and consequent pulmonary embolism. Endotoxic shock and renal necrosis are likely to cause fatalities.[18] Puerperal sepsis can also lead to chronic pelvic inflammatory disease, ectopic pregnancies and secondary infertility. It has been estimated that the condition results in 3–25 cases of infertility per 1000 women aged 15–45 years.[30] The depopulation of an indigenous people in Borneo has even been ascribed to post-pregnancy infections leading to infertility.[31]

Infection control measures relevant to puerperal sepsis

Recent pandemics of infections, emerging antibiotic resistance and awareness of the burden of disease resulting from infection have led to a revival of general interest in infection control.[32] The concept of infection control encompasses a range of technologies, interventions and strategies of varying complexity. These measures aim to avoid infection (primary prevention), detect early infections (secondary prevention), reduce complications (tertiary prevention) or aid in diagnosis and treatment (Table 8.4). Infection control measures of current interest that have particular relevance to puerperal sepsis are discussed below. Many advances in this area of work have been from outside maternity and obstetric care. Specific technologies applicable to puerperal sepsis have been detailed in other reviews.[33,34]

Hand hygiene

The transmission of puerperal sepsis through the delivery attendants' hands was discovered by Semmelweis in 1847. Hand hygiene is promoted as a simple, effective measure to prevent infection[35] although high-grade evidence linking specific hand hygiene interventions with prevention of nosocomial infections is lacking.[36] In 2005, an infection control campaign 'Clean Care is Safer Care' was launched by WHO as part of its Global Patient Safety Challenge.[37] The infection control campaign placed hand hygiene as its first priority and, as an underlying action, promoted clean products (such as blood), practices (including surgical site preparation), equipment (instruments and syringes) and environment (water, waste and sanitation) in health care.[38] Guidelines in hand hygiene have been developed using recommendations based on evidence.[39]

Products used for hand washing and hand disinfection are broadly divided into plain soaps, antimicrobial soaps and alcohol-based antiseptics. Studies have shown that washing hands with waterless antiseptic agents is more efficacious than soap, although most studies test use of the product for over 30 seconds rather than the less than 15 seconds that most health workers spend washing their hands.[40] Alcohol-based hand rubs are now recommended as the method of choice for routine clinical hand disinfection unless hands are visibly dirty.[41] Alcohol rubs have been shown to be cost-effective[42] and suitable for use where water and sanitation systems are suboptimal. They can also be made more easily available at the patient's bedside and as dispensers for personal use.[41,43] The alternative to alcohol-based hand rubs for routine clinical use is to wash hands with an antimicrobial soap and water.[40]

The effectiveness of gloves in preventing contamination has been widely confirmed. However, a number of studies have suggested that wearing of gloves may actually reduce compliance with standard hand hygiene procedures. Defects in gloves and contamination during glove removal add to the need to comply with hand hygiene procedures.[40]

Table 8.4 Infection control in puerperal sepsis

Purpose	Infection control measures	Key findings on effectiveness
Avoidance of infection	Identification and correction of risk factors predisposing to infection	Specific to risk factor
	Hand hygiene and related products	Systematic review has revealed lack of rigorous evidence on the link with prevention of healthcare-associated infections;[36] waterless antiseptic agents are more efficacious than soap[40]
		2 minutes hand washing combined with superior antiseptic products recommended[36]
		Increased bed numbers increases risk of infections[43]
	Surgical asepsis	Women using home delivery kit were 32 times less likely to develop puerperal sepsis than women without kit[45]
	Environmental improvements	
	Clean equipment	Routine use in caesarean sections will decrease infection rate by at least two-thirds[63]
	Antibiotic prophylaxis	Conflicting findings for vitamin A;[60] zinc and other supplements show promise[62]
	Micronutrient supplements	
	Vaginal antisepsis	No evidence of effect in preventing puerperal sepsis[50]
	Training of traditional birth attendants	Conflicting findings[47,48]
Early detection of infection	Clinical monitoring of temperature, uterine involution, tenderness and vaginal discharge	None found
	Screening and treatment for group B streptococci colonisation	Main outcome of interest is on neonatal sepsis
	Screening and treatment of bacterial vaginosis	Beneficial effects on risk of postpartum endometritis in high-risk women[65]
	Treatment of chorioamnionitis before and during labour	Routine antibiotics for term prelabour rupture of membranes may reduce the risk of infection of the uterus[85]
Reduction of complications	Barrier nursing of infected individuals	Transfer of bacteria via clothes is a significant route of infection[43]
	Antibiotics	Widely recognised
	Treatment of septic shock	Various regimens described, not specific to puerperal sepsis
Diagnosis and treatment	Antibiotics	Widely recognised
	Drainage and irrigation of local wound infections	Not effective as a routine procedure[86]
	Microbiological diagnostic techniques	None found
Behavioural and organisational change	Issue of guidelines	No change in hand hygiene compliance[71]
	Training and feedback	Handwashing compliance increased from 23% to 65%, infection rates decreased from 5 to 3 per 100 patient days[72]
	Senior management support, hand hygiene product distribution and education	Hand hygiene compliance increased from 48% to 66%; infection rates decreased from 17% to 10%[42]
	Surveillance and infection control	A maximum decrease in infection rates by 32% if all components implemented[73]
	Audit/quality improvement	Largest observed increase in administering of antibiotic prophylaxis from 36% to 89%, with downward trend in surgical site infection rate[75]
	Opinion leaders	Systematic review on general quality improvement (not specific to puerperal sepsis) found to be more effective than feedback and didactic educational meetings[76]

Equipment and clean delivery kits

The cleaning, sterilisation and storage of equipment is an important part of infection control procedures. Instruments used to provide delivery care, whether for normal or complicated deliveries, require functioning autoclave equipment linked to reliable power supplies. Some instruments, such as vacuum extractors, have several removable parts and may need particular care to maintain and keep clean.

The distribution of delivery kits has been used to encourage clean practices during childbirth. Several studies on the use of such kits for home birth in low-resource settings have been conducted. In Nepal, the kits were observed to encourage birth attendants to adopt more hygienic practices, such as hand washing with soap. Numbers of infections in babies were reduced as a result of the kits but the study did not look at infections in the mothers.[44] In Tanzania, the provision of clean delivery kits for home birth was associated with a three-fold reduction in puerperal sepsis.[45] There has been interest in promoting the use of clean delivery kits in health facilities but the effects of such an intervention have not yet been evaluated.

Training and education of traditional birth attendants

The need to wash hands during delivery is not universally known or practised by traditional birth attendants.[46] For more than 20 years, there has been debate about the possible role of traditional birth attendants in reducing maternal mortality through prevention of infection and by training to conduct safer, clean deliveries. Trained traditional birth attendants have been observed to be more likely to practise hygienic delivery than their untrained counterparts, yet no significant difference in the levels of puerperal sepsis was seen when comparing groups of trained and untrained attendants.[47] In another study,[48] however, training and issuing traditional birth attendants with disposable delivery kits seemed to lower the risk of maternal mortality in Pakistan (odds ratio [OR] 0.74; 95% CI 0.45–1.23), with rates of maternal sepsis significantly lower compared with other complications (OR 0.17; 95% CI 0.13–0.23). Educating traditional birth attendants is not a key priority today as there is a greater focus on trained health professionals.

Vaginal antisepsis

The use of chlorhexidine as a vaginal or perineal cleansing solution showed promising findings in reducing puerperal sepsis in a Malawian hospital setting,[49] but a Cochrane review[50] was unable to find a relationship between chlorhexidine and a reduction in maternal sepsis. The review was based on three randomised studies, all of which were conducted in healthcare facilities in resource-rich countries, so it could be argued that chlorhexidine's role in reducing puerperal sepsis in low-resource settings and for use in home deliveries needs further exploration.[34,51] A hospital-based study in Egypt[52] using chlorhexidine has also shown reductions in infection rates. Chlorhexidine vaginal washes have also been tried in women's homes in Pakistan, where it was found to be safe and acceptable although effects on health outcome were inconclusive.[53]

Surgical asepsis

Caesarean sections are thought to be required as a life-saving procedure in at least 5% of deliveries. However, it is also a procedure that is associated with an increased risk of puerperal sepsis and that could potentially double the risk of maternal infection.[16,17,54]

Up to 50% of healthcare-associated infections in developing countries are thought to be surgical site infections,[55] so surgical aseptic practices are key to infection control in health facilities. Surgical personnel were traditionally advised to use a brush to scrub their hands before surgery. However, current evidence suggests that neither a brush or sponge are required and a minimum of 2 minutes of hand washing with a chlorhexidine or povidone-iodine product followed by application of an alcohol hand rub produces acceptable bacterial counts on the hands of surgical staff.[40] Shortened scrub times together with superior antiseptic products may contribute to improving compliance and effectiveness of infection control strategies.

Micronutrient supplementation

For nearly 80 years, malnutrition has been known to be linked to puerperal sepsis,[56] and it has been acknowledged that micronutrients can influence immune function.[57] Vitamin A or beta-carotene supplements, especially in undernourished women, were thought to be a potential means of reducing maternal deaths from infection and other causes. Such supplementation was associated with a 40% reduction in all-cause maternal mortality ratios (from 645 to 385 deaths per 100000 live births) in Nepal[58] and with a 78% reduction in maternal infections elsewhere.[59] A systematic review[60] of the effects of vitamin A was, however, inconclusive. A recent trial from Ghana[61] showed no maternal benefits. There is thus currently no reason to introduce vitamin A supplementation programmes to reduce maternal mortality.

It has been suggested that other supplements may be protective against puerperal sepsis. Different groups of women in Nepal were randomised in a study[62] to receive either a placebo or one of the following preparations: folic acid, folic acid/iron, folic acid/iron/zinc or folic acid/iron/zinc with 11 other micronutrients. All preparations, including the placebo, contained vitamin A. Significant reductions were observed for preparations containing iron, with or without zinc, and in one group receiving the 11 micronutrients. The largest reduction was seen in the group receiving zinc.

Antibiotics

Routine antibiotic prophylaxis during caesarean section reduces endometritis by at least two-thirds and is currently recommended practice.[63] For other high-risk situations, such as in vacuum or forceps vaginal delivery, current data are insufficient to make recommendations on the routine use of prophylactic antibiotics.[64] Emerging concerns of bacterial vaginosis and group B streptococcus colonisation of the genital tract have led to consideration of routine antibiotic prophylaxis for all pregnant women. Individual studies have shown conflicting findings. A Cochrane review of six randomised controlled trials suggests that antibiotic prophylaxis during the second or third trimester of pregnancy is effective in reducing postpartum endometritis for women with a history of previous preterm births (OR 0.46; 95% CI 0.24–0.89) but the effect in unselected women or those where risk was not specified is less clear (OR 0.49; 95% CI 0.23–1.06). Prophylaxis is therefore not recommended for routine use in all pregnant women.[65] In poorly resourced health systems, the feasibility of identifying women at high risk is, in any case, limited by poor quality of services, lack of laboratory facilities and difficulty in following women up during antenatal care. However, much can be gained by introducing changes to practices where the evidence is clear and the intervention straightforward. For example, the impact of wasteful administering of antibiotics was studied in Mozambique,[66] where it was estimated that ten-fold savings could be achieved with single-dose, prophylactic antibiotic administration before caesarean section compared with the week-long, postoperative regimen that was standard practice.

In terms of treatment of puerperal sepsis with antibiotics, broad-spectrum treatment without identification of the infective agent is widely practised in many developing countries.[67] The treatment of puerperal sepsis according to antibiotic sensitivity is constrained by poor diagnostic and laboratory facilities in these settings. Laboratory and technological advances to improve microbiological assessment, such as the use of disc diffusion methods with antibiotic impregnation of paper discs[68] by non-specialist health workers, have not been widely implemented.

Behavioural and organisational change

Motivational, behavioural or organisational change underlies most, if not all, of the infection control measures described. Even for apparently simple interventions such as hand washing, behavioural and organisational implications have been found to be important. For example, compliance rates with hand hygiene procedures of less than 50% have been reported in healthcare workers when factors such as irritation of hands, lack of time, placement of sinks, detergent or towels, and lack of role models are not addressed.[69] Physicians and nursing assistants have been found to be poorer hand washers than nurses. The higher the need for hand hygiene, the lower the adherence, and poor compliance is more common in intensive care units, during procedures where the risk of contamination is high, during weekdays and when wearing gloves and gowns.[40] Many of these factors have specific relevance to delivery care and should be addressed as part of any infection control measure. For developing countries, key elements for any infection control strategy will require modification of health systems, including:[43,67,70]

- procurement policies to enable use of new hand cleaning products with introduction of antibiotic prophylaxis
- human resource interventions such as changes in nurse : patient ratios, training, monitoring and performance feedback
- organisational interventions to review ward layout, develop posters and promote involvement of managers and opinion leaders.

Evaluation of behavioural change strategies needs to account for the way in which specific interventions included in the strategy interact. Many strategies incorporate both individual behaviour change and organisational changes. Education and feedback, written reminders, use of protocols, administrative sanctions and organisational changes such as increasing convenience of hand hygiene facilities and avoiding overcrowding or understaffing have been investigated.[40] Improvements in infection rates have been shown in both developed and developing countries when comprehensive approaches involving various levels within the organisation, education of health personnel and feedback mechanisms are incorporated.[71–75] (Table 8.4) The effect of opinion leaders has been assessed in a few studies on general quality-improvement literature related to maternity care and found to be more effective than feedback and didactic educational meetings.[76]

Behavioural change strategies are not confined to those involving health professionals. Training of traditional birth attendants has been discussed earlier. Understanding the beliefs and behaviours of women in relation to childbirth is also important. Various ethnographic studies have been done to understand and incorporate the beliefs of rural women into infection control measures. One commonly held belief is that childbirth is physically and spiritually polluting. Cleaning the surroundings and items used for cutting the cord before delivery can seem illogical when all the equipment would have to be physically (and spiritually) cleansed again after childbirth.[77] Bathing practices may be of interest as women who bathe before labour have been found to have lower rates of cord infection and puerperal sepsis.[45] Women also prefer health workers to have an appreciation of their cultural beliefs[77] and this may encourage care-seeking behaviours that minimise risk of infection and reporting of symptoms during the postpartum period.

Why is puerperal sepsis a continuing problem?

Given the knowledge on puerperal sepsis summarised in this chapter, why do so many deaths from puerperal sepsis continue to occur in low- and middle-income settings? There are many possible ways of describing the root causes, which may stem from biomedical reasons such as poor nutrition and virulence of various pathogens, or from social and cultural factors and those related to unresponsive and poorly functioning health systems. Three major problems have been highlighted in this chapter:

- lack of accurate data relevant to puerperal sepsis
- the need to improve understanding of organisational and behavioural change
- related to both these issues, poor visibility of the burden of puerperal sepsis.

Lack of accurate data

Problems in defining cases of puerperal sepsis and poor use of standard definitions have led to difficulties in accurately estimating incidence and case fatality rates. Microbiological confirmation remains unfeasible for low-resource settings in the short to medium term. Surveys may under- or overestimate the condition. Puerperal sepsis, unlike other major causes of maternal mortality, is more likely to manifest itself many days after delivery. Under-reporting is likely because of poor follow-up during the puerperium. Puerperal sepsis may resolve spontaneously, also leading to under-reporting. Even when the condition spontaneously resolves, women may experience long-term morbidities, some of which can be life threatening, such as ectopic pregnancies. The attributing of puerperal sepsis to such long-term morbidities is, as yet, poorly quantified. Increasing trends for deliveries in health facilities and the rise in rates of caesarean section in some settings, such as in Latin America, without concurrent improvements in quality of care and infection control have the potential to result in aggravation of the risk of infections during the postpartum period.

The lack of information on emerging antibiotic resistance is another key consideration. Use of broad-spectrum antibiotics and unnecessary and non-evidence-based practices (for example, the routine administering of antibiotics to women after delivery) is common in many settings where infection control practices are poor. The lack of microbiological diagnostic facilities has not allowed tracking of changing patterns of resistance in many low-resource settings.

Understanding organisational and behavioural factors

Late recognition of sepsis, severe complications and health facility-acquired infections are thought to explain higher morbidity and mortality in developing country settings.[78] Behavioural and organisational change is required to improve some of these factors. Much can be learnt from lessons on the use of behavioural and systems change in other medical disciplines to control infection but a better evidence base on effective measures specific to delivery care needs to be developed. Information on the cost-effectiveness of various preventive and curative strategies is also necessary. In the USA, it has been estimated that infection prevention would have to reduce infections by only 6% for the costs of the programme to be offset by the savings from reduced hospitalisation.[73,79] Wasteful practices and unnecessary use of antibiotics in developing countries have been documented and are only adding to the constraints of the health system in many low- and middle-income settings.[43,67]

Poor visibility of the burden of puerperal sepsis

> …then, as now, advances in, and acceptance of, medical progress depends largely on political context.[80]

The two names most closely associated with historical discoveries on puerperal sepsis are those of Alexander Gordon (1752–99) and Ignac Semmelweis (1818–65). Both failed to effectively communicate their findings and died with their discoveries unacknowledged and unaccepted.[81,82] The story of their lives provides stark lessons on how political change underlies advances in health outcome and how effective communication and advocacy is an important part of scientific advancement.

The lack of accurate epidemiological and biomedical data and the uncertainty about the effectiveness of behavioural and organisational change interventions are at least partially responsible for the poor visibility of puerperal sepsis as a key cause of maternal deaths. Better data on the burden of disease and the effect on interventions could be used to advocate for and improve the visibility of puerperal sepsis as an unnecessary cause of death today.

Looking ahead

Reducing puerperal sepsis for many low- and middle-income countries will require a concerted and multifaceted approach. Historical data have shown that, where puerperal sepsis is common, steep declines in maternal mortality can result from effective interventions.[4] Despite current knowledge on the aetiology of puerperal sepsis and effectiveness of infection control measures, case fatality rates for puerperal sepsis in some countries are today still as high as those seen in the past. New technologies and evidence-based practices alone will not be enough to reduce maternal mortality rates. Three key strategies for reducing unnecessary deaths from puerperal sepsis are proposed.

Build a stronger knowledge base on puerperal sepsis and infection control in childbirth

Studies are needed to quantify the disease burden related to puerperal sepsis. The effectiveness of interventions, particularly those that comprise multiple components related to influencing behaviour and creating improvements in the health system, should be rigorously tested. Evidence on cost effectiveness will help to inform decisions for investment in prevention and diagnosis rather than treatment. The understanding of social and cultural aspects surrounding puerperal sepsis should also be developed.

Current evidence on effectiveness of infection control strategies is limited by variations in settings, nature and components of the various strategies and the use of quasi-experimental designs with no controls. The studies that are conducted should provide high-quality evidence, focusing on labour and delivery in settings when the risk of introducing infection is high.

Interventions to reduce puerperal sepsis must take health system factors into account

The multifaceted components necessary to implement an effective infection control strategy reflect the many structural elements of the health system. Although there is some high-quality evidence available on a few specific interventions to reduce puerperal sepsis, it is unlikely that successful infection control will be achieved solely through single technological advances.[32] Strategies to change behaviour and improve systems will need to be multifaceted, drawing from psychological, educational, organisational, administrative, technological and medical perspectives.

Create political change

There is an urgent need to improve the visibility of infection as a major cause of maternal death in the postpartum period. A number of opportunities exist today to catalyse interest in this area of work, including the concerted efforts to reach the MDGs, increased global interest in infection pandemics and cross-disciplinary efforts such as the Global Patient Safety Alliance. Effective communication of information and messages to profile the importance of puerperal sepsis is required. Advocates for maternal mortality reduction, including obstetricians, should engage and become involved in an invigorated global effort to making puerperal sepsis a tragedy of the past.

Acknowledgements

This work was undertaken as part of Immpact (www.immpact-international.org). The authors are funded by the University of Aberdeen and are grateful to the MacArthur Foundation for allowing the use of materials generated through an infection control study funded by the Foundation. Sheetal Sharma helped to conduct literature searches on infections in pregnancy and on the microbiology of puerperal sepsis. The funding agencies have no responsibility for the information provided or the views expressed in this chapter. The views expressed herein are solely those of the authors.

References

1. World Health Organization. *The Global Burden of Disease: 2004 Update*. Geneva: WHO; 2008.
2. Lewis G, editor. *Saving Mothers' Lives: Reviewing Maternal Deaths to Make Motherhood Safer 2003–2005. The Seventh Report on Confidential Enquiries into Maternal Deaths in the United Kingdom.* London: CEMACH; 2007.
3. Loudon I. *Death in Childbirth: An International Study of Maternal Care and Maternal Mortality 1800–1950.* Oxford: University Press; 1992.
4. Loudon I. *The Tragedy of Childbed Fever.* Oxford: University Press Oxford; 2000.
5. World Health Organization. *International Statistical Classification of Diseases and Related Health Problems.* ICD-10 [apps.who.int/classifications/apps/icd/icd10online].
6. Dolea C, Stein C. *Global Burden of Maternal Sepsis in the Year 2000.* Global Burden of Disease 2000. Evidence and Information for Policy (EIP). Geneva: World Health Organization; 2003 [www.who.int/healthinfo/statistics/bod_maternalsepsis.pdf].
7. Mantel GD, Buchmann E, Rees H, Pattinson RC. Severe acute maternal morbidity: a pilot study of a definition for a near miss. *BJOG* 1998;105:985–90.

8. Brentlinger PE, Capps L. Pregnancy outcomes in El Salvador during the post-war period. *Int J Gynaecol Obstet* 1998;61:59–62.

9. Prual A, Bouvier-Colle MH, de Bernis L, Bréart G. Severe maternal morbidity from direct obstetric causes in West Africa: incidence and case fatality rates. *Bull World Health Organ* 2000;78:593–602.

10. Seale AC, Mwaniki M, Newton CR, Berkley JA. Maternal and early onset neonatal bacterial sepsis: burden and strategies for prevention in sub-Saharan Africa. *Lancet Infect Dis* 2009;9:428–38.

11. Lagro M, Liche A, Mumba T, Ntebeka R, van Roosmalen J. Postpartum health among rural Zambian women. *Afr J Reprod Health* 2003;7:41–8.

12. Sebitloane HM, Moodley J, Esterhuizen TM. Prophylactic antibiotics for the prevention of postpartum infectious morbidity in women infected with human immunodeficiency virus: a randomized controlled trial. *Am J Obstet Gynecol* 2008;198:189.e1–6.

13. Khan KS, Wojdyla D, Say L, Gülmezoglu AM, Van Look PF. WHO analysis of causes of maternal death: a systematic review. *Lancet* 2006;367:1066–74.

14. McKibben L, Horan T, Tokars JI, Fowler G, Cardo DM, Pearson ML, *et al.* Guidance on public reporting of healthcare-associated infections: recommendations of the healthcare infection control practices advisory committee. *Am J Infect Control* 2005;33:217–26.

15. de Bernis L, Dumont A, Bouillin D, Gueye A, Dompnier JP, Bouvier-Colle MH. Maternal morbidity and mortality in two different populations of Senegal: a prospective study (MOMA survey). *BJOG* 2000;107:68–746.

16. Newton ER, Prihoda TJ, Gibbs RS. A clinical and microbiologic analysis of risk factors for puerperal endometritis. *Obstet Gynecol* 1990;75:402–6.

17. Vacca A, Henderson A. Puerperal sepsis in Port Moresby. Papua New Guinea. *P N G Med J* 1980;23:120–5.

18. Maharaj D. Puerperal pyrexia: a review. Part I. *Obstet Gynecol Surv* 2007;62:393–9.

19. Romero R, Nores J, Mazor M, Sepulveda W, Oyarzun E, Parra M, *et al.* Microbial invasion of the amniotic cavity during term labor. Prevalence and clinical significance. *J Reprod Med* 1993;38:543–8.

20. Guaschino S, De Seta F, Piccoli M, Maso G, Alberico S. Aetiology of preterm labour: bacterial vaginosis. *BJOG* 2006;113 Suppl 3:46–51.

21. Muller AE, Oostvogel PM, Steegers EA, Dörr PJ. Morbidity related to maternal group B streptococcal infections. *Acta Obstet Gynecol Scand* 2006;85:1027–37.

22. Larsen JW, Sever JL. Group B Streptococcus and pregnancy: a review. *Am J Obstet Gynecol* 2008;198:440–8.

23. Mason PR, Katzenstein DA, Chimbira TH, Mtimavalye L. Vaginal flora of women admitted to hospital with signs of sepsis following normal delivery, cesarean section or abortion. The Puerperal Sepsis Study Group. *Cent Afr J Med* 1989;35:344–51.

24. Dare FO, Bako AU, Ezechi OC. Puerperal sepsis: a preventable post-partum complication. *Trop Doct* 1998;28:92–5.

25. Perine PL, Duncan ME, Krause DW, Awoke S. Pelvic inflammatory disease and puerperal sepsis in Ethiopia. I. Etiology. *Am J Obstet Gynecol* 1980;138:969–73.

26. Omu AE, Ajabor LN. Contribution of endotoxic shock to gynaecological and maternal morbidity and mortality. *J Obstet Gynaecol East Cent Africa* 1983;2:41–5.

27. Kampikaho A, Irwig LM. A randomized trial of penicillin and streptomycin in the prevention of post-partum infection in Uganda. *Int J Gynaecol Obstet* 1993;41:43–52.

28. Dan M, Maximova S, Siegman-Igra Y, Gutman R, Rotmensch HH. Varied presentations of sporadic group A streptococcal bacteremia: clinical experience and attempt at classification. *Rev Infect Dis* 1990;12:537–42.

29. Ooe K, Udagawa H. A new type of fulminant group A streptococcal infection in obstetric patients: report of two cases. *Hum Pathol* 1997;28:509–12.

30. Abouzahr CL. Lessons on safe motherhood. *World Health Forum* 1998;19:253–60.

31. Polunin I. The Muruts of North Borneo and their declining population. *Trans R Soc Trop Med Hyg* 1959;53:312–26.

32. Pittet D. Infection control and quality health care in the new millennium. *Am J Infect Control* 2005;33:258–67.

33. Hussein J, Fortney JA. Puerperal sepsis and maternal mortality: what role can new technologies play? *Int J Gynaecol Obstet* 2004;85 Suppl 1:S52–61.

34. Tsu VD, Coffey PS. New and underutilised technologies to reduce maternal mortality and morbidity: what progress have we made since Bellagio 2003? *BJOG* 2009;116:247–56.

35. Pittet D. Improving adherence to hand hygiene practice: a multidisciplinary approach. *Emerg Infect Dis* 2001;7:234–67.

36. Backman C, Zoutman DE, Marck PB. An integrative review of the current evidence on the relationship between hand hygiene interventions and the incidence of health-care-associated infections. *Am J Infect Control* 2008;36:333–48.

37. Pittet D, Donaldson L. Clean Care is Safer Care: a worldwide priority. *Lancet* 2005;366:1246–7.

38. Pittet D, Allegranzi B, Storr J, Donaldson L. 'Clean Care is Safer Care': the Global Patient Safety Challenge 2005–2006. *Int J Infect Dis* 2006;10:419–24.

39. Allegranzi B, Storr J, Dziekan G, Leotsakos A, Donaldson L, Pittet D. The First Global Patient Safety Challenge 'Clean Care is Safer Care': from launch to current progress and achievements. *J Hosp Infect* 2007;65 Suppl 2:115–23.

40. Boyce JM, Pittet D. Guideline for hand hygiene in health-care settings. *Am J Infect Control* 2002;30:1–46.

41. Pittet D, Allegranzi B, Storr J, Nejad SB, Dziekan G, Leotsakos A, *et al.* Infection control as a major World Health Organization priority for developing countries. *J Hosp Infect* 2008;68:285–92.

42. Pittet D, Hugonnet S, Harbarth S, Mourouga P, Sauvan V, Touveneau S, *et al.* Effectiveness of a hospital-wide programme to improve compliance with hand hygiene. *Lancet* 2000;356:1307–12.

43. Hambraeus A. Lowbury Lecture 2005: Infection control from a global perspective. *J Hosp Infect* 2006;64:217–23.

44. Tsu V. *Nepal Clean Home Delivery Kit: Evaluation of the Health Impact.* Seattle: PATH Publications; 2000 [www.path.org/publications/details.php?i=711].

45. Winani S, Wood S, Coffey P, Chirwa T, Mosha F, Changalucha J. Use of a clean delivery kit and factors associated with cord infection and puerperal sepsis in Mwanza, Tanzania. *J Midwifery Womens Health* 2007;52:37–43.

46. Beun MH, Wood SK. Acceptability and use of clean home delivery kits in Nepal: a qualitative study. *J Health Popul Nutr* 2003;21:367–73.

47. Goodburn EA, Chowdhury M, Gazi R, Marshall T, Graham W. Training traditional birth attendants in clean delivery does not prevent postpartum infection. *Health Policy Plan* 2000;15:394–9.

48. Jokhio AH, Winter HR, Cheng KK. An intervention involving traditional birth attendants and perinatal and maternal mortality in Pakistan. *N Engl J Med* 2005;352:2091–9.

49. Taha TE, Biggar RJ, Broadhead RL, Mtimavalye LA, Justesen AB, Liomba GN, *et al.* Effect of cleansing the birth canal with antiseptic solution on maternal and newborn morbidity and mortality in Malawi: clinical trial. *BMJ* 1997;315:216–19.

50. Lumbiganon P, Thinkhamrop J, Thinkhamrop B, Tolosa JE. Vaginal chlorhexidine during labour for preventing maternal and neonatal infections (excluding Group B Streptococcal and HIV). *Cochrane Database Syst Rev* 2004;(4):CD004070.

51. Goldenberg RL, McClure EM, Saleem S, Rouse D, Vermund S. Use of vaginally administered chlorhexidine during labor to improve pregnancy outcomes. *Obstet Gynecol* 2006;107:1139–46.

52. Bakr AF, Karkour T. Effect of predelivery vaginal antisepsis on maternal and neonatal morbidity and mortality in Egypt. *J Womens Health (Larchmt)* 2005;14:496–501.

53. Saleem S, Reza T, McClure EM, Pasha O, Moss N, Rouse DJ, *et al.* Chlorhexidine vaginal and neonatal wipes in home births in Pakistan: a randomized controlled trial. *Obstet Gynecol* 2007;110:968–9.

54. Yokoe DS, Christiansen CL, Johnson R, Sands K, Livingston J, Shtatland ES, *et al.* Epidemiology of and surveillance for postpartum infections. *Emerg Infect Dis* 2001;7:837–41.

55. Pittet D, Donaldson L. Clean Care is Safer Care: The first global challenge of the WHO World Alliance for Patient Safety. *Am J Infect Control* 2005;33:476–9.

56. Green HN, Pindar D, Davis G, Mellanby E. Diet as a prophylactic agent against puerperal sepsis. *Br Med J* 1931;2:595–8.

57. Keen CL, Clegg MS, Hanna LA, Lanoue L, Rogers JM, Daston GP, *et al.* The plausibility of micronutrient deficiencies being a significant contributing factor to the occurrence of pregnancy complications. *J Nutr* 2003;133(5 Suppl 2):1597S–605S.

58. West KP, Katz J, Khatry SK, LeClerq SC, Pradhan EK, Shrestha SR, *et al.* Double blind, cluster randomised trial of low dose supplementation with vitamin A or beta-carotene on mortality related to pregnancy in Nepal. *BMJ* 1999;318:570–5.

59. Hakimi M, Dibley MJ, Suryono A, Nurdiati D, Th Ninuk SH, Dawiesah Ismadi S. Impact of vitamin A and zinc supplements on maternal post partum infections in rural central Java, Indonesia. In: *Report of the XIX International Vitamin A Consultative Group Meeting.* 8–11 March 1999, Durban, South Africa. Washington, DC: ILSI Press; 1999. p. 34.

60. Van DE, Kulier R, Gülmezoglu AM, Villar J. Vitamin A supplementation during pregnancy. *Cochrane Database Syst Rev* 2002;(4):CD001996.

61. Kirkwood B, ObaapaVitA Trial Team. The ObaapaVitA Trial: impact of weekly vitamin A supplementation (VAS) on pregnancy related mortality in Ghana. The Second Annual Meeting of the Micronutrient Forum, 12–15 May 2009, Beijing, China. Abstract.

62. Christian P, Khartry S, LeClerq S, Dali SM. Effects of prenatal micronutrient supplementation on complications of labor and delivery and puerperal morbidity in rural Nepal. *Int J Gynaecol Obstet* 2009;106:3–7.

63. Hofmeyr GJ, Smaill FM. Antibiotic prophylaxis for cesarean section. *Cochrane Database Syst Rev* 2002;(3):CD000933.

64. Liabsuetrakul T, Choobun T, Peeyananjarassri K, Islam QM. Antibiotic prophylaxis for operative vaginal delivery. *Cochrane Database Syst Rev* 2004;(3):CD004455.

65. Thinkhamrop J, Hofmeyr GJ, Adetoro O, Lumbiganon P. Prophylactic antibiotic administration in pregnancy to prevent infectious morbidity and mortality. *Cochrane Database Syst Rev* 2002;(4):CD002250.

66. Kayihura V, Osman NB, Bugalho A, Bergström S. Choice of antibiotics for infection prophylaxis in emergency cesarean sections in low-income countries: A cost–benefit study in Mozambique. *Acta Obstet Gynecol Scand* 2003;82:636–41.

67. Shears P. Poverty and infection in the developing world: healthcare-related infections and infection control in the tropics. *J Hosp Infect* 2007;67:217–24.

68. Talaat M, Kandeel A, Rasslan O, Hajjeh R, Hallaj Z, El-Sayed, N, *et al.* Evolution of infection control in Egypt: Achievements and challenges. *Am J Infect Control* 2006;34:193–200.

69. Posfay-Barbe KM, Pittet D. New concepts in hand hygiene. *Semin Pediatr Infect Dis* 2001;12:147–53.

70. Lynch P, Pittet D, Borg MA, Mehtar S. Infection control in countries with limited resources. *J Hosp Infect* 2007;65 Suppl 2:148–50.

71. Larson EL, Quiros D, Lin SX. Dissemination of the CDC's Hand Hygiene Guideline and impact on infection rates. *Am J Infect Control* 2007;35:666–75.

72. Rosenthal VD, Guzman S, Safdar N. Reduction in nosocomial infection with improved hand hygiene in intensive care units of a tertiary care hospital in Argentina. *Am J Infect Control* 2005;33:392–7.

73. Haley RW, Culver DH, White JW, Morgan WM, Emori TG, Munn VP, *et al.* The efficacy of infection surveillance and control programs in preventing nosocomial infections in US hospitals. *Am J Epidemiol* 1985;121:182–205.

74. Yealy DM, Auble TE, Stone RA, Lave JR, Meehan TP, Graff LG, *et al.* Effect of increasing the intensity of implementing pneumonia guidelines: a randomized, controlled trial. *Ann Intern Med* 2005;143:881–94.

75. Weinberg M, Fuentes JM, Ruiz AI, Lozano FW, Angel E, Gaitan H, *et al.* Reducing infections among women undergoing cesarean section in Colombia by means of continuous quality improvement methods.. *Arch Intern Med* 2001;161:2357–65.

76. Althabe F, Buekens P, Bergel E, Belizan JM, Campbell MK, Moss N, *et al.* A behavioral intervention to improve obstetrical care. *N Engl J Med* 2008;358:1929–40.

77. Adams V, Miller S, Chertow J, Craig S, Samen A, Varner M. Having a 'safe delivery': conflicting views from Tibet. *Health Care Women Int* 2005;26:821–51.

78. Baccar K, Baffoun N, Zaghdoudi Z, Abassi S, Magouri M, Souissi R, *et al.* Severe sepsis and septic shock during pregnancy and puerperium: The incidence, the etiology, and the outcome. *J Critical Care* 2008;23:267.

79. Haley RW, Quade D, Freeman HE, Bennett JV. Study on the efficacy of nosocomial infection control (SENIC Project): summary of study design. *Am J Epidemiol* 1980;111:472–85.

80. Pittet D. The crusade against puerperal fever. *Lancet* 2004;363:1331–2.

81. Lowis GW. Epidemiology of puerperal fever: the contributions of Alexander Gordon. *Med Hist* 1993;37:399–410.

82. Nuland SB. *The Doctors' Plague – Germs, Childbed Fever and the Strange Story of Ignac Semmelweis.* New York: WW Norton and Company; 2003.

83. World Health Organization, Maternal Health and Safe Motherhood Programme. *Mother–Baby Package: Implementing Safe Motherhood in Countries.* Geneva: WHO; 1994.

84. World Health Organization, International Confederation of Midwives. *Managing Puerperal Sepsis.* Geneva: WHO; 2008.

85. Flenady V, King JF. Antibiotics for prelabour rupture of membranes at or near term. *Cochrane Database Syst Rev* 2002;(3):CD001807.

86. Ochsenbein-Imhof N, Huch A, Huch R, Zimmermann R. No benefit from post-caesarean wound drainage. *Swiss Med Wkly* 2001;131:246–50.

Chapter 9

Unsafe abortion and strategies to reduce its impact on women's lives

Caitlin Shannon and Beverly Winikoff

Introduction

Harrowing stories of women seeking abortion are universal and commonplace. Take, for example, the story of a Nicaraguan girl who, at 8 years old, became pregnant, raped by her neighbour.[1] Without the help of her family, international attention and several months of hard fighting, this young girl could have become another faceless statistic in the pandemic of unsafe abortion. The outrage many feel in reaction to this and other similar stories has been insufficient to end the political struggle over abortion. What is more, that young girl was fortunate, as one woman dies every 8 minutes from an unsafe abortion somewhere in the world, most likely south of the equator. The greatest tragedy is that unsafe abortion is largely, if not entirely, preventable and yet remains one of the most neglected public health challenges.

Millennium Development Goal (MDG) 5, announced in 2001, is an internationally agreed-upon imperative to reduce maternal mortality by 75% from its 1990 level by the year 2015. As a significant proportion of mortality is due to unsafe abortion, this goal probably cannot be met without specific and direct programmatic efforts to reduce the impact of unsafe abortion. Thousands of publications trace efforts to reduce mortality due to other significant contributors, yet few, if any, papers highlight efforts designed specifically and directly to reduce the impact of unsafe abortion. Additionally, many Safe Motherhood Initiatives ignore altogether the problem of unsafe abortion because of the difficult political issues involved.

Despite the continued absence of abortion in serious policy discussion, a common goal has been to make abortion 'safe, legal and rare'.[2] Global statistics published in 2007[3] showed that it is possible to reduce the need for abortion by wider access to contraception. However, while the need for abortion can be reduced, it can never be eliminated entirely, as there will always be circumstances in which even wanted pregnancies cannot be carried to term. Nonetheless, nearly half of all countries still highly restrict abortion, often including pregnancies arising from rape. Even where abortion is legal, the procedure can remain highly inaccessible and unavailable, regardless of its technical legality.

By and large, the reasons why unsafe abortions happen are known, if not perfectly, at least to a degree sufficient for developing effective interventions. Given the complicated and often opposing forces affecting global abortion provision, what are the appropriate and sufficient means to stem the pandemic? What are the consequences of failing to do so? This chapter proposes some answers to these perplexing questions.

The problem of unsafe abortion

Prevalence and distribution

The World Health Organization (WHO)[4] defines unsafe abortion as a procedure for terminating a pregnancy either by people that lack the necessary skills or in an environment that lacks the minimal medical standards, or both. Data for 2003[5] show that each year approximately 210 million women become pregnant and of these pregnancies an estimated 80 million are unplanned. About 42 million of these unplanned pregnancies are terminated intentionally, at a rate of 29 abortions per 1000 women of reproductive age. In low-resource countries, only one in three abortions is legal, and 98% of all unsafe abortions occur in these low-resource countries.[5] Nearly half of all abortions, or approximately 19–20 million per year, are estimated to be unsafe.[3] This means that in low-resource countries a woman can expect to experience one unsafe abortion in her lifetime.[6] In contrast, it is rare that a woman in a developed country will undergo an unsafe abortion.

The majority of unsafe procedures are performed where abortion is legally restricted. However, the rate of unsafe abortion in some countries where abortion has been liberalised for decades is still quite high, for example in India, Armenia and Zambia.[5] Therefore, legality is not the only significant contributor to unsafe abortion. Other primary (individual-level) and secondary (systemic) determinants include where a woman lives (urban versus rural), a woman's financial resources, and the availability and quality of abortion and post-abortion services.

Mortality and morbidity

Approximately 70000 women die each year as a result of unsafe abortion, the overwhelming majority of them in low-resource countries.[5] Deaths from unsafe abortion account for approximately 13% of maternal mortality worldwide but this varies by country from negligible to over 30%.[7] The mortality rate for an abortion done safely is less than 1 per 100000 procedures for all abortions and may be as low as 1 per 1000000 procedures for early first-trimester procedures.[8] However, the mortality rate in regions where unsafe abortion is commonplace is very much higher: 350 deaths per 100000 procedures in low-resource countries overall and, specifically in Africa, 680 per 100000 procedures.[3]

Global estimates of the disability burden of unsafe abortion show a loss of approximately 5 million years of productive life each year, representing an estimated 14% of all annual disability from pregnancy-related conditions.[9] However, researchers believe the impact of abortion to be underestimated because of the clandestine nature of some procedures and limitations of measuring abortion disability.[10] Abortion complications are the cause of major morbidities such as pelvic inflammatory disease and other infections of the reproductive tract, secondary infertility, ectopic pregnancy, mid-trimester miscarriage and preterm labour. For example, it is estimated that 1.7 million women each year suffer secondary infertility as a consequence of unsafe abortion. Furthermore, unsafe abortion contributes to the development of chronic reproductive tract infections in an estimated 3 million women per year.[5] The rate and severity of complications are related to the quality of health care for abortion and management of complications, including the skill of providers, the method of abortion used, and the availability and use of antibiotics. Individual-level factors include the health of the woman, genital tract anomalies, reproductive health infections, female circumcision and gestational age at the time of the procedure.

Economic and social costs

The combined regional annual cost of unsafe abortion in Latin America and Africa was estimated in 2009 to be between US$159 million and US$333 million.[11] In comparison with the cost of providing legal, safe abortion, this economic burden is inordinately high. Data from Uganda,[12] Nigeria,[13] Brazil[14] and Mexico[15] show that the cost of post-abortion care is several times that of providing safe abortion with manual vacuum aspiration. A theoretical costing study estimated that the cost of post-abortion care in tertiary facilities is ten times more than elective abortion by mid-level providers in primary centres; this finding is similar to the results of country-level studies.[12] In Tanzania,[16] it is estimated that the cost of treating a complicated abortion is seven times the annual per person expenditure for health care. Data from Mexico City published in 2009[17] showed that management of severe sepsis costs almost ten times more than manual vacuum aspiration. Together, these data support not only improved services for managing complications but also legalisation of abortion, because of the tremendous cost savings.

The cost of unsafe abortion is also high because its occurrence and complications are so common. Estimates in 2006[9] from 13 low-resource countries indicated that between three and 15 per 1000 women of reproductive age are hospitalised each year for post-abortion care. In some countries, the burden of these hospitalisations accounts for almost 50% of hospital budgets for obstetrics and gynaecology.[18]

The high level of morbidity and mortality associated with unsafe abortion also translates to indirect economic and social costs that are difficult to quantify. 'Indirect' economic costs are related to loss of productivity and increased health problems for those women who survive. The non-economic costs are related to the impact on the children and the extended family of a woman. An estimated quarter to half a million children lose their mothers each year as a result of unsafe abortion;[19] those children are more likely than children with two parents to receive inadequate health care and social services such as education and are more likely to die at an early age.[20]

Pathways to unsafe abortion

Unwanted pregnancy, the necessary (but insufficient) step

Unwanted pregnancy is an extremely common phenomenon, affecting approximately 80 million women each year.[5] Women may know that they do not want a new pregnancy but be unable to exercise choice over conception because of insufficient access to or information about contraception, incorrect and inconsistent contraceptive use, or an inability to exercise autonomy over their own bodies, including being subject to rape. For other women, a pregnancy that was not necessarily unwanted may become unwanted because of changes in life circumstances, including:

- abandonment by spouse
- risk to her life or health
- fetal malformation
- inability to care for an additional child.

Contraceptive use is clearly a critical determinant of abortion. In fact, abortion is lowest where contraceptive use is high, despite the fact that abortion services also may be legal and widely available. For example, the abortion rate is low at 10 per 1000 women of reproductive age in Belgium, Germany and the Netherlands, where access to safe abortion is widespread and modern contraceptive use is high.[3] In contrast, in Africa, rates of modern contraceptive use are low, at approximately 30%, and abortion rates are high, at 30 per 1000 women of reproductive age, despite the legal restrictions on abortion.[3,21] What is more, the cost of providing effective family planning is significantly lower than providing either abortion or post-abortion care services. For example, a study in Nigeria published in 2007[22] estimated that the cost of contraceptive services that would have enabled women to avoid the unintended pregnancies that ended in unsafe abortions would have been one-quarter that of the post-abortion care provided by health facilities. Yet, since 1995, funding for family planning programmes has been drastically reduced.[23]

Desired fertility also plays a critical role in the link between contraception and abortion.[24] Low desired fertility increases the likelihood that any given pregnancy will be unwanted, a phenomenon that occurs more frequently in the absence of universal access to safe and effective methods of contraception.[25] The attitudes and education of providers and women affect whether women adopt modern methods, even where access is universal or near universal.

Legal environment

Approximately 60% of women in the world live in countries where abortion is legal for at least one reason.[26] Most countries allow abortion to save a woman's life. More than half permit it to preserve physical and mental health, and roughly half specify rape or incest as accepted grounds. A minority of countries allow abortion for fetal impairment and for economic or social reasons. Far fewer women in low-resource countries than in developed countries live where abortion in the first trimester is available, regardless of reason. In countries that restrict the legality of abortion, unsafe abortions are far more common than in countries where abortion is more freely available. Moreover, where women may need abortion the most – as a result of poverty and lack of access to contraception – they typically face the most restrictions. In some places, providers may be willing to provide abortions regardless of the law, yet such clandestine services are often of questionable quality, frequently resulting in tragically poor outcomes.

Liberalisation of abortion laws can have a dramatic impact on reducing mortality and morbidity related to unsafe abortion. Documented examples in South Africa and in Romania demonstrate this impact. In Romania, maternal mortality increased dramatically between 1960 and 1990, peaking in 1989 at an estimated 170 deaths per 100 000 live births, reflecting the restrictive abortion and contraception laws implemented by Ceauşescu.[6] This rate declined rapidly to 40 per 100 000 births in 1999 following his ejection from office and the restoration of access to abortion and contraception. South Africa liberalised its abortion laws in 1996 and subsequently the incidence of infection resulting from abortion declined by 52% and the maternal mortality rate declined by 92%.[27,28]

Although some have argued that legal liberalisation increases recourse to abortion, evidence for such a trend is weak at best. Certainly, the advent of legal and available services may increase the count of procedures as, previously, clandestine acts were always under-reported. In addition, the extent of unsatisfied demand may become clearer immediately after legalisation. Yet, when contraceptive use increases and fertility levels stabilise, abortion rates tend to decrease where abortion services are legal and available. Global abortion statistics demonstrate that, in developed countries, the rate of abortion decreased from 39 to 26 per 1000 women of reproductive age between 1995 and 2003 – a decline that was even more marked in the countries of the former Soviet Union, where the rate has declined nearly 50% to 44 per 1000 women of reproductive age.[9]

Liberalisation of abortion, however, is not completely predictive of access to abortion, especially in low-resource countries. The translation of law to policy is a necessary step that can have a critical impact on the level of unsafe abortion in a country or municipality. The law on the books is not always the law in practice, often because political will and commitment to ensuring the availability of services is lacking. Indeed, the willingness and ability of health systems to make available services for legal indications affects availability and consequently recourse to unsafe abortion. For example, in India,[29] despite liberalisation of abortion in 1971, the law restricts who can provide abortion, how abortion can be provided and where abortion can be provided – all of which have been translated to policies that restrict access. Also, although abortion is widely available in the private sector, those services are primarily located in urban centres and are expensive, especially in comparison with the free services offered at public clinics. As a result, approximately 40% of the 6.7 million abortions that occur each year in India are unsafe.[30]

Both provider and public awareness of the law, imperative to achieving access to safe services, can be driven by national and local policies. Provider knowledge of the law and willingness to provide abortion for legal indications also directly influences the availability of safe services. At the same time, women's knowledge affects their decisions to seek safe versus unsafe procedures.

Health system constraints

The burden of unsafe abortion on health systems is great, given both the scale of the problem and the high cost of treating complications. An estimated 5 million women are hospitalised each year for treatment of abortion-related complications, such as haemorrhage or sepsis.[31] In many low-resource countries, incomplete abortion is both one of the leading obstetric emergencies and the most common cause of hospital admission.

The rate of hospitalisation for abortion complications often reflects the relative safety of abortion in a particular locality. For example, in Bangladesh, where the rate of abortion remains relatively high, the rate of hospitalisations is fairly low, probably attributable to a widespread, well-developed system of menstrual regulation services.[9] In contrast, in countries where abortion is highly restricted and few services are available, such as the Dominican Republic, Chile, Peru or Egypt, women are forced to resort to unsafe abortion and the proportion hospitalised may be greater than in Bangladesh.

In many countries, in addition to limited health infrastructure, there is a shortage of well-trained healthcare providers. The lack of appropriately trained providers adds yet another barrier to accessing safe procedures. Even where abortion services are available, providers often use outmoded, risky and expensive techniques, both for induction and for treatment of complications. For example, in South Africa, a study in 2000[32] on the management of incomplete abortion in public hospitals showed that the majority of evacuation procedures were done with sharp curettage as well as general anaesthesia or sedation.

Finally, when women have serious complications from unsafe abortion they may also have trouble accessing appropriate and timely treatment.[33] In most low-resource countries, only tertiary-level facilities have the resources and skilled providers necessary to manage complications such as sepsis and uterine perforation. Therefore, the majority of women at risk of such complications are miles from treatment. Even when women with serious complications reach a tertiary facility, there is no guarantee that the providers will have the necessary training and resources to manage the complication.

Economic and geographic barriers

Poverty is associated with women's inability to access safe abortion services. Two studies, one in Nigeria[34] and one in Tanzania,[35] found that poor women were more than twice as likely to seek abortion services from non-professional providers. Poor women seek recourse to unsafe abortion because they are less likely to be educated, to know their rights under the law and to have the resources to pay for safe services. Additionally, women who are poor have difficulty paying for the travel that is usually required to access services, even unsafe services. Where women work or are primary caregivers, inability to afford the time to seek services is an additional barrier. Moreover, the time it might take a poor women to raise the funds for an abortion further delays the procedure, which becomes riskier with advancing gestational age. Poor women are also more likely to live in countries where abortion is restricted and, thus, where safe services are hard to find.

Ironically, poor women are willing and do pay significant sums of money for services, regardless of safety. A study in one of the poorest districts in Thailand[36] showed that women paid one to two months' salary for an unsafe abortion. In contrast, safe procedures such as manual vacuum aspiration or medical abortion could be provided for far lower cost, if providers were trained, if services were accessible, and if women were knowledgeable about the safety and accessibility of those procedures. Again, this reality highlights the benefit of introducing these simple technologies at all levels of the healthcare system. The cost is far less than developing higher order surgical services or services for managing obstetric trauma and, therefore, the benefit can be more widely shared.

Whether a woman lives in an urban or rural setting is also predictive of access to safe abortion. For example, a study in India[37] demonstrated that women in the rural areas of Uttar Pradesh rarely seek services for abortion complications in secondary or tertiary facilities; rather, they typically obtain care at the village level, where there are no doctors and few skilled healthcare providers. Several factors were found to contribute to this pattern of healthcare-seeking:

- women believed the local providers to be skilled
- few women were willing to expose themselves to the perceived risk of seeking care at referral facilities
- women were unlikely to have resources to seek higher level care.

An additional contributing factor was that rural providers did not necessarily refer women to higher level care when indicated. This research demonstrates that the situation of rural women, the majority of them poor, can prolong resolution of complications, worsen the outcome and increase the cost to women. The study highlights the need to develop linkages between village-level (primary) care facilities and higher level facilities. It also suggests that providers who are less skilled should receive training and women should be educated on how to manage abortion and its complications.

Cultural constraints

Provider

Physicians play a critical role in expanding the accessibility and availability of safe abortion, both where legal and where restricted. Opinions, knowledge and training affect providers' willingness to provide abortion services and their ability to perform high-quality procedures. A 2001–02 survey of Brazilian obstetricians and gynaecologists[38] demonstrated that confusion and misperception were widespread about the legal indications for abortion. Surveys of providers in countries with similar restrictions, such as Nigeria,[39] show comparable results. Moreover, where knowledge is low and the legal environment highly restrictive, providers are more likely to use substandard methods and thus to cause more serious complications.[13,35]

Even in countries where abortion is legally permitted, physicians act as gatekeepers for abortion provision. Since the rise of medicine as a profession, healthcare services by non-physicians, including abortion practice, have been constrained globally. Owing largely to economic and health worker constraints, many countries and localities have had to rethink such laws and policies restricting practice by non-physician health providers. Yet despite the expanding role of mid-level providers and community health workers in the delivery of health services generally, in many, if not most, countries, physicians remain the only providers allowed to perform abortions.

Women's status in society

Unsafe abortion is perpetuated principally by ideologies and power dynamics that undermine women's right to life and health. These ideologies and dynamics shape policies concerning contraceptives, abortion, sexuality education and, most importantly, women's ability to make independent choices. In patriarchal structures, which are predominant in the low-resource countries of Africa, Latin American and Asia, the male norm drives policies and the distribution of resources. Thus, the female perspective is absent and needs rooted in the women's experiences are not priority areas for law and policy. In this manner, women become second-class citizens – either by law or in reality – and, practically speaking, their diminished status contributes directly to low levels of contraceptive use and high levels of unwanted pregnancy and unsafe abortion. While liberalisation of abortion laws and scaling up contraceptive access is an important step to reversing the impact of unsafe abortion, it cannot be reduced sustainably without the inclusion of women's voices in public decision making.

Stigma

In most places, especially where unsafe abortion is most common, abortion is highly stigmatised. As a result, women do not talk about their experiences: they seek services without good advice, and, when they experience complications, they may delay seeking treatment. Providers also face stigma and either do not share their experiences in providing abortion or shy away from providing it altogether. In addition, because people do not talk openly about abortion, misinformation is rampant. For example, women who self-induce abortion often use ineffective methods, such as herbal remedies, because they are misinformed about the best way to induce an abortion. Added to the desperation felt by women with unwanted pregnancies, misinformation can cause women to expose themselves to unnecessary risk as a result of unsafe abortion. These contributing factors affect poor and uneducated women disproportionately.

Strategy priorities to reduce the impact of unsafe abortion

Liberalise laws and policies currently restricting abortion provision

Restrictive abortion laws contribute directly to the pandemic of unsafe abortion and thus liberalisation is imperative to improving this situation. While it is possible to mitigate the impact of unsafe abortion in legally restricted environments by improving post-abortion care, such efforts are unduly burdened, costly and inefficient compared with the high impact of making services legal first and then accessible. Indeed, efforts to 'mop up' the effects of unsafe abortion – by expanding post-abortion care programmes – fail to address the most severe and costly complications, as women suffering those consequences rarely reach services. Even when such women manage to reach services, they usually require interventions that are far beyond the scope of basic post-abortion care services. Additionally, expanding post-abortion care will do nothing to address the irreducible need for safe services. Safety valves sometimes exist in places where abortion is legally restricted, allowing some women access to safe but illegal procedures or high-quality post-abortion care. These safety valves are not sufficient. More importantly, as a matter of public policy, reliance on informal mechanisms to mitigate unsafe abortion ensures that inequalities become further entrenched, as these services tend to be available disproportionately to the wealthy and well-educated.

Public health and human rights arguments for liberalisation or decriminalisation of abortion can help to marshal the necessary political will for change. Although not ideal, liberalisation in steps may be the best and most feasible approach in some environments. Even where consensus for abortion on request is lacking and would be difficult to achieve immediately, consensus on abortion for specific indications could result in more liberal laws more swiftly and, in turn, more quickly improve access to safe services.

Scale up the availability of safe and appropriate services

Scaling up health services, including through decentralisation of systems from tertiary to primary levels, has been a critical element of the MDG initiative. Nevertheless, abortion services in many settings fall far behind the norms, policies and guidelines established by international treaties, national laws, professional associations and, in some cases, even ministries of health. Both abortion and post-abortion services have been inadequately integrated into comprehensive efforts to improve maternal health care. To this end, reducing the impact of unsafe abortion will require a significant investment of resources. Important questions remain as to how to achieve better services and to improve resource allocation, including how to ensure that providers are trained, that women are knowledgeable and that the safe, appropriate services can be accessed, even where legally restricted. Generally speaking, there is a need for more trained providers, more points-of-service and more cost-effective means of delivering those services. To achieve these goals will require training and educating providers on modern abortion practice and its complications. Ensuring the use of appropriate technologies can improve services, expand access and save money. The following are priorities for scaling up the delivery of safe services:

1. replace first-trimester dilatation and curettage with manual or electric vacuum aspiration or mifepristone–misoprostol medical abortion, as appropriate

2. replace outmoded second-trimester procedures with dilatation and evacuation or mifepristone–misoprostol medical abortion, as appropriate

3. implement medical abortion services more widely, including replacing a large percentage of early surgical abortions with medical abortions, especially where physicians and surgical services are lacking

4. simplify surgical services, by reducing or eliminating the use of general anaesthesia

5. decentralise services to outpatient and primary care settings

6. train providers at all levels, most importantly, mid-level providers

7. improve post-abortion care by upgrading clinical care (including misoprostol) and expanding access (including by decentralisation and use of mid-level providers or community health workers)

8. provide integrated comprehensive contraceptive and family planning services.

Medical abortion service alternatives

Expanding the implementation of medical alternatives to surgery must be a critical aspect of future interventions aimed at reducing the impact of unsafe abortion. These methods are highly safe and effective means of delivering both abortion and post-abortion care services. Additionally, they are cost-effective, in large part because services can be provided by a range of less-skilled health professionals and because they require less infrastructure to deliver.

Misoprostol – a synthetic analogue of the E_1 class of prostaglandins, a group of chemicals occurring naturally in the human body – has been invaluable in the development of such non-surgical alternatives. The stability of misoprostol at room temperature and its low cost make it an ideal treatment in low-resource settings. It is not surprising, therefore, that misoprostol is an essential component of all commonly used medical abortion regimens and has been recommended for abortion induction both as a standalone method and in combination with other medications, such as mifepristone or methotrexate.

The combined use of mifepristone and misoprostol has become the 'gold standard' for abortion induction up to 9 weeks' amenorrhoea and has been approved in over 40 countries.[40] Regimens of mifepristone (200 mg) followed by oral, buccal, sublingual or vaginal misoprostol (400–800 μg) are 92–99% effective.[41] Mifepristone in combination with misoprostol has also been recommended by the Royal College of Obstetricians and Gynaecologists for late first-trimester abortion.[42] In the second trimester, mifepristone in combination with misoprostol has been shown to be highly effective at inducing abortion and is the standard of care in many jurisdictions. However, while combined mifepristone–misoprostol regimens should be considered as first-line treatments, methotrexate–misoprostol or misoprostol-alone regimens may be preferable in some delivery settings and to some women because they may be easier to use and/or less costly. Furthermore, in many jurisdictions, mifepristone is not available. In the first trimester, the use of misoprostol-alone for pregnancy termination is 80–90% effective among women up to 8 weeks' amenorrhoea. Methotrexate can be used in combination with misoprostol up to 8 weeks' amenorrhoea, with reported success rates of 85–95%. The reported success of second-trimester abortion with misoprostol-alone varies widely by regimen and has been reported to be as high as 95% and as low as 40%.[41]

Additionally, misoprostol treatment for incomplete abortion could revolutionise post-abortion care. Until recently, the only available treatment for incomplete abortion was dilatation and curettage, which was then replaced by the equally effective but cheaper and safer manual vacuum aspiration. Unfortunately, manual vacuum aspiration is not always available in low-resource settings, because it requires special equipment and training for use. Furthermore, surgical methods generally have increased risks associated with instrumentation of the uterus: infection, cervical tears, uterine perforation, bleeding and reactions to anaesthesia, among others. In low-resource settings, the highest risk of infection with miscarriage occurs as a result of uterine instrumentation rather than the failure to evacuate the products of conception promptly.

More than a dozen randomised or comparative trials showed that misoprostol has a success rate of 71–100% for treatment of incomplete abortion and miscarriage.[41] Infrequent complications reported in over 20 publications documenting use over 2000 women show it is also highly safe. Moreover, in 2009, WHO added misoprostol for treatment of incomplete abortion to its Essential Medicines List, recommending a single-dose regimen of either 400 μg sublingual or 600 μg oral misoprostol.[43]

Designing effective service-based interventions where abortion is legally restricted

Legal restrictions to abortion complicate the issue of whether and how to train providers and educate women, as in some places such activities may put educators and advocates in legal peril. However, successful programmes have been developed to increase the safety of abortion provided in illegal settings. In such settings, interventions to update medical education about unsafe abortion, new technologies, family planning and reduction of the stigma of abortion may be the most effective means of addressing the problem of access to safe services.

Two novel programmes have been developed recently, one involving telemedicine and the other a harm-reduction approach. Both show promise in more effectively getting at the heart of the problem of unsafe abortion in legally restricted environments. 'Women on Web' provides medical abortion information via the internet (www. womenonweb.org) and services for women up to 9 weeks pregnant via telemedicine. This novel method of delivering accurate information and good services provides a safety net for women who would otherwise resort to riskier procedures. Women are educated on eligibility criteria and contraindications to the procedure, asked to seek a medical evaluation from a doctor to confirm they are eligible, and, if eligible, are sent the required medication. They are asked to follow up via the internet and educated on when to seek care for possible complications. The outcomes of this service after a year are comparable to other services – more than three-quarters sought follow-up care and 6.8% of those reported needing an aspiration procedure.[44]

In Uruguay, Iniciativas Sanitarias has taken a unique approach to reducing the harm caused by unsafe abortion in a legally restrictive environment.[45] With the understanding that, in the absence of legal and policy change, women will continue to expose themselves to risk by seeking unsafe abortions, this initiative strives to provide women who are determined to abort with ready access to reliable information and compassionate counselling before and after their attempts to seek an illegal abortion. The programme emphasises the use of scientific information and preabortion counselling to mitigate the risks of unsafe abortion. In the year after the programme was implemented in one hospital, there were no maternal deaths reported, compared with four over the 3 years preceding this programme; the number of women with post-abortion sepsis also decreased.[46] This initiative, which began in one hospital, is now being expanded throughout Uruguay.

Close the information gap

Abortion provider shortages are acute; geographically and socially marginalised women continue to seek recourse to unsafe abortion services; services remain under-resourced; and legal and policy reform have failed to make inroads. Information is an essential element to reversing all of these trends, yet it remains inadequate or inadequately used. Several factors contribute to the information gap, and programmatic and policy development will have limited success if they fail to address this issue.

To close the existing gap in information, we must facilitate open scientific exchange, stimulate public discourse and education, and improve provider training and patient education. Information must be accurate and widely available. Appropriate and up-to-date information is critical to improving the quality of abortion services. Leaders in the field can facilitate a culture of open scientific interchange, which is largely prohibited where abortion is legally restricted or highly stigmatised and where, as a result, misinformation tends to be pervasive. Additionally, attention must be paid to getting new technologies and other innovations out to where they are most critically needed. Where open interchange is lacking, innovations may not be adequately disseminated.

Conclusion

MDG 5 is a call to improve the health of women, primarily by reducing maternal mortality and ensuring universal access to contraception. Before that, the International Conference on Population and Development in Cairo in 1994 and the Fourth World Conference on Women in Beijing in 1995 recognised the health impact of unsafe abortion and the moral and public health imperative to address it. Nevertheless, more than a decade later, the problem of unsafe abortion persists at levels that are virtually unchanged. This trend highlights the reality that unsafe abortion will continue to be a major public health problem if not addressed with more direct and comprehensive interventions. Thus, we emphasise the responsibility of all health professionals, including public health professionals and researchers, for the provision of safe, high-quality abortion services. Further, we highlight the imperative of education – through the engagement of civil society – to ensure that the general public is aware of abortion services permitted by law and is able to access them. Above all, the value of sustainable access to high-quality services and appropriate technologies cannot be overestimated.

References

1. McNaughton Reyes HL, Hord CE, Mitchell EM, Blandon MM. Invoking health and human rights to ensure access to legal abortion: the case of a nine-year-old girl from Nicaragua. *Health Hum Rights* 2006;9:62–86.
2. Grimes S. Legal, safe, and rare? *Lancet* 2007;370:1309.
3. Sedgh G, Henshaw S, Singh S, Ahman E, Shah IH. Induced abortion: estimated rates and trends worldwide. *Lancet* 2007;370:1338–45.
4. World Health Organization, *The Prevention and Management of Unsafe Abortion*. Geneva: WHO; 2003.

5.   World Health Organization. *Unsafe Abortion: Global and Regional Estimates of the Incidence of Unsafe Abortion and Associated Mortality in 2003.* Geneva: WHO; 2007.

6.   Grimes DA, Benson J, Singh S, Romero M, Ganatra B, Okonofua FE, *et al.* Unsafe abortion: the preventable pandemic. *Lancet* 2006;368:1908–19.

7.   Khan KS, Wojdyla D, Say L, Gülmezoglu AM, Van Look PF. WHO analysis of causes of maternal death: a systematic review. *Lancet* 2006;367:1066–74.

8.   World Health Organization. *Safe Abortion: Technical and Policy Guidance for Health Systems.* Geneva: WHO; 2003.

9.   Singh S. Hospital admissions resulting from unsafe abortion: estimates from 13 developing countries. *Lancet* 2006;368:1887–92.

10.   Fu H, Darroch JE, Henshaw SK, Kolb E. Measuring the extent of abortion underreporting in the 1995 National Survey of Family Growth. *Fam Plann Perspect* 1998;30:128–33,138.

11.   Vlassoff M, Walker D, Shearer J, Newlands D, Singh S. Estimates of health care system costs of unsafe abortion in Africa and Latin America. *Int Perspect Sex Reprod Health* 2009;35:114–21.

12.   Johnston HB, Gallo MF, Benson J. Reducing the costs to health systems of unsafe abortion: a comparison of four strategies. *J Fam Plann Reprod Health Care* 2007;33:250–7.

13.   Henshaw SK, Adewole I, Singh S, Bankole A, Oye-Adeniran B, Hussain R. Severity and cost of unsafe abortion complications treated in Nigerian hospitals. *Int Fam Plan Perspect* 2008;34:40–50.

14.   Fonseca W, Misago C, Fernandes L, Correia L, Silveira D. [Use of manual vacuum aspiration in reducing cost and duration of hospitalization due to incomplete abortion in an urban area of northeastern Brazil]. *Rev Saude Publica* 1997;31:472–8. Portuguese.

15.   Hu D, Grossman D, Levin C, Blanchard K, Goldie SJ. Cost-effectiveness analysis of alternative first-trimester pregnancy termination strategies in Mexico City. *BJOG* 2009;116:768–79.

16.   Mpangile GS, Leshabari MT, Kihwele DJ. Induced abortion in Dar es Salaam, Tanzania: the plight of adolescents. In: Mundigo AI, Indriso C, editors. *Abortion in the Developing World.* New Delhi: World Health Organization; 1999. p. 387–403.

17.   Levin C, Grossman D, Berdichevsky K, Diaz C, Aracena B, Garcia SG, *et al.* Exploring the costs and economic consequences of unsafe abortion in Mexico City before legalisation. *Reprod Health Matters* 2009;17:120–32.

18.   Guttmacher Institute. *Sharing Responsibilities: Women, Society and Abortion Worldwide.* New York: Guttmacher Institute; 1999.

19.   Vlassoff M, Singh S, Darroch JE, Carbone E, Bernstein S. *Assessing Costs and Benefits of Sexual and Reproductive Health Interventions.* Occasional report no. 11. New York: Guttmacher Institute; 2004.

20.   Safe-Motherhood Inter-Agency Group. *Maternal Health: A Vital Social and Economic Investment.* New York: Family Care International; 1998.

21.   Singh S, Wulf D, Hussain R, Bankole A, Sedgh G. *Abortion Worldwide: A Decade of Uneven Progress.* New York: Guttmacher Institute; 2009.

22.   Bankole A, Singh S, Vlassoff M, Woog V. Estimating the cost of post-abortion care in Nigeria: a case study. In: Lule E, Singh S, and Chowdhury SA, editors. *Fertility Regulation Behaviors and Their Costs: Contraception and Unintended Pregnancies in Africa and Eastern Europe & Central Asia.* Washington, DC: World Bank; 2007. p. 65–92.

23.   United Nations Population Fund (UNFPA). *Financing the ICPD Programme of Action: Data for 2005; Estimates for 2007.* New York: UNFPA; 2008.

24.   Bongaarts J, Westoff CF. The potential role of contraception in reducing abortion. *Stud Fam Plann* 2000, 31:193–202.

25.   Åhman E, Shah IH. Contraceptive use, fertility, and unsafe abortion in developing countries. *Eur J Contr Reprod Health Care* 2006;11:126–31.

26.   United Nations Population Division, Department of Economic and Social Affairs. *World Abortion Policies; 2007.* New York: United Nations; 2007.

27.   Bateman C. Maternal mortalities 90% down as legal TOPs more than triple. *S Afr Med J* 2007;97:1238–42.

28.   Jewkes RJ, Brown HC, Dickson-Tetteh K, Levin J, Rees H. Prevalence of morbidity associated with abortion before and after legalisation in South Africa. *BMJ* 2002;324:1252–3.

29.   Hirve SS. Abortion law, policy and services in India: a critical review. *Reprod Health Matters* 2004;12(24 Suppl):114–21.

30. Duggal R, Barge S. *Abortion Services in India: Report of a Multicentric Enquiry. Abortion Assessment Project – India*. Mumbai: CEHAT and HealthWatch; 2004.

31. Guttmacher Institute. *Abortion: Worldwide Levels and Trends*. New York: Guttmacher Institute; 2007.

32. Brown HC, Jewkes R, Levin J, Dickson-Tetteh K, Rees H. Management of incomplete abortion in South African hospitals. *BJOG* 2003:110:371–7.

33. Kayongo M, Rubardt M, Butera J, Abdullah M, Mboninyibuka D, Madili M. Making EmOC a reality – CARE's experiences in areas of high maternal mortality in Africa. *Int J Gynaecol Obstet* 2006;92:308–19.

34. Bankole A, Sedgh G, Oye-Adeniran B A, Adewole I F, Hussain R, Singh S. Abortion-seeking behaviour among Nigerian women. *J Biosoc Sci* 2008;40:247–68.

35. Rasch V, Kipingili R. Unsafe abortion in urban and rural Tanzania: method, provider and consequences. *Trop Med Int Health* 2009;14:1128–33.

36. Whittaker A. Reproducing inequalities: abortion policy and practice in Thailand. *Women Health* 2002;35:101–19.

37. Johnston HB, Ved R, Lyall N, Agarwal K. Where do rural women obtain postabortion care? The case of Uttar Pradesh, India. *Int Fam Plan Perspect* 2003;29:182–7.

38. Goldman LA, Garcia SG, Diaz J, Yam EA, Brazilian obstetrician-gynaecologists and abortion: a survey of knowledge, opinions and practices. *Reprod Health* 2005;2:10.

39. Okonofua FE, Shittu SO, Oronsaye F, Ogunsakin D, Ogbomwan S, Zayyan M. Attitudes and practices of private medical providers towards family planning and abortion services in Nigeria. *Acta Obstet Gynecol Scand* 2005;84:270–80.

40. Gynuity Health Projects. *Map of Mifepristone Approval*. New York: Gynuity Health Projects; 2008.

41. Clark W, Shannon C, Winikoff B. Misoprostol for uterine evacuation in induced abortion and pregnancy failure. *Expert Rev Obstet Gynecol* 2007;2:67–108.

42. Royal College of Obstetricians and Gynaecologists. *Care of Women Requesting Induced Abortion*. London, RCOG Press; 2004.

43. Gynuity Health Projects. *Proposal for the Inclusion of Misoprostol in the WHO list of Essential Medicines*. New York: Gynuity Health Projects; 2009.

44. Gomperts RJ, Jelinska K, Davies S, Gemzell-Danielsson K, Kleiverda G. Using telemedicine for termination of pregnancy with mifepristone and misoprostol in settings where there is no access to safe services. *BJOG* 2008;115:1171–5.

45. Briozzo L,editor. *Iniciativas Sanitarias Contra el Aborto Provocado en Condiciones de Riesgo*. Montevideo: ARENA; 2007.

46. Faúndes A, Rao K, Briozzo L. Right to protection from unsafe abortion and postabortion care. *Int J Gynaecol Obstet* 2009;106:164–7.

Chapter 10
HIV and tuberculosis

James McIntyre

HIV, tuberculosis and the Millennium Development Goals

An estimated 33 million people worldwide were living with HIV at the end of 2007, almost half of whom were women, with 2.7 million new HIV infections and 2 million HIV-related deaths in that year. Two-thirds of people living with HIV are in sub-Saharan Africa, where around 60% of infections are in women, and where 75% of AIDS-related deaths occur. The southern African sub-region is the most severely affected, where 35% of the global HIV infections and 38% of AIDS deaths occurred in 2007.[1] Worldwide, 45% of the estimated 2.7 million new infections annually occur in young people aged 15–24 years, an age group in which young girls are particularly susceptible to infection and in which pregnancy is common. The number of children younger than 15 years living with HIV has continued to increase from 1.6 million in 2001 to 2.0 million in 2007. While new infections in children have shown some decline with increased access to strategies to prevent mother-to-child transmission, an estimated 370 000 children younger than 15 years still became infected with HIV in 2007. This remains a predominantly African problem, with 90% of infections and over 90% of an estimated 270 000 HIV-related deaths in the region in 2007.[1,2]

HIV is the strongest link between the Millennium Development Goals (MDGs) 4, 5 and 6. A response to the global HIV/AIDS pandemic is in itself a major component of the MDGs, with MDG 6 specifically addressing the HIV epidemic. MDG 6 has targets of achieving universal access to treatment for HIV/AIDS by 2010 and of halting and reversing the spread of HIV/AIDS by 2015.[3] Such is the impact of HIV on maternal and child mortality, especially in Africa, that an effective and successful response to HIV is essential to the achievement of MDGs 4 and 5.

While progress towards the MDGs is being made in some sectors and some regions, African countries in general are not on track to meet MDGs 4, 5 and 6 on reducing child mortality, improving maternal health and combating infectious disease, respectively.[3,4] This is largely due to the impact of HIV and AIDS. Although the effective use of anti-retrovirals for the prevention of mother-to-child transmission has made HIV infection in children a rare event in well-resourced settings, AIDS continues to be a significant cause of child mortality in high HIV prevalence settings, killing an estimated 270 000 HIV-infected children younger than 15 years in 2007.[1] Nearly half of all deaths of children under the age of 5 years occur in sub-Saharan Africa[5] and, in the highest prevalence countries in southern Africa, HIV is the underlying reason for more than one-third of all under-five deaths.[6] MDG6 sets targets to halt and begin to reverse the spread of HIV/AIDS by 2015, and to achieve universal access to treatment for HIV/AIDS for all those who need it by 2010.[3] Most countries are not on track to achieve this, despite remarkable progress in providing anti-retroviral treatment over the past 5 years.[5,7] Significant progress has been made in expanding access to anti-retroviral treatment for those in need, with over 3 million people now receiving anti-retroviral treatment worldwide.[8] By the end of 2008, an estimated 4 million people were receiving anti-retroviral therapy in low- and middle-income countries. This global number being treated rose by over 1 million during 2008 and represents a ten-fold increase from the numbers being treated 5 years previously, largely owing to financial support from the Global Fund to Fight AIDS, Tuberculosis and Malaria (the Global Fund) and the United States President's Emergency Plan for AIDS Relief (PEPFAR). Despite these dramatic improvements in access to care, fewer than half of the estimated 9.5 million people in need of treatment are receiving anti-retrovirals.[8,9]

Tuberculosis and HIV

HIV and tuberculosis (TB) form a lethal combination, with each infection increasing the consequences of the other. The adverse effects of HIV and TB overlap most in the least-resourced areas of the world, with 95% of people with TB and 98% of deaths due to TB occurring in the third of the world's population living in resource-limited settings.[10-12] HIV infection accounts for much of the increased global incidence of TB seen over the past two decades. The World Health Organization (WHO) estimated in 2007 that there were an estimated total of 13.7 million people with TB (206 per 100 000 population). Of these, 9.27 million were new cases of TB occurring in 2007, increasing from 9.24 million cases in 2006 and from only 6.6 million cases in 1990. An estimated 1.37 million (15%) of the TB infections were in HIV-positive people; 79% of these HIV-positive cases were in the African region and 11% were in the South East Asia region. The deadly synergy between TB and HIV is reflected in death rates. There were an estimated 1.77 million deaths (including 456 000 people with HIV) in 2007, making TB one of the major global causes of death. One-quarter of the estimated 2 million HIV deaths were associated with TB co-infection.[13] MDG6 sets a goal to have halted by 2015 and begun to reverse the incidence TB. Globally, TB incidence rates have stabilised, except in Africa and Eastern Europe, and regions other than these are on track to reach the MDG goals of halving TB prevalence and deaths by 2015. The multifaceted 'Stop TB' strategy of WHO is helping to achieve these TB reduction goals and incorporates six major components for TB services:[13]

- the expansion and enhancement of high-quality directly observed therapy (DOTS)
- addressing the link between HIV and TB, multi-drug-resistant TB and the needs of poor and vulnerable populations
- contributing to health systems strengthening based on primary health care
- engaging all service providers
- empowering people with TB and communities through partnership
- enabling and promoting research.

Saving children

MDG4 targets a reduction by two-thirds between 1990 and 2015 in the under-five mortality rate.[3] While HIV infections, and their consequences, are now rare events in well-resourced settings, HIV remains a major contributor to child mortality in areas of high prevalence, especially in Africa. The Joint United Nations Programme on HIV/AIDS (UNAIDS) estimates that around 370 000 children were newly infected with HIV in 2008, most through mother-to-child transmission and 90% in sub-Saharan Africa.[1] The majority of these infections occur in low-resource settings with high HIV seroprevalence rates, where antenatal care is limited, mothers are often not diagnosed until late in pregnancy, anti-retroviral access is less widespread and replacement feeding of infants of HIV-infected mothers is infrequent. HIV causes substantial mortality in infected infants in low-resource settings, and mortality in HIV-exposed but uninfected infants is also higher than in HIV-unexposed infants.[14,15]

In the past 15 years, mother-to-child HIV transmission rates in well-resourced countries have dropped to 1–2%,[16,17] leading to dramatic reductions in HIV-related child morbidity and mortality. These low transmission rates are a result of the availability and use of continuing combination anti-retroviral therapy in pregnancy for those women who require it and the use of combination anti-retroviral prophylaxis through the pregnancy for those with higher CD4+ cell counts, together with the use of replacement feeding. Estimates of transmission in low-resource settings without access to this level of care are much higher, with an estimated average rate of 26% in the 33 most affected countries – more than ten-fold more than the rates in better-resourced settings.[7] These infection rates, of approximately one child infected every second day in the USA, one every day in Europe, two a week in Asia and close to 1000 a day in Africa, in turn impact adversely on child mortality.[7,18]

The 2006 WHO guidelines[19] for the prevention of mother-to-child transmission (PMTCT) of HIV lay out an international consensus for low-resource settings. This includes the provision of anti-retroviral therapy for pregnant women who require treatment for their own health, the provision of an appropriate anti-retroviral prophylactic regimen to reduce the risk of transmission to the infants of mothers for those who do not yet need continuing treatment, and the appropriate adaptation of infant feeding practices, depending on the circumstances of the HIV-positive woman. Anti-retroviral treatment should be provided for pregnant women who meet the clinical or immunological criteria for treatment in adults, including symptoms of advanced HIV disease or CD4+ cell counts below 350/mm³. For women who do not yet need to start anti-retrovirals, a prophylactic anti-retroviral regimen must be provided to reduce the risk of transmission to their infants. The recommended first-line regimen for these women is zidovudine from 28 weeks of pregnancy, intrapartum nevirapine and 1 week of zidovudine and lamivudine to mothers postnatally, with single-dose nevirapine and a week of zidovudine to infants. This regimen can reduce transmission rates to less than 5% in non-breastfed infants.[20] Substantial data from Africa have shown the efficacy of short-course anti-retroviral regimens in these settings.[21,22] The use of more complex combination anti-retroviral prophylaxis is likely to increase in these settings as anti-retroviral treatment access improves. The use of PMTCT regimens to reduce mother-to-child transmission has been estimated to have averted over 30 000 infections in infants in 2004 and 2005, and this figure is likely to be considerably higher with the increased access to PMTCT interventions in the past 5 years.[23]

Prevention of transmission through breast milk remains an important issue in reducing the number of HIV-infected infants as this route of transmission contributes significantly to infant HIV infection, with about 150 000 new infant infections every year occurring through breastfeeding, mainly in low-resource settings.[24] WHO has recommended that HIV-infected women should avoid breastfeeding where replacement feeding (the use of milk formula rather than breast milk) is 'acceptable, feasible, affordable, sustainable and safe' (the AFASS criteria).[19] The reality is that this is not possible for many women in the poorest settings, where the use of milk formula carries a significant risk of morbidity and mortality to the baby, mainly through diarrhoeal and respiratory infections.[25,26] In such settings, exclusive breastfeeding carries a lower risk of HIV transmission than mixed feeding (where mothers give other foods in addition to breast milk) and is the recommended option.[27,28]

Anti-retroviral prophylaxis through the breastfeeding period, either to mother or child, has been suggested as a mechanism to retain the benefits of breastfeeding while reducing the risk of transmission. The Post-Exposure Prophylaxis of Infant (PEPI) study in Malawi showed that an extended 14-week course of nevirapine, with or without added zidovudine, commenced at birth, in HIV-exposed infants reduced the risk of HIV transmission by as much as 50% at 9 months compared with the standard regimen of single-dose nevirapine and 1 week of zidovudine.[29] The benefit of this 14-week dosing was, however, lost beyond 12 months where mothers continued to breastfeed. The Six Week Extended-Dose Nevirapine (SWEN) study, conducted in Ethiopia, India and Uganda, showed that there was a significant difference in HIV transmission rates at 6 weeks between HIV-exposed infants who received a single postpartum dose of nevirapine and those who received an extended regimen of daily nevirapine for 6 weeks. At 6 weeks of age, 5.27% of children in the single-dose group and 2.53% in the extended-dose group were HIV positive (relative risk [RR] 0.54; 95% CI 0.34–0.85; $P = 0.009$).[30] However, at 6 months the difference was not significant. Further research on longer infant prophylaxis will provide more necessary information on this strategy.[31]

Observational studies investigating the use of combination anti-retroviral therapy in breastfeeding women who do not yet require treatment for their own health also suggest that this could reduce breast milk transmission.[32–34] Concerns remain about the feasibility of such an approach and the impact of prolonged use of combination anti-retroviral therapy for prophylaxis and subsequent treatment interruption after cessation of breastfeeding. This is based on the findings from other studies that anti-retroviral treatment interruption in individuals with high CD4+ cell counts appears to be associated with an increased risk of HIV disease progression and death.[35] Recommendations about the prophylactic use of combination anti-retroviral therapy for mothers during breastfeeding are yet to be made but this area holds promise for further reductions in HIV infection in infants by minimising viral load during this period.

Early diagnosis of HIV infection in infants is an essential component of care. Without anti-retroviral treatment, HIV progression in children may be very rapid, with early death.[36–38] The Children with HIV Early Antiretroviral Therapy (CHER) study in South Africa[39] demonstrated that, with early diagnosis of HIV-infected infants, immediate initiation of anti-retroviral treatment resulted in a 75% reduction in mortality compared with deferring treatment until the children reached clinical or immunological criteria for treatment. These results have led to a recommendation from WHO[40] to treat all HIV-infected infants in the first year of life, and implementation of this policy would save many children's lives. The success of such a policy also depends on increasing access to polymerase chain reaction (PCR) testing for exposed infants, and strategies such as collection of dried blood spot samples can assist in doing this in low-resource settings.

Saving mothers

MDG 5 seeks to reduce by three-quarters the level of maternal mortality by 2015. Of all the MDGs, the least progress has been made on MDG 5, with the maternal mortality ratio (MMR) declining by less than 1% per year between 1990 and 2005.[5] This lack of progress is due to many factors, not least the lack of political will to address the issue of women's health.

Up to 10 000 women still die every week in developing countries from treatable complications of pregnancy and childbirth. Although most regions are not on track to meet MDG 5, sub-Saharan Africa is the worst, with the highest MMR at 900 deaths per 100 000 live births, a figure 20 times higher than in Europe. This represents the biggest differential on any health indicator between well-resourced and poorly resourced settings. Maternal deaths can be reduced by improving access to skilled personnel for delivery, providing antenatal care and reducing the number of unplanned pregnancies,[5] but AIDS also needs to be addressed to have a major impact on the rates in Africa.

AIDS and HIV infection are major contributing factors to maternal mortality in high HIV prevalence areas, especially in sub-Saharan Africa.[41] The worst-affected region for maternal mortality is also the region with the highest HIV prevalence and largest effect of AIDS on mortality. The true contribution of HIV/AIDS to maternal mortality is difficult to measure accurately as the HIV status of pregnant women is not always known, and collected mortality data are likely to underestimate the role of HIV infection.[42,43] Even with this under-reporting of HIV, there is increasing evidence that HIV/AIDS-related maternal deaths have increased considerably, and AIDS has overtaken direct obstetric causes as the leading cause of maternal mortality in some African settings. HIV impacts on direct obstetric causes of maternal mortality by an associated increase in pregnancy complications such as anaemia, postpartum haemorrhage and puerperal sepsis. HIV is also a major indirect cause of maternal mortality by an increased susceptibility to opportunistic infections such as pneumonia, TB and malaria.[44,45] As the HIV epidemic matures in sub-Saharan Africa, more women become pregnant in the later stages of the disease and are more vulnerable to complications.

Data from several African countries have demonstrated the impact of HIV and AIDS on maternal mortality. Several studies from Africa and Asia in the 1990s demonstrated the increasing role of AIDS and related illnesses as causes of maternal mortality, with MMRs ranging from 400 to over 900 per 100 000 live births. In Zambia,[46] rates of maternal mortality increased eight-fold in the 1980s and 1990s, despite better obstetric services. Indirect causes of maternal mortality were responsible for 58% of deaths, with malaria and AIDS-related TB the most common of these. In the Rakai district of Uganda in the early 1990s,[47] maternal mortality was five times higher in HIV-positive women than HIV-negative women, reaching rates of over 1600 per 100 000 live births in the infected group. In Malawi and Zimbabwe,[48] pregnancy-related mortality has increased 1.9 and 2.5 times in parallel with the increasing AIDS epidemic, while in Brazzaville in the Congo,[49] AIDS-related deaths were the primary cause of death in mothers as early as 1993. In a Tanzanian district in the mid-1990s,[50] AIDS was the fourth highest cause of maternal mortality. In Durban, South Africa, between 1998 and 2004,[51] the most common cause of death related to HIV was WHO Stage 4 HIV disease, followed by pneumonia (bacterial and *Pneumocystis carinii* pneumonia), pregnancy-related sepsis and pulmonary tuberculosis.

Despite the much improved access to anti-retroviral treatment in many African countries, AIDS continues to be a leading cause of maternal mortality. Recent data from two centres in Kenya[52,53] and one in Uganda[54] have shown that HIV is becoming a major cause of maternal mortality and deaths in the first year postpartum. A study from nine hospitals in central Malawi over a 1-year period[55] showed that AIDS was a major cause of indirect maternal mortality (16.3%).

South Africa provides the most striking evidence for the impact of AIDS on maternal mortality. With very high prevalence rates in women of reproductive age, about 30% nationally, HIV is a major concern in pregnant women.[56] A national confidential enquiry into maternal deaths in South Africa was instituted in 1998. AIDS was the second most common cause of maternal death in 1998, accounting for 13% of all deaths.[57] In the years 1999–2001,[58] AIDS was the listed cause of death in 17% of cases, although this figure may be considerably underestimated as HIV status was known in only 36% of maternal deaths. By the 2002–04 triennial enquiry,[59] non-pregnancy-related infections were the most common cause of death, being responsible for 37.8% of deaths. AIDS was the single biggest cause of death at 20.1% of all deaths, higher than any direct obstetric cause. In the triennium 2005–07,[60] there was a 20% increase in the number of deaths reported compared with the previous 3-year period, and non-pregnancy-related infections, mainly AIDS, were responsible for 43.7% of deaths.

More evidence of the impact of HIV is provided in a 5-year review of maternal mortality at a tertiary level hospital in Johannesburg, South Africa.[61] In this setting, MMRs in HIV-infected women were 776 per 100 000 live births (95% CI 591–1000 per 100 000 live births) and 124 per 100 000 live births in HIV-uninfected women (95% CI 72–199 live births). This 6.2-fold increase was despite major increases in HIV testing of pregnant women and despite increased access to anti-retroviral therapy in the latter years of the survey.

Reducing HIV-related maternal mortality

Achieving MDG 5 requires concerted effort in sub-Saharan Africa to reduce the impact of HIV on pregnant women. This requires increased access to and uptake of HIV testing in antenatal services. The global coverage of PMTCT services has improved in recent years but remains suboptimal.[8] In 2008, an estimated 21% of pregnant women in low- and middle-income countries received an HIV test, showing a steady increase from 18% in 2007, and estimates of 16% in 2006 and 10% in 2004 and 2005.[9] This lack of testing is despite 105 of 123 countries reporting the implementation of provider-initiated testing and counselling in all or in some antenatal service sites. Programmes in several African countries have demonstrated that provider-initiated testing, where all pregnant women are routinely offered an HIV test, can dramatically increase the uptake of antenatal HIV testing.[12,62] Antenatal HIV testing in Botswana increased from 75% to 95% within 6 months of the introduction of routine provider-initiated testing.[63]

Identification of pregnant women who are infected with HIV allows both for appropriate strategies to prevent mother-to-child transmission and to provide appropriate care for the mother. Increased access to appropriate anti-retroviral therapy started in pregnancy could reverse the toll of HIV-related maternal mortality. All international guidelines[19,64,65] recommend that combination anti-retroviral therapy for HIV-infected pregnant women who need it for their own health should be started as soon as possible in pregnancy, to benefit the mother and because these women are also the group most likely to transmit HIV to their infants. The WHO guidelines,[19] in common with others, suggest that continuing anti-retroviral therapy should be initiated at a CD4+ count of less than $350/mm^3$, or late-stage clinical AIDS, where this is possible. If CD4+ testing is not available, as is the case in many resource-limited settings, clinical staging alone is used to determine when to start therapy. The increased provision of CD4+ counts for all HIV-infected pregnant women would greatly assist in guiding the provision of appropriate treatment, as there are better maternal and fetal outcomes if a CD4+ threshold of $350/mm^3$ is used for starting combination therapy in pregnancy. WHO reports that only around 34%% of HIV-infected pregnant women were assessed for their eligibility to receive anti-retroviral therapy, according to country level data in 2008, either clinically through a symptom assessment or immunologically by CD4+ count, although this had increased from 12% in 2007.[8,9] This lack of identification of women in need of treatment and care directly impacts on HIV-related maternal mortality.

HIV, TB and pregnancy

Tuberculosis is a leading infectious cause of death in women of reproductive age globally and the most common HIV-related opportunistic infection in resource-poor settings.[12,46,66–68]

Globally, the prevalence of TB is higher in adult men than women, but prevalence rates have risen in women in concert with the rising HIV epidemic. In sub-Saharan Africa, women of reproductive age have disproportionately higher rates, with TB prevalence rates 1.5- to two-fold higher than women aged over 44 years.[10] These women also have higher rates of progression from infection to disease than similarly aged men,[68,69] and 80% of TB mortality in women occurs in this age group.[11,35]

HIV and TB infections in pregnancy are independent risk factors for maternal mortality and concurrent infection is especially dangerous.[11,70] A South African study conducted in Durban[71] investigated 101 maternal deaths occurring in 50 518 deliveries. In this series, the MMR was 323 per 100 000 live births for HIV-infected mothers and 148 per 100 000 live births for HIV-negative mothers. The mortality rate for HIV and TB co-infection was 121 per 1000, three times that of TB without concurrent HIV infection, and 54% of maternal deaths due to TB were attributable to HIV infection. An increase in maternal mortality from TB was reported from Zambia in 1999[46] and these data showed that TB was the cause of one-quarter of non-obstetric-related maternal deaths, with most of these in women with HIV infections.

Strategies to reduce maternal mortality in settings with high prevalence of TB and HIV must include screening of all pregnant women for TB symptoms during antenatal care, consideration of preventive therapy for HIV-infected pregnant women after exclusion of active TB, treatment of active TB and links to local TB services for longer-term care.[10,11,68]

Maternal TB infection also places the newborn at risk. Mother-to-child transmission of TB can occur *in utero* (through haematogenous spread), intrapartum (through infected amniotic fluid or genital secretions) or postpartum (either through infectious respiratory secretions from the mother or ingestion of infected milk in the presence of a TB breast abscess).[72,73] While data for the risk of transmission are few, the transmission rate in a study in Durban[74] was 15%, with higher risk associated with late diagnosis of TB in the mother and pulmonary TB compared with extra-pulmonary manifestations. An Indian study[75] showed transmission of 9% in pregnant women with incident TB. Maternal TB infections during pregnancy have been associated with increases in preterm birth and abortion rates. Congenital TB infection has high mortality rates, of up to 38%, while postnatal TB infection is associated with rapidly progressive and fatal disease.[73] In Pune, India,[75] concurrent TB infection increased the risk of death by 2.2 times for HIV-infected women and 3.4 times for the infants of these women, compared with HIV-positive women without TB and their infants.

TB screening and active case finding

The identification and appropriate management of women infected with TB are central to reducing the risk of mortality and have wider benefits in reducing morbidity in families, communities and health facilities.[10,76] Although the development of new TB diagnostic technologies is a key area of need, relatively simple case-finding strategies can be very successful. In a study in Soweto, South Africa, lay counsellors screened pregnant women with HIV for TB symptoms using a simple 3-minute symptom-screening questionnaire. Of 370 women screened, 120 (32%) had symptoms and eight (2.1%) were diagnosed with active TB by sputum culture; all cases were sputum smear negative.[77] Another study in the same setting[78] used tuberculin skin tests (TST) to screen pregnant women for TB and active TB was found in 11% of those completing screening. TST has lower sensitivity in HIV-infected individuals, especially with low CD4+ counts, and requires additional visits and burden on the health services. New diagnostic technologies would assist greatly in simplifying screening. Antenatal services provide an underused opportunity to extend TB screening in both HIV-infected and -uninfected women.

Pregnant women with HIV must be clinically assessed for active TB disease and provided with multi-drug TB therapy if needed. In women in whom active TB has been excluded, isoniazid preventive therapy (IPT) should be considered.[79]

Reducing the impact of HIV

Reducing the impact of HIV on MDGs 4 and 5 requires a multifaceted approach to improve services and increase access to life-saving anti-retroviral therapy. An integrated and successful response to AIDS will have benefits far beyond control of the disease itself, with impact on child and maternal health. The focus on health services that has come about as a result of the increased push for anti-retroviral access in resource-limited settings has already helped to strengthen weak health service infrastructures and improving human capacity in these services, which will impact beyond AIDS care.[1] Examples of the collaborative linkage of maternal and neonatal health services with HIV/AIDS programmes have demonstrated that this is possible, even in very poorly resourced settings.

A reduction in HIV infections in children is still hampered by the low coverage of PMTCT services, despite extensive knowledge of successful strategies.[7,80] Coverage of anti-retroviral prophylaxis for pregnant women with HIV has increased and improved – from around 10% in 2004 to around 33% in 2007[8] – but two-thirds of women in need are still receiving nothing to reduce the risk of transmission of HIV to their children. Although WHO has recommended the more efficacious regimen of zidovudine with peripartum single-dose nevirapine since 2006, only around one-quarter of women with HIV in sub-Saharan Africa were reported to have received this in 2007, with 50% receiving single-dose nevirapine only and fewer than 10% receiving a triple-combination anti-retroviral regimen (there was some progress towards more use of combination regimens in 2008).[8,9]

WHO has recommended a four-pronged approach to preventing mother-to-child transmission of HIV:[81]

- the prevention of primary infections in mothers
- the provision of appropriate family planning
- the prevention of transmission during pregnancy
- the provision of care and treatment.

Integrating PMTCT services into existing health services and the innovative use of human resources and lay workers add to their sustainability and success.[82] The further involvement of men and communities in general in spreading awareness of and support for PMTCT services is equally important, as is better use of the opportunity to use these programmes as an entry point for care, not only for pregnant women but for their whole families.[83]

Conclusion

Although the expanded access to anti-retrovirals in low-resource, high HIV prevalence settings is already leading to an improvement in the health of women, more integration of treatment and PMTCT programmes with reproductive health services is needed to maximise these benefits. Equally, integration and strengthening of TB services is required, especially in Africa, if the MDG targets are to be met. More widespread implementation of the following will have the greatest impact:

- routine offering of HIV testing in all antenatal care services and appropriate anti-retroviral treatment and prophylaxis for all pregnant women with HIV
- early diagnosis of HIV infection in children, with immediate initiation of anti-retroviral treatment in all children with HIV under 1 year of age
- routine TB screening for both HIV-infected and-uninfected pregnant women in high TB prevalence areas.

HIV diagnosis and management and the prevention of transmission from mother to child remain central to achieving MDGs 4 and 5 and global action is required to ensure that these are provided.

References

1. UNAIDS. *AIDS Epidemic Update 2008*. Geneva: UNAIDS; 2008.
2. UNAIDS. *AIDS Outlook: World AIDS Day 2008*. UNAIDS/08.36E. Geneva: UNAIDS; 2008.
3. United Nations. *The Millennium Development Goals Report 2009*. New York: United Nations; 2009.
4. MDG Africa Steering Group. *Achieving the Millennium Development Goals in Africa. Recommendations of the MDG Africa Steering Group. June 2008*. New York: United Nations; 2009.
5. World Bank. *Global Monitoring Report 2009: A Development Emergency*. Washington, DC: World Bank; 2009.
6. Mason E. WHO's strategy on Integrated Management of Childhood Illness. *Bull World Health Organ* 2006;84:595–6.
7. World Health Organization. *Towards Universal Access: Scaling up Priority HIV/AIDS Interventions in the Health Sector*. 2007 progress report. Geneva: WHO; 2007.
8. World Health Organization. *Towards Universal Access. Scaling up Priority HIV/AIDS Interventions in the Health Sector*. 2008 progress report. Geneva: WHO; 2008.
9. World Health Organization. *Towards Universal Access: Scaling up Priority HIV/AIDS Interventions in the Health Sector*. 2009 progress report. Geneva: WHO; 2009.
10. Deluca A, Chaisson RE, Martinson NA. Intensified case finding for tuberculosis in prevention of mother-to-child transmission programs: a simple and potentially vital addition for maternal and child health. *J Acquir Immune Defic Syndr* 2009;50:196–9.
11. Mofenson LM, Laughon BE. Human immunodeficiency virus, mycobacterium tuberculosis, and pregnancy: a deadly combination. *Clin Infect Dis* 2007;45:250–3.
12. World Health Organization. *TB/HIV: A Clinical Manual*. 2nd ed. Geneva: WHO; 2004.
13. World Health Organization. *Global Tuberculosis Control – Epidemiology, Strategy, Financing*. Geneva: WHO; 2009.
14. Marinda E, Humphrey JH, Iliff PJ, Mutasa K, Nathoo KJ, Piwoz EG, *et al*. Child mortality according to maternal and infant HIV status in Zimbabwe. *Pediatr Infect Dis J* 2007;26:519–26.

15.   Wilfert CM, Fowler MG. Balancing maternal and infant benefits and the consequences of breast-feeding in the developing world during the era of HIV infection. *J Infect Dis* 2007;195:165–7.

16.   European Collaborative Study. The mother-to-child HIV transmission epidemic in Europe: evolving in the East and established in the West. *AIDS* 2006;20:1419–27.

17.   Fowler MG, Lampe MA, Jamieson DJ, Kourtis AP, Rogers MF. Reducing the risk of mother-to-child human immunodeficiency virus transmission: past successes, current progress and challenges, and future directions. *Am J Obstet Gynecol* 2007;197(3 Suppl):S3–9.

18.   McIntyre JA, Lallement M. The prevention of mother-to-child transmission of HIV: are we translating scientific success into programmatic failure? *Curr Opin HIV AIDS* 2008;3:139–45.

19.   World Health Organization. *Antiretroviral Drugs for Treating Pregnant Women and Preventing HIV Infection in Infants in Resource-Limited Settings: Towards Universal Access. Recommendations For a Public Health Approach.* Geneva: WHO; 2006.

20.   Lallemant M, Jourdain G, Le Coeur S, Mary JY, Ngo-Giang-Huong N, Koetsawang S, *et al.* Single-dose perinatal nevirapine plus standard zidovudine to prevent mother-to-child transmission of HIV-1 in Thailand. *N Engl J Med* 2004;351:217–28.

21.   deBruyn M, Stevens M. *Not Vectors but People: Moving from PMTCT to Comprehensive Care for Women with HIV.* [www.rhrealitycheck.org/blog/2009/08/14/not-vectors-but-people-moving-pmtct-comprehensive-care-women-hiv].

22.   Chigwedere P, Seage GR, Lee TH, Essex M. Efficacy of antiretroviral drugs in reducing mother-to-child transmission of HIV in Africa: a meta-analysis of published clinical trials. *AIDS Res Hum Retroviruses* 2008;24:827–37.

23.   Boeke CE, Jackson JB. Estimate of infant HIV-free survival at 6 to 8 weeks of age due to maternal antiretroviral prophylaxis in Sub-Saharan Africa, 2004–2005. *J Int Assoc Physicians AIDS Care (Chic Ill)* 2008;7:133–40.

24.   UNAIDS. *AIDS Epidemic Update: December 2007.* Geneva: UNAIDS and WHO; 2007.

25.   Thior I, Lockman S, Smeaton LM, Shapiro RL, Wester C, Heymann SJ, *et al.* Breastfeeding plus infant zidovudine prophylaxis for 6 months vs formula feeding plus infant zidovudine for 1 month to reduce mother-to-child HIV transmission in Botswana: a randomized trial: the Mashi Study. *JAMA* 2006;296:794–805.

26.   Creek T, Arvelo W, Kim A, Bowen A, Finkbeiner T, Zaks L, *et al.* Role of infant feeding and HIV in a severe outbreak of diarrhea and malnutrition among young children, Botswana, 2006. 14th Conference on Retroviruses and Opportunistic Infections, 25–28 February 2007, Los Angeles, USA. Abstract 770.

27.   World Health Organization. *WHO HIV and Infant Feeding Technical Consultation. Held on Behalf of the Inter-agency Task Team (IATT) on Prevention of HIV Infections in Pregnant Women, Mothers and their Infants. Geneva, October 25–27, 2006.* Consensus Statement. Geneva: WHO; 2006 [www.who.int/child_adolescent_health/documents/pdfs/who_hiv_infant_feeding_technical_consultation.pdf].

28.   Kuhn L, Reitz C, Abrams EJ. Breastfeeding and AIDS in the developing world. *Curr Opin Pediatr* 2009;21:83–93.

29.   Kumwenda NI, Hoover DR, Mofenson LM, Thigpen MC, Kafulafula G, Li Q, *et al.* Extended antiretroviral prophylaxis to reduce breast-milk HIV-1 transmission. *N Engl J Med* 2008;359:119–29.

30.   Six Week Extended-Dose Nevirapine (SWEN) Study Team, Bedri A, Gudetta B, Isehak A, Kumbi S, Lulseged S, *et al.* Extended-dose nevirapine to 6 weeks of age for infants to prevent HIV transmission via breastfeeding in Ethiopia, India, and Uganda: an analysis of three randomised controlled trials. *Lancet* 2008;372:300–13.

31.   Mofenson LM. Antiretroviral prophylaxis to reduce breast milk transmission of HIV type 1: New data but still questions. *J Acquir Immune Defic Syndr* 2008;48:237–40.

32.   Palombi L, Marazzi MC, Voetberg A, Magid NA. Treatment acceleration program and the experience of the DREAM program in prevention of mother-to-child transmission of HIV. *AIDS* 2007;21 Suppl 4:S65–71.

33.   Thomas T, Masaba R, Ndivo R, Zeh C, Borkowf C, Thigpen M, *et al.* Prevention of mother-to-child transmission of HIV-1 among breastfeeding mothers using HAART: The Kisumu Breastfeeding Study, Kisumu, Kenya, 2003–2007. 15th Conference on Retroviruses and Opportunistic Infections, 3–6 February 2008, Boston, MA, USA. Abstract 45aLB.

34. Kilewo C, Karlsson K, Ngarina M, Massawe A, Lyamuya E, Lipyoga R, et al. Prevention of mother-to-child transmission of HIV-1 through breastfeeding by treating mothers prophylactically with triple antiretroviral therapy in Dar es Salaam, Tanzania – the MITRA PLUS study. 4th IAS Conference on HIV Pathogenesis, Treatment and Prevention, 22–25 July 2007, Sydney, Australia. Abstract TUAX101.2007.

35. Tripathy SN, Tripathy SN. Tuberculosis and pregnancy. *Int J Gynaecol Obstet* 2003;80:247–53.

36. Newell ML, Brahmbhatt H, Ghys PD. Child mortality and HIV infection in Africa: a review. *AIDS* 2004;18 Suppl 2:S27–34.

37. Brahmbhatt H, Kigozi G, Wabwire-Mangen F, Serwadda D, Lutalo T, Nalugoda F, et al. Mortality in HIV-infected and uninfected children of HIV-infected and uninfected mothers in rural Uganda. *J Acquir Immune Defic Syndr* 2006;41:504–8.

38. Taha TE, Graham SM, Kumwenda NI, Broadhead RL, Hoover DR, Markakis D, et al. Morbidity among human immunodeficiency virus-1-infected and -uninfected African children. *Pediatrics* 2000;106:E77.

39. Violari A, Cotton MF, Gibb DM, Babiker AG, Steyn J, Madhi SA, et al; CHER Study Team. Early antiretroviral therapy and mortality among HIV-infected infants. *N Engl J Med* 2008;359:2233–44.

40. World Health Organizaton. *WHO Paediatric Treatment Recommendations.* Geneva: WHO; 2008.

41. Mataka E. Maternal health and HIV: bridging the gap. *Lancet* 2007;370:1290–1.

42. Sebitloane HM, Mhlanga RE. Changing patterns of maternal mortality (HIV/AIDS related) in poor countries. *Best Pract Res Clin Obstet Gynaecol* 2008;22:489–99.

43. McIntyre J. Maternal health and HIV. *Reprod Health Matters* 2005;13:129–35.

44. Berer M. HIV/AIDS, pregnancy and maternal mortality and morbidity: implications for care. In: Berer M, Ravindran TKS, editors. *Safe Motherhood Initiatives: Critical Issues.* London: Reproductive Health Matters; 1999. p. 198–210.

45. McIntyre J. Mothers infected with HIV. *Br Med Bull* 2003;67:127–35.

46. Ahmed Y, Mwaba P, Chintu C, Grange JM, Ustianowski A, Zumla A. A study of maternal mortality at the University Teaching Hospital, Lusaka, Zambia: the emergence of tuberculosis as a major non-obstetric cause of maternal death. *Int J Tuberc Lung Dis* 1999;3:675–80.

47. Sewankambo NK, Wawer MJ, Gray RH, Serwadda D, Li C, Stallings RY, et al. Demographic impact of HIV infection in rural Rakai district, Uganda: results of a population-based cohort study. *AIDS* 1994;8:1707–13.

48. Bicego G, Boerma JT, Ronsmans C. The effect of AIDS on maternal mortality in Malawi and Zimbabwe. *AIDS* 2002;16:1078–81.

49. Iloki LH, G'Bala Sapoulou MV, Kpekpede F, Ekoundzola JR. [Maternal mortality in Brazzaville (1993–1994).] *J Gynecol Obstet Biol Reprod (Paris)* 1997;26:163–8.

50. MacLeod J, Rhode R. Retrospective follow-up of maternal deaths and their associated risk factors in a rural district of Tanzania. *Trop Med Int Health* 1998;3:130–7.

51. Ramogale MR, Moodley J, Sebitloane MH. HIV-associated maternal mortality – primary causes of death at King Edward VIII Hospital, Durban. *S Afr Med J* 2007;97:363–6.

52. Ziraba AK, Madise N, Mills S, Kyobutungi C, Ezeh A. Maternal mortality in the informal settlements of Nairobi city: what do we know? *Reprod Health* 2009;6:6.

53. Chersich MF, Luchters SM, Yard E, Othigo JM, Kley N, Temmerman M. Morbidity in the first year postpartum among HIV-infected women in Kenya. *Int J Gynaecol Obstet* 2008;100:45–51.

54. Paal LV, Shafer LA, Mayanja BN, Whitworth JA, Grosskurth H. Effect of pregnancy on HIV disease progression and survival among women in rural Uganda. *Trop Med Int Health* 2007;12:920–8.

55. Kongnyuy EJ, Mlava G, van den Broek N. Facility-based maternal death review in three districts in the central region of Malawi: an analysis of causes and characteristics of maternal deaths. *Womens Health Issues* 2009;19:14–20.

56. Department of Health. *The National HIV and Syphilis Prevalence Survey, South Africa 2007.* Pretoria: Department of Health; 2008.

57. National Committee on Confidential Enquiries into Maternal Deaths. A review of maternal deaths in South Africa during 1998. *S Afr Med J* 2000;90:367–73.

58. National Committee on Confidential Enquiries into Maternal Deaths. *Saving Mothers 1999–2001.* Pretoria: Department of Health; 2003.

59. National Committee on Confidential Enquiries into Maternal Deaths. *Saving Mothers – Report on Confidential Enquiries into Maternal Deaths in South Africa 2002–2004.* Pretoria: Department of Health; 2006.

60. National Committee on Confidential Enquiries into Maternal Deaths. *Saving Mothers 2005–2007: Fourth Report on Confidential Enquiries into Maternal Deaths in South Africa.* Pretoria: Department of Health, South Africa; 2009.

61. Black V, Brooke S, Chersich MF. Effect of human immunodeficiency virus treatment on maternal mortality at a tertiary center in South Africa: a 5-year audit. *Obstet Gynecol* 2009;114(2 Pt 1):292–9.

62. Chandisarewa W, Stranix-Chibanda L, Chirapa E, Miller A, Simoyi M, Mahomva A, *et al.* Routine offer of antenatal HIV testing ('opt-out' approach) to prevent mother-to-child transmission of HIV in urban Zimbabwe. *Bull World Health Organ* 2007;85:843–50.

63. Creek TL, Ntumy R, Seipone K, Smith M, Mogodi M, Smit M, *et al.* Successful introduction of routine opt-out HIV testing in antenatal care in Botswana. *J Acquir Immune Defic Syndr* 2007;45:102–7.

64. Perinatal HIV Guidelines Working Group. *Public Health Service Task Force Recommendations for Use of Antiretroviral Drugs in Pregnant HIV-Infected Women for Maternal Health and Interventions to Reduce Perinatal HIV Transmission in the United States.* [aidsinfo.nih.gov/ContentFiles/PerinatalGL.pdf].

65. Clumeck N, Pozniak A, Raffi F. European AIDS Clinical Society (EACS) guidelines for the clinical management and treatment of HIV-infected adults. *HIV Med* 2008;9:65–71.

66. Corbett EL, Marston B, Churchyard GJ, De Cock KM. Tuberculosis in sub-Saharan Africa: opportunities, challenges, and change in the era of antiretroviral treatment. *Lancet* 2006;367:926–37.

67. Corbett EL, Steketee RW, ter Kuile FO, Latif AS, Kamali A, Hayes RJ. HIV-1/AIDS and the control of other infectious diseases in Africa. *Lancet* 2002;359:2177–87.

68. Adhikari M. Tuberculosis and tuberculosis/HIV co-infection in pregnancy. *Semin Fetal Neonatal Med* 2009;14: 234–40.

69. Diwan VK, Thorson A. Sex, gender, and tuberculosis. *Lancet* 1999;353:1000–1.

70. Pillay T, Khan M, Moodley J, Adhikari M, Padayatchi N, Naicker V, *et al.* The increasing burden of tuberculosis in pregnant women, newborns and infants under 6 months of age in Durban, KwaZulu-Natal. *S Afr Med J* 2001;91:983–7.

71. Khan M, Pillay T, Moodley JM, Connolly CA. Maternal mortality associated with tuberculosis-HIV-1 co-infection in Durban, South Africa. *AIDS* 2001;15:1857–63.

72. Skevaki CL, Kafetzis DA. Tuberculosis in neonates and infants: epidemiology, pathogenesis, clinical manifestations, diagnosis, and management issues. *Paediatr Drugs* 2005;7:219–34.

73. Adhikari M, Pillay T, Pillay DG. Tuberculosis in the newborn: an emerging disease. *Pediatr Infect Dis J* 1997;16:1108–12.

74. Pillay T, Sturm AW, Khan M, Adhikari M, Moodley J, Connolly C, *et al.* Vertical transmission of *Mycobacterium tuberculosis* in KwaZulu Natal: impact of HIV-1 co-infection. *Int J Tuberc Lung Dis* 2004;8:59–69.

75. Gupta A, Nayak U, Ram M, Bhosale R, Patil S, Basavraj A, *et al.* Postpartum tuberculosis incidence and mortality among HIV-infected women and their infants in Pune, India, 2002–2005. *Clin Infect Dis* 2007;45:241–9.

76. Golub JE, Mohan CI, Comstock GW, Chaisson RE. Active case finding of tuberculosis: historical perspective and future prospects. *Int J Tuberc Lung Dis* 2005;9:1183–203.

77. Kali PBN, Gray GE, Violari A, Chaisson RE, McIntyre JA, Martinson NA. Combining PMTCT with active case finding for tuberculosis. *J Acquir Immune Defic Syndr* 2006;42: 379–81.

78. Nachega J, Coetzee J, Adendorff T, Msandiwa R, Gray GE, McIntyre JA, *et al.* Tuberculosis active case-finding in a mother-to-child HIV transmission prevention programme in Soweto, South Africa. *AIDS* 2003;17:1398–400.

79. Kaplan JE, Benson C, Holmes KH, Brooks JT, Pau A, Masur H. Guidelines for prevention and treatment of opportunistic infections in HIV-infected adults and adolescents: recommendations

from CDC, the National Institutes of Health, and the HIV Medicine Association of the Infectious Diseases Society of America. *MMWR Recomm Rep* 2009;58(RR-4):1–207.

80. Spensley A, Sripipatana T, Turner AN, Hoblitzelle C, Robinson J, Wilfert C. Preventing mother-to-child transmission of HIV in resource-limited settings: the Elizabeth Glaser Pediatric AIDS Foundation experience. *Am J Public Health* 2009;99:631–7.

81. World Health Organization. *Strategic Approaches to the Prevention of HIV Infection in Infants.* Report of a WHO meeting, Morges, Switzerland, 20–22 March 2002. Geneva: WHO; 2002.

82. Global Partners Forum. *Achieving Universal Access to Comprehensive PMTCT Services.* 2007 [www.procaare.org/archive/procaare/200711/msg00013.php].

83. Abrams EJ, Myer L, Rosenfield A, El-Sadr WM. Prevention of mother-to-child transmission services as a gateway to family-based human immunodeficiency virus care and treatment in resource-limited settings: rationale and international experiences. *Am J Obstet Gynecol* 2007;197(3 Suppl):S101–6.

Chapter 11
A pragmatic approach to safe anaesthesia

Kate Grady and Catriona Connolly

Background

An estimated 536 000 women die each year owing to complications arising from pregnancy and childbirth.[1] Eighty percent of maternal deaths are due to haemorrhage, sepsis, eclampsia, obstructed labour and complications of abortion.[2] A larger number of women survive with residual complex physical and emotional health problems as a result of such complications. Neonatal welfare is inextricably dependent on maternal welfare. An estimated 4 million neonatal deaths occur each year,[3,4] three-quarters of which occur in sub-Saharan Africa and South Asia.[1,5] Inexpensive and simple medical and surgical interventions are recognised to be life saving in the management of these conditions.

The impact and importance of safe anaesthesia in obstetric care

The optimal management of potentially life-threatening complications of childbirth and pregnancy requires anaesthesia or anaesthetic-related skills. In the UK, anaesthetists are involved in the care of over 50% of women in a typical delivery unit.[6]

The most obvious role of the anaesthetist in the obstetric care of women is in the provision of anaesthesia for caesarean section and epidural analgesia for labour but the role goes far beyond this. Anaesthesia may be required to facilitate surgery to gain control of life-threatening haemorrhage that otherwise could become catastrophic, as in women with uterine atony, ruptured uterus, retained placenta or genital tract trauma. Anaesthesia is needed to manage other life-threatening obstetric conditions such as prolapsed cord, obstructed labour and drainage of a septic focus.

The anaesthetist also has an important role outside the obstetric operating theatre. The importance of pre- and postoperative care is often underestimated. The best chance of survival from surgery is with preoperative optimisation of physiological disturbance. Equally, successful surgery must be followed by expert postoperative care. The anaesthetist has an advanced understanding of perioperative physiology and therefore makes a valuable contribution to management of postoperative fluid balance, analgesia and management of cardiorespiratory complications.

Anaesthetic knowledge and skills are essential for supervision and delivery of high-dependency care to ensure that an understanding of pathophysiology, timely institution and interpretation of invasive monitoring and guidance on appropriate treatment are available for the most seriously ill women. Intensive care is a core component of all anaesthetists' training and intensive care units are, in the main, directed and staffed by anaesthetists. As a result, the anaesthetist may start intensive care management of a seriously ill woman in the operating theatre, manage the physiological changes during surgery and implement safe transfer to the intensive care unit. The anaesthetist takes the lead in maternal resuscitation and can have a useful role in resuscitation and care of the newborn. The anaesthetist also has an integral role in antenatal care, assessing and planning management of high-risk and complex cases with the obstetrician.

Analgesia is a key component of anaesthesia. Provision of effective analgesia relieves maternal distress and thereby restores dignity to women. There is a wider role to be fulfilled: education, participating in 'fire drills', drawing up guidelines, linking and liaising with other medical specialities, and reflecting on maternal morbidity and mortality. Today's low-resource countries could potentially benefit from Western modern medicine's experience and circumvent the need to develop anaesthetic techniques, drugs and equipment. A great gift for low-resource parts of the world would be the benefits of Western medicine's experience and attention to detail in reducing maternal mortality. This experience does, however, have to be transferred properly through good teaching and training, and with adequate resources and support.

No anaesthesia versus substandard anaesthesia

Where there is no provision of anaesthesia or where that provision is patchy or its quality very poor, the conclusion can be drawn that this is a causative factor in maternal deaths.[7,8] However, anaesthesia carries its own risks. By definition, general anaesthesia causes unconsciousness and cessation of spontaneous respiration. General or regional anaesthesia can cause cardiovascular instability if not properly conducted and can harm the woman over and above her existing condition. Obstetric anaesthesia is recognised as a highly specialist sub-branch of anaesthetics and more high risk than other areas of anaesthetic practice. Anaesthesia, particularly substandard anaesthesia, is in itself a killer of mothers. This is recognised not only in low-resource parts of the world but also in the UK.[9] The medical principle *primum non nocere* (first, do no harm) has to be upheld. Death and morbidity from anaesthesia can be minimised by continuous and long-term attention to detail and by effective training. In countries where there is an anaesthetic training programme (for example, Malawi), the anaesthetists can work to protocols and become highly skilled very quickly, thus preventing some maternal deaths.

Non-doctor anaesthesia – a possible solution?

Historically, anaesthesia was administered by the operator surgeon or their assistant. There has been a move away from this and the medical specialty of anaesthesia has become independent, distinct and respected, particularly in the UK. Anaesthetists are fully qualified doctors who have undertaken a minimum further 7 years of a rigorous specified training programme, with close clinical supervision throughout.

In some parts of the world, such as the USA, the Netherlands and Sweden, anaesthetics are administered by non-doctor anaesthetists working under the direct supervision of doctor anaesthetists. The ratio of more than one non-doctor anaesthetist to each doctor anaesthetist confers an economic advantage.

This system has set the precedent of a move away from the 'anaesthesia only by anaesthetists' paradigm and embracement of the non-doctor anaesthetist's professional role. The concept of the non-doctor anaesthetist is a venture away from the 'individual highest quality care' model towards treating a greater number overall with a greater number of survivors.

In sub-Saharan Africa and South Asia, the doctor can be a rare commodity and delivery of medical care across various medical specialties can fall to non-doctors. It is unlikely that a doctor who has been adequately trained and is dedicated to the administration of anaesthetics would be a frequently available resource, particularly in rural settings.[8] Anaesthesia is instead delivered by non-doctor anaesthetists. McAuliffe and Henry, in a survey of 200 countries,[10] found that 107 of them employed non-doctor anaesthetists.

Non-doctor anaesthetists form a more permanent resource as they are less likely to be poached or lured to well-resourced countries for exchange placements or postgraduate training or by financial incentives. A significant proportion of local doctors readily move into alternative or combined careers in medical management or government positions, creating further deficiencies in the doctor workforce in the clinical enviroment.[11]

The concept of task shifting has been comprehensively addressed by the World Health Organization (WHO) in their document *Global Recommendations and Guidelines: Rational Redistribution of Tasks among Health Workforce Teams*.[12] The emphasis is on its application to tackle health worker shortages. It is recognised that task shifting will be needed to meet the Millennium Development Goals (MDGs) and, although the document's focus is on access to HIV services, it provides strategies that are applicable across wider aspects of health care. Task shifting is the movement of specific tasks, where appropriate, from the remit of highly qualified health workers to health workers who have received shorter training and have fewer qualifications. The WHO document makes 22 recommendations to ensure a safe, effective, equitable and sustainable approach and it can be considered as an authoritative text. It emphasises that task shifting be adopted or expanded alongside other strategies for healthcare improvement and that it will require significant specific investment and planning. Task shifting must be a quality-assured exercise and not simply a cheap, easy, ineffective 'tick box' exercise implemented as a 'quasi' solution. The WHO has also addressed the issue of the exodus of trained personnel to better opportunities; it suggests approaches to retention in its 'Treat, Train, Retain' philosophy.[13]

The serious limitations of non-doctor anaesthesia

While it is recognised that the skills of non-doctor anaesthetists can be adequate and, in the experience of the authors, non-doctor anaesthetists are knowledgeable, dedicated and extremely keen to learn, they do not match those of trained doctor anaesthetists who have completed a postgraduate specialist training programme as outlined above. The doctor anaesthetist has superior knowledge, an understanding of applied pharmacology and physiology – particularly to patients with co-morbidities – and a mental bank of medical information to draw upon. Where resources can possibly allow, the doctor anaesthetist is always preferential and the concept of anaesthesia being delivered by doctors should be promoted.

Continuing professional development

In the UK, continuing professional development (CPD) for doctors is compulsory and integral to the practice of all medical specialties, including anaesthesia. It is invariably absent in any degree of formality in low-resource countries. The non-doctor anaesthetist does not command the same professional respect and is less likely than his/her medical counterpart to be able to access CPD. In reality, CPD is more necessary for the lesser-qualified non-doctor anaesthetist but is, in fact, less available.

Preoperative preparation

The wider skills and potential of the anaesthetist outside the operating theatre can go unrecognised or be ignored. Non-doctor anaesthetists often have no opportunity to make a preoperative assessment and optimise women before surgery. In some situations, lack of preoperative resuscitation is a major contributor to intraoperative death. There are anecdotal reports of significant anxiety among non-doctor anaesthetists when they are not given the opportunity to see the woman before she enters the operating theatre, with the expectation from colleagues that the woman should be immediately anaesthetised. This practice is deemed unacceptable in well-resourced countries, where the anaesthetist is an integral member of the multidisciplinary team, usually directing the preoperative optimisation effort and fully involved in the timing of surgery before the woman is transferred to theatre. The non-doctor anaesthetist has little control over this attitude and practice. Where non-doctor anaesthetists are working with doctors, medical hierarchy and cultural practice usually dictate that the non-doctor anaesthetist must comply with the wishes and instructions of the doctors present, even though those doctors may not have the understanding of the principles of anaesthesia that the non-doctor anaesthetist has. Examples reported to the authors as commonplace include obstetricians insisting on performing caesarean sections immediately on seriously hypertensive eclamptic women instead of stabilising them first, despite advice from the non-doctor anaesthetist to the contrary. It is impossible in a hierarchical society for the non-doctor anaesthetist to insist that their opinion is correct.

Anaesthetic assistance

The practice of anaesthesia in parts of the world where it is well respected attracts skilled assistance for the anaesthetist, which is available for the whole of the intraoperative period. In the UK, the presence of a skilled assistant is an absolute national requirement; this is because when things go wrong, they do so extremely quickly and valuable competent assistance makes a difference to outcome. In the resource-poor world, it is likely that skilled assistance for the anaesthetist will be unavailable.

Postoperative recovery

In well-resourced countries, women are transferred from the operating theatre to a recovery room for observation by trained staff during the immediate postoperative period. This is an integral component of safe perioperative care. In resource-poor countries, the recovery room staff are often not appropriately skilled in recovery from anaesthesia, so the anaesthetist must spend more time in the recovery room until the woman is sufficiently well recovered to be safely left with such staff. This impedes the anaesthetist's ability to treat another woman or may tempt the anaesthetist to leave the woman sooner than is ideal. Under-trained recovery staff do not have the skills to observe and interpret the early physiological changes of complications such as haemorrhage and thus to seek intervention from the anaesthetist and obstetrician in a timely fashion.

Monitoring equipment and drugs

Monitoring equipment is in great shortage, further compromising the delivery of safe anaesthesia, postoperative care and high-dependency care. In resource-poor countries, the supply of essential anaesthetic and emergency medicine drugs that are 'in date' is poor. Anaesthetists are often forced to use donated drugs (often past the expiry date) whose pharmacology may be unpredictable if the drug is a long time past its expiry date.

Pain control

In well-resourced countries, anaesthetists play a leading role in management of pain. In resource-poor countries, however, pain control is not the domain of the anaesthetist and can be very poor. The role of the anaesthetist in this area is undervalued and unrecognised. The anaesthetist is skilled in the provision of pain relief and could educate, change attitudes and allay anxieties and reservations about the administration of analgesics, if given the opportunity; the non-doctor anaesthetist cannot be assertive in this regard.

Learning from clinical disasters

It is important to be realistic and face the absolute blame culture and associated humiliation that can exist in poorly resourced parts of the world. There are anecdotal reports of non-doctor anaesthetists being relocated to different parts of the country because they have been ostracised in their village over a maternal death or death of a child.

Most countries do not have a robust perioperative morbidity and mortality recording system in place. There are no root-cause analysis sessions and no formalised reflection so little is gained from adverse experiences. Thus, there is no potential for system change after a clinical catastrophe. The non-doctor anaesthetist often works in relative professional isolation. Clearly, there is great difficulty in discussing difficult cases and debriefing after disasters, and this is very hard on morale.

Training of non-doctor anaesthetists

The non-doctor anaesthetist resource is itself scarce. The need for anaesthesia is recognised by midwives and obstetricians but demand for anaesthesia outstrips availability and this imbalance results in death and morbidity.[8] This must be corrected and, where non-doctor anaesthetists are required, training programmes should be introduced and conducted with adherence to the principles of adult education. There are many continuing initiatives[8,14] supported by the Crisp report[15] and several models to be considered:

- training for those with no professional background
- training for those from the professional backgrounds of nursing, clinical officers and medical officers
- updating courses for existing anaesthetic clinical/medical officers and nurse anaesthetists.

One example of an excellent programme of education of non-doctor anaesthetists exists in Malawi. If selected, general clinical officers or nurses do an 18-month programme to become an anaesthetic clinical officer (ACO). After that, they may work in a district hospital with one or, at best, two other ACOs. Some work alone in departments, covering on a 24-hour, 7-day-a-week basis. To cope in this relative isolation, it is important that ACOs have training not only in technical skills but also leadership, team-work, effective communication and other managerial competencies.

Within the UK, major contributions to advocacy and training in anaesthesia are made by the Association of Anaesthetists of Great Britain and Ireland (AAGBI), the Obstetric Anaesthetists' Association (OAA) and the Royal College of Anaesthetists. The AAGBI was a founder member and has a major role in the activities of the World Federation of Societies of Anaesthesiologists (WFSA). The WFSA is very active in the fields of education and training, including the running of training centres, writing and distributing publications, safety and quality, and professional wellbeing, and has its own scientific committee. The World Anaesthesia Society (WAS) is a specialist society of the AAGBI and coordinates like-minded specialists to contribute to the development of anaesthesia worldwide through dissemination of teaching materials, website discussion groups and local support. The Royal College of Anaesthetists works to address the status of anaesthesia worldwide, to provide training for its own Fellows in the delivery of health care to the resource-poor world, to support non-medically qualified anaesthesia, to offer expertise in training and assessment, to ensure equity between medical disciplines, to agree international standards and to offer expertise in the writing of clinical guidelines.

The WHO document on task shifting[12] can be adopted as both a practical guide and an authoritative text on training and the wider aspects of non-doctor anaesthesia. It can be used to support national consultation and endorsement, to encourage situation analysis, to create enabling regulatory frameworks or to adjust existing regulations at senior level and offer quality analysis, standards, supportive supervision, assessment and certification.

The absence of CPD training for anaesthetists in resource-poor countries could be covered by internet or distance packages. However, in district hospitals in particular, the only reliable form of communication is mobile phone. Internet access is available in theory but, in reality, the computer is often in the office of the regional medical officer and usually not accessible to the clinical officers. This hinders access to online education packages that have been specifically designed for practitioners in resource-poor countries who have little access to textbooks or postgraduate training.

Face-to-face teaching sessions composed of different components have been delivered throughout Africa by various UK-based anaesthetists. The following list is not exhaustive but gives a few examples of countries where teaching is being provided by UK anaesthetists in sub-Saharan Africa: Ethiopia, Liberia, Malawi, Somaliland, Tanzania and Uganda. Comprehensive training has also been developed in Bangladesh.[7] In all of these examples, courses that are tailored to the local needs have been developed by the individuals involved.

Summary

The authors endorse increased provision of doctor-provided obstetric anaesthesia where possible, and enhanced international training of non-doctor anaesthetists in obstetric anaesthesia where doctors are not available. Wider coordination of the commendable efforts being made at grass-roots level is likely to make them more effective, more efficient and more attractive to funding. From the outset, it is essential to decide on the process indicators to be applied to any endeavours.

With the 2015 target date for achieving MDGs 4 and 5 fast approaching, 'quick wins' and therefore workable, practical solutions have to be identified. Training programmes must be provided where there are deficiencies and enhanced where they are in existence:

- Exemplary 'off-the-shelf' training programmes are suggested, where anaesthetists are trained to a structure and clinical guidelines. These should be available to be applied in appropriate settings by a defined faculty.
- Such programmes would be supported by CPD opportunities, with integrated mentoring and development incentives, which should guard against decay in skills and knowledge.
- The programmes must have rigorous monitoring and evaluation (see Box 11.1),[16] and quality assurance.

Box 11.1   Monitoring and evaluation structures for non-doctor anaesthetists' training programmes

Kirkpatrick[16] developed a four-level model for determining the effectiveness of training programmes. It has been in use for four decades and has retained its relevance over this period. The four levels are:
1. Reaction: a measure of learner satisfaction – it uses visual analogue scores and focus group discussion
2. Learning: measured through before and after knowledge multiple choice questions and skills tests
3. Behaviour: a log book kept by the learner of how workplace behaviour has improved
4. Results: identification of changes in outcomes within institutions and within society.

- It is proposed that such programmes would create an international standard of achievement and training and, in time, lead to an international qualification and accreditation.
- The programmes would impart skills in non-technical areas such as leadership and team-work and the principles of being a good instructor for informal teaching and training in the workplace.

Enhanced training opportunities must be supported by endeavours to have the non-doctor anaesthetist accepted, well positioned and respected as an essential member of a multidisciplinary maternity team; in this respect, the support of WHO and its task-shifting document are invaluable.[12] Suggested aims would be to:

- provide advocacy, recognition and support through visiting and distance mentoring
- address deficiencies in equipment and drug provision, engaging with partners at government and international level (a list of drugs essential to the practice of safe obstetric anaesthesia is provided in Box 11.2)

Box 11.2   Advocacy drug list to facilitate the practice of safe obstetric anaesthesia

The following drugs are considered essential to the practice of safe obstetric anaesthesia:
- thiopental sodium
- propofol
- suxamethonium (needs fridge)
- atracurium (needs fridge)
- vecuronium
- neostigmine
- ketamine
- atropine
- ephedrine
- phenylephrine or metaraminol or methoxamine
- adrenaline/epinephrine
- antibiotics: co-amoxiclav, cefuroxime, metronidazole, flucloxacillin
- oxytocin (Syntocinon®; Alliance)
- ergometrine
- ergometrine maleate (Syntometrine®; Alliance)
- carboprost
- local anaesthetics – lidocaine, bupivacaine (heavy, if available) or ropivacaine
- analgesics – paracetamol, diclofenac, codeine (if available)
- controlled drugs such as fentanyl and morphine, although there are probably restrictions and legislative and cultural issues to be overcome.

- campaign for skilled assistance for the anaesthetist (including the non–doctor anaesthetist) intraoperatively and during recovery
- create a culture and introduce methods of professional reflection and move away from a culture of immediate blame
- offer international senior, large-scale advocacy and support for training and status.

References

1. World Health Organization. *Maternal Mortality in 2005. Estimates Developed by WHO, UNICEF, UNFPA and the World Bank.* Geneva: WHO; 2007.
2. Khan KS, Wojdyla D, Say L, Gülmezoglu AM, Van Look PFA. WHO analysis of causes of maternal death: a systematic review. *Lancet* 2006;367: 1066–74.
3. Lawn JE, Cousens S, Bhutta ZA, Darmstadt GL, Martines J, Paul V, *et al.* Why are 4 million newborn babies dying each year? *Lancet* 2004;364:399–401.
4. Black RE, Morris SS, Bryce J. Where and why are 10 million children dying every year? *Lancet* 2003;361:2226–34.
5. Hill K, Thomas K, AbouZahr C, Walker N, Say L, Inoue M, *et al.* Estimates of maternal mortality worldwide between 1990 and 2005: an assessment of available data. *Lancet* 2007;370:1311–19.
6. *OAA/AAGBI Guidelines for Obstetric Anaesthesia Services.* Revised edition. London: Association of Anaesthetists of Great Britain and Ireland and Obstetric Anaesthetists' Association; 2005.
7. Edwards CH, Cave WP, Greene K, *et al.* Non-physician Anaesthetists – an Appropriate Use of Personnel for Delivery of Comprehensive Emergency Obstetric Care. ICDDR,B – Knowledge for Global Life Saving Solutions, March 2007, Dhaka. Poster presentation.
8. Zimmerman M, Lee M, Retnaraj S. Non-doctor anaesthesia in Nepal; developing an essential cadre. *Trop Doct* 2008;38:148.
9. Lewis G, editor. *Saving Mothers' Lives: Reviewing Maternal Deaths to Make Motherhood Safer 2003–2005. The Seventh Report on Confidential Enquiries into Maternal Deaths in the United Kingdom.* London: CEMACH; 2007.
10. McAuliffe MS, Henry B. Nurse anesthesia practice and research – a worldwide need. *CRNA* 2000;11:89–98.
11. Zijlstra EE, Broadhead RI. The College of Medicine of Malawi: towards sustaining improvement. *Human Resour Health* 2007;5:1–5.
12. World Health Organization. *Task Shifting: Rational Redistribution of Tasks among Health Workforce Teams: Global Recommendations and Guidelines.* Geneva: WHO; 2008.
13. World Health Organization. *Treat, Train, Retain: The AIDS and Healthcare Workforce Plan.* Report on the Consultation on AIDS and Human Resources for Health. Geneva: WHO; 2006.
14. Beed M. Links with Ethiopia. *Anaesthesia News* 2009;262:16–19.
15. Crisp N. *Global Health Partnerships: the UK Contribution to Health in Developing Countries.* London: Central Office of Information; 2007.
16. Kirkpatrick DL, Kirkpatrick JD. *Evaluating Training Programmes: the Four Levels.* 3rd edition. San Francisco: Berrett–Koehler; 2006.

Section 3

Clinical problems and solutions – neonatal

Chapter 12
Innovations for improving newborn survival in developing countries: do integrated strategies for maternal and newborn care matter?

Zulfiqar Bhutta, Saad Seth and Noureen Afzal

Introduction

Each year millions of women, newborns and children die from preventable diseases. Worldwide, more than 60 million women deliver at home every year without a skilled birth attendant[1] and about 530 000 women die from pregnancy-related complications, with about 68 000 of these deaths resulting from unsafe abortion.[2] About 4 million babies die within the first month of life and more than 3 million are stillborn. An estimated 9.2 million children die under the age of five,[3] of which 40% of deaths occur during the neonatal period.[4] Three-quarters of all neonatal deaths (3 million) occur within the first week of life and at least 1 million babies die on their first day of life.[4] With only 5 years left to achieve the Millennium Development Goals (MDGs), many obstacles stand in the way. Inequality, poverty, illiteracy, civil unrest and the absence of good-quality care are the major obstacles in progressing towards better health of mothers and children, a key component of the MDGs. Achieving MDG 4 to reduce the under-five mortality by two-thirds from the level in 1990 by the year 2015 is not only critically dependent on a substantial reduction in neonatal mortality but also on measures to address high burdens of maternal morbidity and mortality, which also have a major effect on newborn survival and child health.

Achieving MDG 5 of reducing the maternal mortality by three-quarters from the level in 1990 by 2015 requires concrete measures that may go way beyond the health sector. Strategies to improve the health care, socio-economic status and education of women in low-resource communities and countries are also expected to improve both pregnancy and neonatal health outcomes.[5] In poor communities, a mother's death during childbirth means that her newborn will have a very high risk of dying and that her older children are more likely to suffer from disease and poor growth. When mothers are malnourished, sick or receive inadequate health care, their newborns face a higher risk of disease and premature death.[6] Maternal and child health policies and programmes to date tend to address the maternal and the child health issues in discrete silos, resulting in gaps in care that especially affect babies during the perinatal period. Maternal programmes mainly emphasise facility-based and emergency obstetric care, while newborn and child healthcare programmes increasingly concentrate on community-based strategies. There is thus no consistent strategy for addressing the major health issues of mothers, newborn and children, which are actually closely intertwined and for effective results have to be addressed together, preferably through a common platform.

Why integrated maternal and neonatal health?

There is an urgent need to build linkages between maternal, newborn and child healthcare strategies based on the best possible evidence so that effective and practical models of care can be created and recommended for implementation in those communities most in need.

Integration of maternal, newborn and child health care can build linkages between maternal, newborn and child healthcare strategies and programmes in order to reduce maternal, neonatal and child mortality and morbidity. Saving maternal and newborn lives depends on high coverage and high quality of integrated service-delivery packages throughout the continuum of care. This continuum of care for maternal, neonatal and child health requires access to care provided by families and communities, by outpatient and outreach services, and by clinical services throughout the lifecycle, including adolescence, pregnancy, childbirth, the postnatal period and childhood. These integrated services should also have functional linkages between levels of care in the health system and between service-delivery packages, so that the care provided at each time and place contributes to the effectiveness of all the linked programmes.[7]

Why integrate in primary care settings?

Integration aims to blend the various components into a functioning whole. Although there are a host of definitions of integration and, as indicated by Briggs and Garner,[8] integration of primary health care is 'a variety of managerial or operational changes to health systems to bring together inputs, delivery, management and organization of particular service functions' with the aim of improving service in relation to efficiency and quality and maximising use of resources and opportunities.

Integration of healthcare services is happening across the globe, although the patterns of integration and the issues related to the integration process are different in high- and in low- or middle-income countries. The concept of integrating healthcare services at the primary healthcare level emerged out of health sector reform policies supported by the World Bank in the 1990s.[9] These policies were created in response to problems faced by national health sectors, such as demands for decentralisation of services, calls for adopting a market approach and reductions in government funding for health care. Although the concept of integration is part of the policy agenda in developing countries, there is often a lack of capacity within the health systems to formulate elaborate integration processes and strategies, to coordinate all the required inputs and to provide the necessary support to the local managers, especially in under-resourced settings and in the context of decentralised health systems.

In most low- and middle-income countries, health programmes are delivered independently of each other in a vertical fashion and are designed to target a specific disease or health problem. Such specialised, separate, vertical programmes ensure technical supervision to focus and deliver health services to a specific target population. The widespread notion is that such an approach will ensure delivery of health services but it is not without its disadvantages. The more obvious disadvantages are service duplication, inefficiency and service fragmentation.[8] While it allows each programme to focus on a particular disease or intervention, such an approach may not be the wisest and most efficient, as it demands more resources. Integrated approaches to provision of health services emerge as obvious solutions to ensure efficient use of resources and better provision of quality services.

The goal of integration is to deliver quality health services efficiently, using resources and opportunities to the maximum. This approach is beneficial for both the service provider and the consumer. It provides various health services or interventions packaged together in one composite programme delivered through a single platform. For example, trained staff in primary health care can cure patients (using drugs and procedures, etc.), provide reproductive health services (family planning services, treatment of sexually transmitted diseases, antenatal care, etc.) and child and newborn care (postnatal care and immunisations, etc.). The outcome is improved efficiency and better quality of health services, and thus there is better health for everyone. Integration also provides the opportunity to deliver a wider range of health services. It is expected to bridge the gap in access and use of health services between geographical and socio-economic groups.[8]

Integrating maternal and newborn health in primary care settings

Integration of maternal and newborn health interventions can improve the:[10]

- efficiency and productivity of delivery of health services
- health status of the community
- user satisfaction and convenience
- equity of health services.

The proximity and intimacy of the relationship of the mother and her newborn and the mother and her child offers an opportunity to deliver better health to both through composite health packages consisting of interventions for both age groups, using the same infrastructure and delivery platform. The intertwined health needs of mother, newborn and child are approached as a continuum, as has been proposed by the World Health Organization (WHO): 'The core principle underlying the strategies to develop maternal, newborn and child health (MNCH) programmes is the 'continuum of care" (Figure 12.1). This expression has two meanings:[9]

- care has to be provided as a continuum throughout the lifecycle, including adolescence, pregnancy, childbirth and childhood
- care has to be provided in a seamless continuum that spans the home, the community, the health center and the hospital.

Recent years have seen a major emphasis on the persisting burden of maternal, child and newborn mortality globally, with a particular focus on the MDGs for maternal and child health. Issues pertaining to the burden of this mortality and on interventions to reduce it have been the subject of several recent *Lancet* series on child (2003), newborn (2005) and maternal survival (2006). These series have been complemented by series on reproductive health (2006), child development (2007) and maternal and childhood under-nutrition (2008). All of these series provided estimates of disease burden and described a wide array of effective interventions that could make a difference.

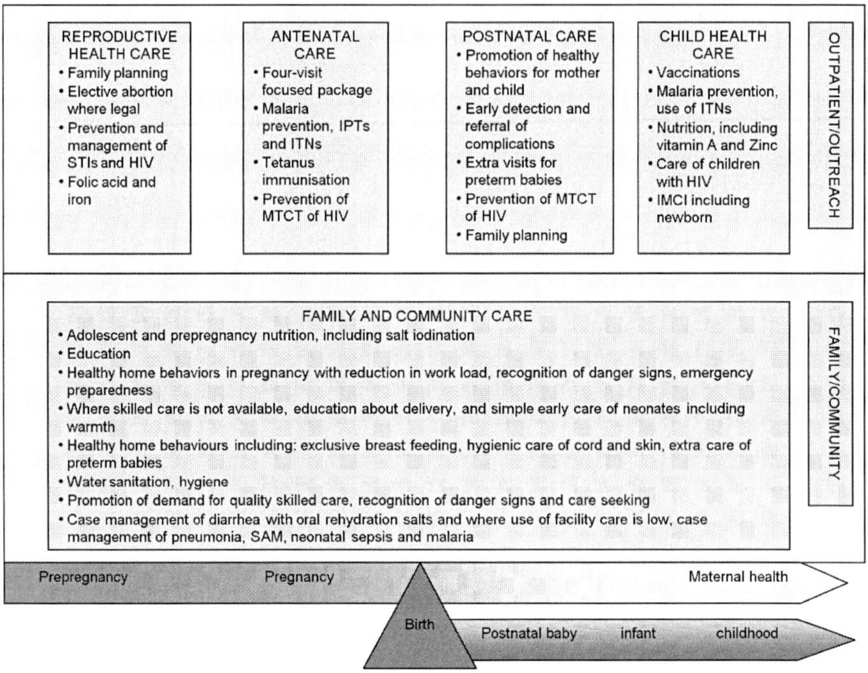

Figure 12.1 Interventions spanning the continuum of maternal, newborn and child health; IMCI = integrated management of childhood illness, IPT = intermittent preventive treatment, ITN = insecticide-treated bed net, MTCT = mother-to-child transmission, SAM = severe acute malnutrition, STI = sexually transmitted infection; reproduced with permission from Kerber *et al.*[7]

A recent evaluation of intervention coverage from 68 countries with 97% of the global burden of maternal and child deaths revealed that the implementation and uptake of interventions and the extent to which their distribution is equitable vary greatly (Figure 12.2).[11] It is uncertain whether any attempts have been made to integrate MNCH interventions at primary care level and a 2006 Cochrane review[8] revealed that few studies had attempted to do so, none including efforts at community level for demand generation. These findings are a major cause for concern and reflection. More than three decades after the Alma-Ata Declaration, the state of primary care for mothers, newborns and children remains poor and as a result only 16 countries are on track to reach MDG 4 of reducing child mortality, while data from which to estimate maternal mortality trends reliably simply do not exist.[8]

Some of the factors associated with this include lack of coordination between various programmes (both vertical and horizontal) and existing health workers, and critical shortages of trained health staff in primary care settings in populations at risk. These problems are exacerbated by a lack of common measures, messages and targets across the continuum of care for MNCH and by sometimes strongly conflicting views with regard to the optimal balance between community-, outreach- and facility-based intervention strategies.[12] For example, there has been an understandable emphasis on facility-based care and emergency obstetric care from those concerned with maternal health, while advocacy for newborn and child health has placed more emphasis on

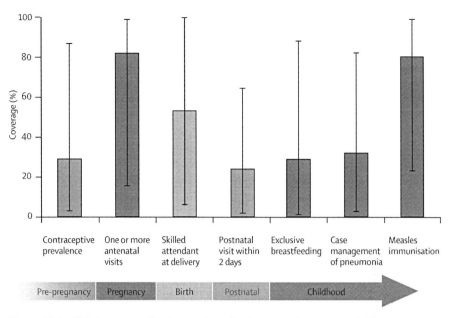

Figure 12.2   Global coverage of key interventions affecting maternal, newborn and child health in 68 Countdown countries; reproduced with permission from Bryce *et al.*[11]

community-based strategies. There is a real concern that, despite the proliferation of recent evidence reviews, no clear, consistent and generally agreed strategy for integrated MNCH care at primary care level, where the greatest need exists, has emerged. The evidence base for the types of interventions that a range of primary healthcare workers such as medical and paramedical staff, community health workers and other private sector care providers can deliver, together with complementary community and health system support strategies, is poor. In general, previous studies[13] and reviews[14] of community-based interventions have largely addressed care at household level without clear linkages and complementarities with the health system facilities. While several attempts have been made to package interventions for newborn and child survival, comparable efforts for understanding the evidence base for suitable and scalable maternal health interventions in primary care settings have lagged behind.

This gap of inefficient delivery of health services can be bridged by upgrading and implementing integrated MNCH interventions as health programmes at primary care level in low-income countries, which carry the major burden of maternal, newborn and child mortality. Needless to say, a good and well-developed health system and society infrastructure is fundamental to delivering quality health care and uplifting the health status of citizens. However, most developing nations lack such infrastructure. Until such a time that more stable infrastructure is built within developing, low-income countries, interventions delivered at the primary care level via existing cadres of health workers can help achieve the MDG targets. Integration is a more cost-effective, efficient and intelligent way to deliver health services and it is what is needed now when it comes to primary care.

Literature review of MNCH interventions

Selection criteria for interventions

Interventions with the potential to affect MNCH outcomes were included in this review, with a focus on studies undertaken in primary care settings in low- and middle-income countries. Primary care settings and interventions were defined as those that included:

- family and community interventions (largely at household or domiciliary level)
- interventions through outreach services including community health workers operating from village health outposts or first-level facilities
- interventions suitable for application in first-level facilities
- interventions to improve the continuity of care within and between these levels.

We also reviewed interventions that, although indirect, could potentially influence care-seeking behaviours and outcomes in primary care settings, including those that addressed women's empowerment and relevant poverty alleviation initiatives such as conditional cash transfers, vouchers and microcredit schemes.

Where the intervention was biologically plausible and feasible in primary care settings but evidence was unavailable from developing country settings, we also considered trials conducted in facility-based settings.

Search methods employed

The following databases were searched: MEDLINE, Cochrane Database of Systematic Reviews, Medcaribe, WHOLIS, PAHO, LILACS (Literatura Latino Americana e do Caribe em Ciências da Saúde) and SciELO (Scientific Electronic Library Online). Additional studies were obtained through handsearching of references from identified studies. Unpublished data were requested, when possible, from authors who reported having measured one of our outcomes of interest.

Evidence from the Cochrane Database of Randomised Controlled Trials (RCTs) and PubMed was also evaluated. Although our principal focus was information from RCTs, we extended the evaluation and included studies with a variety of alternative designs, especially large-scale or well-designed observational studies.

Interventions that work

Promotion of early and exclusive breastfeeding

Some of the most promising interventions may be delivered at the household level, with limited need for external material inputs. Among many others, promotion of exclusive breastfeeding is one such intervention. There is extensive evidence of both short- and long-term benefits of breastfeeding for the infant and the mother.[15] Epidemiological evidence suggests that beginning breastfeeding within the first day after birth reduces neonatal mortality.[16] Recent data indicate that very early initiation of breastfeeding within the first few hours after birth may significantly reduce neonatal mortality.[17]

The early initiation of breastfeeding is a cornerstone in any child survival programme. The *Lancet* neonatal survival series had breastfeeding as one of its interventions to reduce neonatal and child mortality.

A meta-analysis by Sheikh *et al.*[18] showed that there was a significant benefit of group counselling versus routine care on exclusive breastfeeding at 1 month (OR 3.95; 95% CI 2.09–7.44). Mothers who were individually counselled on breastfeeding were three times more likely (OR 3.06; 95% CI 2.10–4.45) to be exclusively breastfeeding in the neonatal period.

Possible basic resuscitation strategies in newborn care

Birth asphyxia is defined simply as the failure to initiate and sustain breathing at birth. According to WHO estimates, around 3% of approximately 120 million infants born every year in developing countries develop birth asphyxia requiring resuscitation. It is estimated that about 900 000 of these newborns die each year.[19] A survey of 127 institutions in 16 developed and developing countries found that there was often no basic resuscitation equipment or that it was in poor condition, and that health personnel were not properly trained in newborn resuscitation.[20] Effective basic resuscitation can revive more than three-quarters of newborns with birth asphyxia.[19] Delays in supporting a non-breathing baby to begin ventilation, as may happen in many developing country settings, may worsen hypoxia, increase the need for assisted ventilation and contribute to neonatal morbidity and mortality.

The optimal concentration of oxygen for neonatal resuscitation is uncertain. Evidence from animal studies suggests that room air is as effective as 100% oxygen in resuscitation, Rootwelt *et al.*[21] used a newborn pig model and resuscitated asphyxiated animals with either air or 100% oxygen. Birth asphyxia and the need for neonatal resuscitation are more common in the developing world. The difficulty of providing 100% oxygen is a limiting factor and if air were as effective it would be the preferred gas for neonatal resuscitation. It is vital that resuscitation of the newborn infant is performed efficiently. Determining the concentration of oxygen that maximises efficacy and safety is an important component of efforts to further improve techniques of neonatal resuscitation.[21]

Advanced resuscitation (including chest compressions, endotracheal intubation or medications) is required for less than 1% of all babies born.[22] The majority of newborns who require advanced resuscitation may not survive without continuing ventilation and neonatal intensive care. Thus, basic neonatal resuscitation including bag-and-mask ventilation is enough for most babies who would be saved by resuscitation in settings where resources are low. In a review of the evidence for neonatal resuscitation, Newton and English[23] concluded that effective resuscitation was possible with basic equipment and skills in low-resource settings.

A total of two reviews and six trials met our inclusion criteria. A Cochrane review by Tan *et al.*[24] compared the resuscitation of newborn with room air versus with 100% oxygen, which is recommended by the International Liaison Committee on Resuscitation (ILCOR), with the outcomes of death and neurological disability. The review included a total of five studies with 1302 neonates (mainly term infants). Pooled analysis of four studies (Ramji *et al.*,[25] Ramji *et al.*,[26] Saugstad[27] and Vento *et al.*[28]) reported the outcome of death at latest follow-up when room air was used versus 100% oxygen in the resuscitation of the newborn. Individual studies found no statistically significant difference between the two groups but the meta-analysis showed a statistically significant reduction in mortality in the group allocated to room air (typical RR 0.71; 95% CI 0.54–0.94). The comparison of room air versus 100% oxygen on the rate of failure of resuscitation in the two groups showed no statistically significant differences between the two groups. (RR 0.96; 95% CI 0.81–1.14).[24]

Cord care in newborn infants

The umbilical cord, which connects the baby and placenta *in utero*, comprises blood vessels and connective tissue. It is covered by a membrane that is bathed in amniotic fluid. After birth, cutting the cord physically and symbolically separates the mother and her baby. The cord stump dries, falls off and the wound heals. The cord usually separates between five and 15 days after birth. Before the separation, the remaining stump can be considered to be a healing wound and thus a possible route for infection through the vessels into the baby's bloodstream.[29] Umbilical cord infection contributes to neonatal mortality and morbidity risk in developing countries but reliable data from low-resource settings have been largely lacking. Cord cutting and care of the umbilical stump varies according to accepted practice and culture. In many parts of the world, the cord is cut with non-sterile tools such as used razors or scissors, after which various substances are applied, including charcoal, grease, cow dung or dried banana, to speed up cord separation. These practices are important sources of bacterial infection and neonatal tetanus.[29]

Contamination of the umbilical cord can lead to omphalitis, characterised by pus, abdominal erythema or swelling. Pathogens can enter the bloodstream through the patent vessels of the newly cut cord and lead to rapid demise, even in the absence of overt signs of cord infection. Hygienic delivery and postnatal care practices are widely promoted as important interventions to reduce risk of omphalitis and death.[30] In developed countries, many studies have shown that single or repeated antiseptic applications to the cord can substantially reduce bacterial colonisation.[30] However, the WHO and others emphasise good hygiene at delivery, and promote good cord care practice,[29] but acknowledge that antiseptics may be helpful when harmful, unhygienic, traditional practices place newborns at increased risk for omphalitis.[31]

Chlorhexidine, a widely used antiseptic, has broad-spectrum activity against Gram-positive (aerobic) and Gram-negative (anaerobic) organisms, especially those that are implicated in perinatal infections.[32]

We included a total of one review and nine RCTs evaluating the beneficial effect of cord care. Zupan et al.[29] conducted a systemic review that included trials comparing topical cord care versus no care. The review included 21 studies, comprising both randomised and quasi-randomised trials. Pooled analysis of nine studies comparing the antiseptics alcohol (Bain et al.,[33] Dore et al.,[34] Medves et al.[35] and Pezzati et al.[36]), triple dye (Barrett et al.,[37] Speck et al.[38] and Wald et al.[39]), silver sulfadiazine (Barrett et al.[37] and Speck et al.[38]), zinc powder (Mugford et al.[40]), chlorhexidine (Meberg et al.[41]), and salicylic sugar powder, green clay powder, katoxin powder and fuschine (Pezzati et al.[36]), versus dry cord care or placebo, showed no statistically significant difference between them (RR 0.53; 95% CI 0.25–1.13).

In Nepal,[30,31] a community-based, cluster-randomised study carried out from November 2002 to March 2005 and including a total of 15 123 infants evaluated the effects of 4.0% chlorhexidine on omphalitis and mortality risk and on the duration of cord separation. It found that cords of infants who received chlorhexidine were 3.6 times more likely to separate after 7 days. The study compared three cord-care regimens, with 4934 infants being assigned to 4.0% chlorhexidine, 5107 to cleansing with soap and water, and 5082 to dry cord care. The results showed a statistically significant reduction of omphalitis in the chlorhexidine group.

Kangaroo mother care

Worldwide, twenty-five million low-birthweight (LBW) infants are born each year, the great majority (96%) of them in developing countries. About two-thirds of all infant deaths in developed countries occur in this group of infants.[42] The care of an

LBW baby is a strategically difficult issue for these countries as the required financial support is scarce, as are the required technologies and the trained personnel.

In 1978, at Instituto Materno Infantil in Santa Fe de Bogotá, Colombia, kangaroo mother care (KMC) was proposed as an alternative to the conventional contemporary method of care for preterm LBW infants. The term KMC is derived from similarities to marsupial care-giving.[42] The mothers are used as 'incubators' and as the main source of food and stimulation for LBW infants until they are mature enough to face extrauterine life in similar conditions as those born at term. The method is applied only after the LBW infant has stabilised and all LBW infants need a variable period of conventional care before being eligible. KMC is based on two key practices:

1. the baby is kept dry and naked attached to the mother's breast in an upright position (day and night)

2. exclusive breastfeeding.

Various modalities of KMC have been adopted around the world, according to the needs of the settings. This diversity includes exclusive and non-exclusive breastfeeding, breast- or gavage (tube) feedings, completely or partially naked, with variable duration of exposure (1–24 hours/day), and early-or-not hospital discharge.[42]

The literature search yielded a total of two reviews and nine trials. Moore et al.[43] reviewed 30 studies, including 29 RCTs, evaluating the potential benefits of the practice of skin-to-skin care. Early skin-to-skin contact (SSC) resulted in statistically significantly better breastfeeding status. Ten RCTs evaluating the effect of SSC versus standard infant care on breastfeeding at 1–4 months had OR 1.82 (95% CI 1.08–3.07) and on exclusive breastfeeding at 4–6 months had OR 5.67 (95% CI 2.27–14.16).

A review by Conde-Agudelo et al.[42] of KMC showed reduced risk of nosocomial infection at 41 weeks' corrected gestational age (RR 0.49; 95% CI 0.25–0.93) and reduced risk of severe illness (RR 0.30; 95% CI 0.14–0.67). The mean hospital stay from randomisation to 41 weeks' corrected gestational age was 4.5 days for KMC infants and 5.6 days for infants in the control group in one study.[44]

Emollient use in newborns

Acquired infection is one of the major preventable causes of global neonatal mortality. The skin of preterm infants is immature and ineffective as an epidermal barrier.[45] Furthermore, preterm infants lack vernix caseosa, which contains microbial polypeptides that protect against invasion by microorganisms.[46] Preterm infants also have weak immune systems. Topical ointment therapy may enhance epidermal barrier function by protecting the stratum corneum, leading to improved skin integrity and less risk of nosocomial infection.[45] Topical oils may also be a nutritional source of essential fatty acids for preterm or LBW infants.[47,48] Few risks have been previously reported with the use of topical ointment, but concern has been expressed that ointment therapy may complicate the use of adhesives needed to secure intravenous catheters or endotracheal tubes.[45]

The literature search yielded one review and two trials meeting our inclusion criteria. The review by Conner et al.[45] assessed the effects of prophylactic application of topical ointment on nosocomial sepsis rates and other complications. Pooled data from the four included trials by Lane and Drost,[49] Nopper et al.,[50] Pabst et al.[51] and Edwards et al.[52] showed no statistically significant difference in the risk of bacterial infection with a known pathogen (RR 0.90; 95% CI 0.63–1.29). Only the trials by Edwards et al.[52] and Pabst et al.[51] provided data on the occurrence of fungal infection:

in the meta-analysis of these two trials, no statistically significant difference was noted between groups in the risk of fungal infection (RR 1.21; 95% CI 0.72–2.02). Conner *et al.*[46] proposed a protocol to assess the effects of topical application of emollients on the incidence of invasive infection in preterm or LBW infants in low- and or middle-income countries.

In a large trial in Bangladesh, Darmstadt *et al.*[53] evaluated sunflower seed oil as skin emollient and found improved skin condition and reduced nosocomial infections (RR 0.59; 95% CI 0.37–0.96) compared with controls. Mortality risk was substantially reduced (RR 0.74; 95% CI 0.55–0.99) among preterm infants receiving sunflower seed oil compared with controls.[54]

Mustard oil is used in a majority of neonates in developing countries, especially in South Asia but it is associated with serious adverse effects, including increased risk of microfissures in the epidermal layer. Traditional massage is often vigorous and involves substantial shear force to the skin, long exposure times and removal of residual vernix. These injurious effects heighten the likelihood of transcutaneous acquisition of invasive pathogens from the environment. Massage of the newborn with mustard oil has been associated with increased risk of umbilical cord sepsis.[55] In community settings, mustard oil is now been replaced by sun flower oil as a skin emollient in neonates.

Community treatment of infection in newborns (including antibiotics for pneumonia and sepsis)

Of the 4 million neonatal deaths in developing countries, a large proportion occur at home, frequently in circumstances where there are few alternative options[56] and where there is no attempt to seek care in the formal health system. There is thus an urgent need to define alternative strategies for care.[56] However, the two critical indicators, maternal and newborn mortality, have hardly changed.[14] Pneumonia still causes around 2 million deaths among children annually (20% of all child deaths). Any intervention that would reduce pneumonia-induced mortality would be of great public health importance.[57] Late-onset sepsis (systemic infection after 48 hours of age) continues to be a significant cause of morbidity and mortality. The incidence of late-onset sepsis increases with both decreasing birth weight and gestational age, and has been reported as occurring in approximately 25% of very LBW infants.[58]

Recommended treatment of serious systemic bacterial infections, including pneumonia, in neonates in developed countries includes parenteral administration of antibiotics in a healthcare facility. Similarly, in developing countries, WHO recommends parenteral antibiotic therapy (for example, benzylpenicillin or ampicillin plus an aminoglycoside such as gentamicin) in a health facility for treatment of serious neonatal infections. The range of organisms causing late-onset sepsis includes Gram-positive and Gram-negative bacteria as well as fungi. As bacterial infections predominate, empirical antibiotic regimens focus on cover for both Gram-positive and Gram-negative bacterial infection.[58] In resource-poor countries, however, the majority of births and neonatal deaths take place in the home, and families are often reluctant to seek care outside the home for neonatal illness.[14] Neonatal care is not available to most neonates in developing countries because hospitals are inaccessible and costly.[59]

Insight into the role of oral antibiotic therapy as a potentially simpler and more feasible regimen for treating serious neonatal infections in situations in which referral to a health facility for quality care and parenteral therapy is not possible may be gained by reviewing pneumonia case-management trials that included treatment of neonates.[14] A paucity of community-based data was found from developing-country studies on health status impact for many interventions currently being considered for inclusion in neonatal health programmes.

We have included six systemic reviews relevant to the topics of community-based treatment of pneumonia and sepsis in our literature review. Meta-analysis in the review by Sazawal et al.[57] evaluating the case-management approach proposed by WHO on the mortality rates due to pneumonia found a reduction in total mortality of 27% (95% CI 18–35%). A review by Gordon and Jeffery[58] compared the effectiveness of various antibiotic regimens for initial treatment of suspected late-onset sepsis (after 48 hours of age) in newborn infants with respect to mortality, septic shock and neurodevelopmental outcome. The review included randomised and quasi-randomised trials. Miall-Allen et al.[60] compared the a beta-lactam antibiotic versus a combination of beta-lactam plus aminoglycosides on the outcome of mortality before discharge and found no statistically significant difference between the two (RR 0.17; 95% CI 0.01–3.23). A review by Mtitimila and Cooke[61] included studies by Miall-Allen[60] and Snelling[62] comparing antibiotic monotherapy versus combination therapy on the outcome of mortality (28 days after birth). There were no deaths in intervention groups in one study[61] but a total of eight deaths in the other study.[62] Three deaths occurred in the monotherapy group (ticarcillin plus clavulanic acid; Timentin®; GSK) and five deaths were in the combination therapy group (piperacillin and gentamicin). A meta-analysis found that there was no statistically significant difference in mortality to 28 days (RR 0.75; 85% CI 0.19–2.9). A review by Rao et al.[63] evaluating the efficacy and safety of one dose per day compared with multiple doses per day of gentamicin in suspected or proven sepsis in neonates showed a statistically significant difference indicating that a once a day regimen is associated with fewer failures than a multiple doses a day regimen (RR 0.22; 95% CI 0.11–0.47).

A review by Shah et al.[64] compared the effectiveness and safety of intraventricular antibiotics (with or without intravenous antibiotics) in neonates with meningitis (with or without ventriculitis) versus conventional treatment with intravenous antibiotics alone. The mortality was statistically significantly higher in the group that received intraventricular antibiotics and intravenous antibiotics compared with the group that received intravenous antibiotics only (RR 3.43; 95% CI 1.09–10.74).

Bhutta et al.[65] reviewed all available observational reports, RCTs, systematic reviews and meta-analyses that addressed the management of serious neonatal infections in primary care settings. Evidence for the benefit of community-based case management of neonatal pneumonia was synthesised in a meta-analysis of five included trials, which were conducted in India, Pakistan, Nepal, Tanzania and Bangladesh. The pooled analysis showed a statistically significant reduction in pneumonia-specific neonatal mortality of 42% (95% CI 22–57%; four trials), as well as a statistically significant reduction in the overall neonatal mortality rate (NMR) of 27% (95% CI 8–35%; five trials).

Our review also included the study by Bartlett et al.[66] on infant pneumonia and/or sepsis in a rural community in Guatemala. Thirty-four infants (10%) developed potentially life-threatening infectious diseases (92% of all serious medical problems encountered) and were treated in the community with various regimens. The overall case fatality was 14%, and none of the babies managed wholly in the community died. An estimated NMR of 6 per 1000 live births was calculated using local population-based data, compared with a historical NMR of 39 per 1000 live births recorded for Guatemala, translating to an 85% reduction in NMR (P<0.001). Bang et al.[13] evaluated a home-based package for neonatal care in rural Gadchiroli, India, an area with an extremely high baseline NMR of almost 100 per 1000 live births. Village heath workers administered home-based treatment using oral co-trimoxazole twice daily and intramuscular gentamicin twice daily for 7 days in full-term babies and 10 days in preterm babies, with support for temperature maintenance and encouragement of breastfeeding, together with follow-up twice daily for 7–10 days. The overall decline in mortality from 62 to 25.5 per 1000 live births represented a 62% reduction relative to baseline control rates ($P<0.001$); sepsis-specific mortality was reduced by 76% from 27.5 to 6.6 per 1000 live births in the intervention area compared with the control ($P<0.005$).

Baqui et al.[67] reviewed an RCT from Sylhet in rural Bangladesh in which 24 clusters (with a population of about 20000 each) were randomly assigned in equal numbers to one of two intervention arms (home care or community care) or to a comparison arm. In the home visits clusters, newborns were assessed on the first, third and seventh day of life, and sick neonates were referred or treated. In the community-care arm, birth and newborn-care preparedness and care-seeking from qualified providers were promoted solely through group sessions held by female and male community mobilisers. The NMRs were 29.2 per 1000, 45.2 per 1000 and 43.5 per 1000 in the home-care, community-care and comparison arms, respectively. Neonatal mortality was reduced in the home-care arm by 34% (adjusted RR 0.66; 95% CI 0.47–0.93) during the last 6 months of the 30-month intervention versus the comparison arm. No mortality reduction was noted in the community-care arm (adjusted RR 0.95; 95% CI 0.69–1.31).

Finally, data were also reviewed from a study of community management of suspected neonatal sepsis in Pakistan[68] that suggested that community health workers could recognise serious neonatal infections and refer newborns for treatment with injectable antibiotics in a primary care community health centre. Among 434 newborn infants with suspected sepsis, an overall 86% success rate was seen for treatment with one of three regimens (daily injectable penicillin and gentamicin or daily injectable ceftriaxone or daily oral co-trimoxazole and injectable gentamicin). The latter regimen was found to be inferior to the penicillin and gentamicin combination and to the ceftriaxone regimen.

Community support groups and packages of care

Six studies evaluating the impact of community-based interventions on perinatal and neonatal outcomes were identified in the literature search. All studies had used a cluster design, with four using a randomised assignment of the intervention. The studies were conducted in developing countries. Table 12.1 presents a summary of the main characteristics of the included studies.

All included studies implemented an intervention package at the community level for improving perinatal and newborn care. Three studies[59,69,70] engaged local community/village health workers who were further trained in essential maternal and newborn care. The preventive intervention package consisted of home visits both in the antenatal and postnatal periods to promote birth and newborn care preparedness. Community-based group counselling was also employed to promote domiciliary care and improved care-seeking. These health workers were also linked up with the traditional birth attendants (TBAs) in the area. Bhutta et al.[65] engaged public sector trained staff (lady health workers; LHWs) who received additional training on essential newborn care. The LHWs were also supported by voluntary community health committees that assisted in community health education group sessions. The

Table 12.1 Studies investigating intervention packages at the community level for improving perinatal and newborn care

Study	Region	Design	Intervention
Baqui *et al.* (2008)[69]	Sylhet, Bangladesh	Cluster RCT	The home-care (HC) intervention consisted of two antenatal and three postnatal home visits, as well as home screening/management of sick children by community health workers, community mobilisation meetings with men and women, orientation of TBAs on newborn care and strengthening of health facilities for routine maternal/neonatal care and management of maternal/newborn complications (represented as 'Baqui hc 2008' in Figure 12.3). The community-care (CC) intervention consisted of community meetings with pregnant women and family members and advocacy meetings with local leaders, TBA training on cleanliness during delivery, maternal danger signs and newborn care; recruitment of volunteer community-resource people to improve attendance at community meetings and care-seeking for maternal and neonatal complications (represented as 'Baqui cc 2008' in Figure 12.4).
Bhutta *et al.* (2008)[65]	Hala, Pakistan	Cluster CT	The LHWs in the intervention clusters received additional training on essential maternal and newborn care, conducted community education group sessions, and were encouraged to link up with local TBAs (dais). The intervention was delivered within the regular government LHW programme and was supported by the creation of a voluntary community health committee.
Kumar *et al.* (2008)[70]	Shivgarh, India	Cluster RCT	Preventive package of essential newborn care (ENC) plus use of ThermoSpot. In the intervention clusters, community health workers delivered the intervention package to target groups (community stakeholders, newborn care stakeholders, households) through group meetings and two antenatal and two postnatal household visits.
Jokhio *et al.* (2005)[71]	Sind, Pakistan	Cluster RCT	TBAs were trained and issued disposable delivery kits; LHWs linked TBAs with established services and documented processes and outcomes, and obstetric teams provided outreach clinics for antenatal care.
Manandhar *et al.* (2004)[72]	Makwanpur, Nepal	Cluster RCT	Female facilitators supported women's groups through an action–learning cycle in which they identified local perinatal problems and formulated strategies to address them.
Bang *et al.* (1999)[59]	Maharashtra, India	Cluster CT	Village health workers trained in neonatal care made home visits and managed birth asphyxia, preterm birth or low birth weight, hypothermia and breastfeeding problems. They diagnosed and treated neonatal sepsis. Assistance by trained TBAs, health education and fortnightly supervisory visits were also provided.

CT = controlled trial; LHW = lady health worker; RCT = randomised controlled trial; TBA = traditional birth attendant

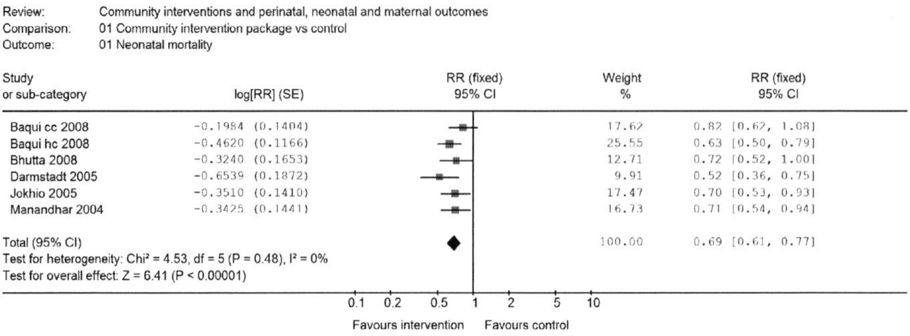

Review: Community interventions and perinatal, neonatal and maternal outcomes
Comparison: 01 Community intervention package vs control
Outcome: 01 Neonatal mortality

Study or sub-category	log[RR] (SE)	RR (fixed) 95% CI	Weight %	RR (fixed) 95% CI
Baqui cc 2008	-0.1984 (0.1404)		17.62	0.82 [0.62, 1.08]
Baqui hc 2008	-0.4620 (0.1166)		25.55	0.63 [0.50, 0.79]
Bhutta 2008	-0.3240 (0.1653)		12.71	0.72 [0.52, 1.00]
Darmstadt 2005	-0.6539 (0.1872)		9.91	0.52 [0.36, 0.75]
Jokhio 2005	-0.3510 (0.1410)		17.47	0.70 [0.53, 0.93]
Manandhar 2004	-0.3425 (0.1441)		16.73	0.71 [0.54, 0.94]
Total (95% CI)			100.00	0.69 [0.61, 0.77]

Test for heterogeneity: Chi² = 4.53, df = 5 (P = 0.48), I² = 0%
Test for overall effect: Z = 6.41 (P < 0.00001)

0.1 0.2 0.5 1 2 5 10
Favours intervention   Favours control

Figure 12.3 Impact of community interventions on neonatal mortality

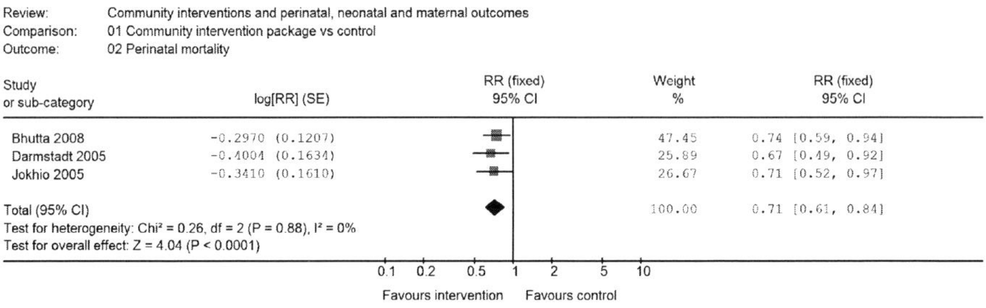

Review: Community interventions and perinatal, neonatal and maternal outcomes
Comparison: 01 Community intervention package vs control
Outcome: 02 Perinatal mortality

Study or sub-category	log[RR] (SE)	RR (fixed) 95% CI	Weight %	RR (fixed) 95% CI
Bhutta 2008	-0.2970 (0.1207)		47.45	0.74 [0.59, 0.94]
Darmstadt 2005	-0.4004 (0.1634)		25.89	0.67 [0.49, 0.92]
Jokhio 2005	-0.3410 (0.1610)		26.67	0.71 [0.52, 0.97]
Total (95% CI)			100.00	0.71 [0.61, 0.84]

Test for heterogeneity: Chi² = 0.26, df = 2 (P = 0.88), I² = 0%
Test for overall effect: Z = 4.04 (P < 0.0001)

0.1 0.2 0.5 1 2 5 10
Favours intervention   Favours control

Figure 12.4 Impact of community interventions on perinatal mortality

TBAs in this study were also offered voluntary training in basic newborn care. Jokhio et al.[71] trained TBAs, who were issued with disposable delivery kits. TBAs were asked to visit women three times during pregnancy to check for danger signs and to encourage women to seek emergency care, if necessary. Manandhar et al.[72] engaged female facilitators who convened women's group meetings with the objective of identifying local perinatal problems and developing strategies to address them through an action–learning cycle. The community workers or TBAs in all studies except two[59,72] were linked with the local health system.

A meta-analysis was undertaken to estimate a summary measure for perinatal, neonatal and maternal outcomes. To control for the cluster design of included studies, data were analysed using a generic inverse variance method. Community-based interventions were associated with a 31% reduction in neonatal mortality (five studies: RR 0.69; 95% CI 0.61–0.77) (Figure 12.3). Analysis for the outcome of perinatal mortality included data from three studies.[65,70,71] The outcome was defined as stillbirths and neonatal deaths in the first week of life by Darmstadt et al.[70] and Bhutta et al.[65] However, the perinatal mortality outcome reported by Jokhio et al.[71] included stillbirths and neonatal deaths in the first month of life. Summary estimates including data from these studies showed a 29% reduction in the risk of perinatal mortality with community-based interventions (three studies: RR 0.71; 95% CI 0.61–0.84) (Figure 12.4).

References

1. Bhutta ZA, Memon Z, Zaidi S, Billoo AG, Hyder A. *Etiology of Perinatal and Neonatal Deaths in a Rural Population of Pakistan: a Verbal Autopsy*. Geneva: WHO (Global Forum For Health Research); 2002.

2. Bhutta ZA, Ali N, Hyder A, Wajid A. Perinatal and newborn care in Pakistan: seeing the unseen. In: Bhutta ZA, editor. *Maternal and Child Health in Pakistan: Challenges and Opportunities*. Karachi: Oxford University Press; 2004. p. 19–46.

3. Child Health Research Project. *Special Report: Reducing Perinatal and Neonatal Mortality*. Report of a meeting. Baltimore, MD: Child Health Research Project; 1999 .

4. Lawn JE, Cousens S, Zupan J; Lancet Neonatal Survival Steering Team. 4 million neonatal deaths: when? Where? Why? *Lancet* 2005;365:891–900.

5. Commission on Social Determinants of Health. *Closing the Gap in One Generation: Health Equity through Action on Social Determinants of Health*. Geneva: World Health Organization; 2008 [www.who.int/social_determinants/thecommission/finalreport/en/index.html].

6. Jamison DT, Shahid-Salles SA, Jamison JS, Lawn JE, Zupan J. Incorporating deaths near the time of birth into estimates of the global burden of disease. In: Jamison DT, editor. *Disease Control Priorities in Developing Countries*. 2nd edition. New York/Washington, DC: Oxford University Press/World Bank; 2006. p. 427–62.

7. Kerber KJ, de Graft-Johnson JE, Bhutta ZA, Okong P, Starrs A, Lawn JE. Continuum of care for maternal, newborn, and child health: from slogan to service delivery. *Lancet* 2007;370:1358–69.

8. Briggs CJ, Garner P. Strategies for integrating primary health services in middle- and low-income countries at the point of delivery. *Cochrane Database Syst Rev* 2006;(2):CD003318.

9. World Health Organization. *World Health Report 2005: Make Every Mother and Child Count*. Geneva: WHO; 2005..

10. World Health Organization. *Strategic Framework for Integrating Additional Child Survival Interventions with Immunization in the African Region*. Geneva; WHO; 2006.

11. Bryce J, Daelmans B, Dwivedi A, Fauveau V, Lawn JE, Mason E, *et al*. Countdown to 2015 for maternal, newborn, and child survival: the 2008 report on tracking coverage of interventions. *Lancet* 2008;371:1247–58.

12. Haines A, Horton R, Bhutta Z. Primary health care comes of age. Looking forward to the 30th anniversary of Alma-Ata: call for papers. *Lancet* 2007;370:911–13.

13. Bang AT, Bang RA, Reddy HM. Home-based neonatal care: summary and applications of the field trial in rural Gadchiroli, India (1993 to 2003). *J Perinatol* 2005;25 Suppl 1:S108–22.

14. Bhutta ZA, Darmstadt GL, Hasan BS, Haws RA. Community-based interventions for improving perinatal and neonatal health outcomes in developing countries: a review of the evidence. *Pediatrics* 2005;115(2 Suppl):519–617.

15. Britton C, McCormick FM, Renfrew MJ, Wade A, King SE. Support for breastfeeding mothers. *Cochrane Database Syst Rev* 2007;(1):CD001141.

16. Jones G, Steketee RW, Black RE, Bhutta ZA, Morris SS. How many child deaths can we prevent this year? *Lancet* 2003;362:65–71.

17. Edmond KM, Kirkwood BR, Amenga-Etego S, Owusu-Agyei S, Hurt LS. Effect of early infant feeding practices on infection-specific neonatal mortality: an investigation of the causal links with observational data from rural Ghana. *Am J Clin Nutr* 2007;86:1126–31.

18. Sheikh SM, Yakoob MY, Haider BA, Bhutta ZA. Effect of individual and group counselling on breastfeeding rates. *BMC Pregnancy Childbirth* (in press).

19. World Health Organization. *Basic Newborn Resuscitation: A Practical Guide*. Geneva: WHO; 1998.

20. Palme C. 'State of the art' in workshop participating countries: a report of a survey. In: Sterky G, Tafari N, Tunell R, editors. *Breathing and Warmth at Birth*. Stockholm: SAREC; 1985. p. 29–32.

21. Rootwelt T, Odden JP, Hall C, Saugstad OD. Regional blood flow during severe hypoxemia and resuscitation with 21% or 100% O2 in newborn pigs. *J Perinat Med* 1996;24(3):227–36.

22. Kattwinkel J, Boyle DW, editors. *Textbook of Neonatal Resuscitation*. 5th ed. Elk Grove Village, IL: American Academy of Pediatrics; 2005.

23. Newton O, English M. Newborn resuscitation: defining best practice for low-income settings. *Trans R Soc Trop Med Hyg* 2006;100:899–908.

24. Tan A, Schulze A, O'Donnell CP, Davis PG. Air versus oxygen for resuscitation of infants at birth. *Cochrane Database Syst Rev* 2005;(2):CD002273.

25. Ramji S, Ahuja S, Thirupuram S, Rootwelt T, Rooth G, Saugstad OD. Resuscitation of asphyxic newborn infants with room air or 100% oxygen. *Pediatr Res* 1993;34:809–12.

26. Ramji S, Rasaily R, Mishra PK, Narang A, Jayam S, Kapoor AN, et al. Resuscitation of asphyxiated newborns with room air or 100% oxygen at birth: a multicentric clinical trial. *Indian Pediatr* 2003;40:510–17.

27. Saugstad OD. Resuscitation with room-air or oxygen supplementation. *Clin Perinatol* 1998;25:741–56,xi.

28. Vento M, Asensi M, Sastre J, Lloret A, Garcia-Sala F, Vina J. Oxidative stress in asphyxiated term infants resuscitated with 100% oxygen. *J Pediatr* 2003;142:240–6.

29. Zupan J, Garner P, Omari AA. Topical umbilical cord care at birth. *Cochrane Database Syst Rev* 2004;(3):CD001057.

30. Mullany LC, Darmstadt GL, Khatry SK, Katz J, LeClerq SC, Shrestha S, et al. Topical applications of chlorhexidine to the umbilical cord for prevention of omphalitis and neonatal mortality in southern Nepal: a community-based, cluster-randomised trial. *Lancet.* 2006;367:910–18.

31. Mullany LC, Darmstadt GL, Khatry SK, LeClerq SC, Katz J, Tielsch JM. Impact of umbilical cord cleansing with 4.0% chlorhexidine on time to cord separation among newborns in southern Nepal: a cluster-randomized, community-based trial. *Pediatrics* 2006;118:1864–71.

32. Lumbiganon P, Thinkhamrop J, Thinkhamrop B, Tolosa JE. Vaginal chlorhexidine during labour for preventing maternal and neonatal infections (excluding Group B Streptococcal and HIV). *Cochrane Database Syst Rev* 2004;(4):CD004070.

33. Bain J. Midwifery: umbilical cord care in preterm babies. *Nurs Stand* 1994;8:32–6.

34. Dore S, Buchan D, Coulas S, Hamber L, Stewart M, Cowan D, et al. Alcohol versus natural drying for newborn cord care. *J Obstet Gynecol Neonatal Nurs* 1998;27:621–7.

35. Medves JM, O'Brien BA. Cleaning solutions and bacterial colonization in promoting healing and early separation of the umbilical cord in healthy newborns. *Can J Public Health* 1997;88:380–2.

36. Pezzati M, Biagioli EC, Martelli E, Gambi B, Biagiotti R, Rubaltelli FF. Umbilical cord care: the effect of eight different cord-care regimens on cord separation time and other outcomes. *Biol Neonate* 2002;81:38–44.

37. Barrett F, Mason E, Fleming D. The effect of three cord care regimens on the bacterial colonization of normal newborn infants. *J Pediatrics* 1979;94:796–800.

38. Speck WT, Driscoll JM, O'Neil J, Rosenkranz HS. Effect of antiseptic cord care on bacterial colonization in the newborn infant. *Chemotherapy* 1980;26:372–6.

39. Wald ER, Snyder MJ, Gutberlet RL. Group B beta-hemolytic streptococcal colonization. Acquisition, persistence, and effect of umbilical cord treatment with triple dye. *Am J Dis Child* 1977;131:178–80.

40. Mugford M, Somchiwong M, Waterhouse IL. Treatment of umbilical cords: a randomised trial to assess the effect of treatment methods on the work of midwives. *Midwifery* 1986;2:177–86.

41. Meberg A, Schoyen R. Bacterial colonization and neonatal infections. Effects of skin and umbilical disinfection in the nursery. *Acta Paediatr Scand* 1985;74:366–71.

42. Conde-Agudelo A, Diaz-Rossello JL, Belizan JM. Kangaroo mother care to reduce morbidity and mortality in low birthweight infants. *Cochrane Database Syst Rev* 2003;(2):CD002771.

43. Moore ER, Anderson GC, Bergman N. Early skin-to-skin contact for mothers and their healthy newborn infants. *Cochrane Database Syst Rev* 2007;(3):CD003519.

44. Charpak N, Ruiz-Pelaez JG, Charpak Y. Rey-Martinez Kangaroo Mother Program: an alternative way of caring for low birth weight infants? One year mortality in a two cohort study. *Pediatrics* 1994;94(6 Pt 1):804–10.

45. Conner J, Soll R, Edwards W. Topical ointment for preventing infection in preterm infants. *Cochrane Database Syst Rev* 2003;(4):CD001150.

46. Yoshio H, Tollin M, Gudmundsson GH, Lagercrantz H, Jornvall H, Marchini G, et al. Antimicrobial polypeptides of human vernix caseosa and amniotic fluid: implications for newborn innate defense. *Pediatr Res* 2003;53:211–16.

47. Lee EJ, Gibson RA, Simmer K. Transcutaneous application of oil and prevention of essential fatty acid deficiency in preterm infants. *Arch Dis Child* 1993;68(1 Spec No):27–8.

48. Solanki K, Matnani M, Kale M, Joshi K, Bavdekar A, Bhave S, *et al.* Transcutaneous absorption of topically massaged oil in neonates. *Indian Pediatr* 2005;42:998–1005.

49. Lane AT, Drost SS. Effects of repeated application of emollient cream to premature neonates' skin. *Pediatrics* 1993;92:415–19.

50. Nopper AJ, Horii KA, Sookdeo-Drost S, Wang TH, Mancini AJ, Lane AT. Topical ointment therapy benefits premature infants. *J Pediatr* 1996;128(5 Pt 1):660–9.

51. Pabst RC, Starr KP, Qaiyumi S, Schwalbe RS, Gewolb IH. The effect of application of aquaphor on skin condition, fluid requirements, and bacterial colonization in very low birth weight infants. *J Perinatol* 1999;19:278–83.

52. Edwards WH, Conner JM, Soll RF. The effect of prophylactic ointment therapy on nosocomial sepsis rates and skin integrity in infants with birth weights of 501 to 1000 g. *Pediatrics* 2004;113:1195–203.

53. Darmstadt GL, Saha SK, Ahmed AS, Chowdhury MA, Law PA, Ahmed S, *et al.* Effect of topical treatment with skin barrier-enhancing emollients on nosocomial infections in preterm infants in Bangladesh: a randomised controlled trial. *Lancet* 2005;365:1039–45.

54. Darmstadt GL, Saha SK, Ahmed ASM, Ahmed S, Chowdhury MAK, Law PA, *et al.* Effect of skin barrier therapy on neonatal mortality rates in preterm infants in Bangladesh: a randomized, controlled, clinical trial. *Pediatrics* 2008;121:522.

55. Mullany LC, Darmstadt GL, Katz J, Khatry SK, LeClerq SC, Adhikari RK, *et al.* Risk factors for umbilical cord infection among newborns of southern Nepal. *Am J Epidemiol* 2007;165:203.

56. Bhutta ZA, Ahmed T, Black RE, Cousens S, Dewey K, Giugliani E, *et al.* What works? Interventions for maternal and child undernutrition and survival. *Lancet* 2008;371:417–40.

57. Sazawal S, Black RE. Effect of pneumonia case management on mortality in neonates, infants, and preschool children: a meta-analysis of community-based trials. *Lancet Infect Dis* 2003;3:547–56.

58. Gordon A, Jeffery HE. Antibiotic regimens for suspected late onset sepsis in newborn infants. *Cochrane Database Syst Rev* 2005;(3):CD004501.

59. Bang AT, Bang RA, Baitule SB, Reddy MH, Deshmukh MD. Effect of home-based neonatal care and management of sepsis on neonatal mortality: field trial in rural India. *Lancet* 1999;354:1955–61.

60. Miall-Allen VM, Whitelaw AG, Darrell JH. Ticarcillin plus clavulanic acid (Timentin) compared with standard antibiotic regimes in the treatment of early and late neonatal infections. *Br J Clin Pract* 1988;42:273–9.

61. Mtitimila EI, Cooke RW. Antibiotic regimens for suspected early neonatal sepsis. *Cochrane Database Syst Rev* 2004;(4):CD004495.

62. Snelling S, Hart CA, Cooke RW. Ceftazidime or gentamicin plus benzylpenicillin in neonates less than forty-eight hours old. *J Antimicrob Chemother* 1983;12 Suppl A:353–6.

63. Rao SC, Ahmed M, Hagan R. One dose per day compared with multiple doses per day of gentamicin for treatment of suspected or proven sepsis in neonates. *Cochrane Database Syst Rev* 2006;(1):CD005091.

64. Shah S, Ohlsson A, Shah V. Intraventricular antibiotics for bacterial meningitis in neonates. *Cochrane Database Syst Rev* 2004;(4):CD004496.

65. Bhutta ZA, Zaidi AK, Thaver D, Humayun Q, Ali S, Darmstadt GL. Management of newborn infections in primary care settings: a review of the evidence and implications for policy? *Pediatr Infect Dis J* 2009;28(1 Suppl):S22–30.

66. Bartlett AV, Paz de Bocaletti ME, Bocaletti MA. Neonatal and early postneonatal morbidity and mortality in a rural Guatemalan community: the importance of infectious diseases and their management. *Pediatr Infect Dis J* 1991;10:752–7.

67. Baqui AH, El-Arifeen S, Darmstadt GL, Ahmed S, Williams EK, Seraji HR, *et al*; Projahnmo Study Group. Effect of community-based newborn-care intervention package implemented through two service-delivery strategies in Sylhet district, Bangladesh: a cluster-randomised controlled trial. *Lancet* 2008;371:1936–44.

68. Zaidi *et al.* (2007), personal communication.

69. Baqui AH, Arifeen SE, Darmstadt GL. Improving newborn survival and changing household essential newborn care practices in rural Bangladesh: The Projahnmo Experience. *Lancet* 2008;371:1936–44.

70. Kumar V, Mohanty S, Kumar A, Misra RP, Santosham M, Awasthi S, *et al*; Saksham Study Group. Effect of community-based behaviour change management on neonatal mortality in Shivgarh, Uttar Pradesh, India: a cluster-randomised controlled trial. *Lancet* 2008;372:1151–62.

71. Jokhio AH, Winter HR, Cheng KK. An intervention involving traditional birth attendants and perinatal and maternal mortality in Pakistan. *N Engl J Med* 2005;352:2091–9.

72. Manandhar DS, Osrin D, Shrestha BP, Mesko N, Morrison J, Tumbahangphe KM, *et al*. Effect of a participatory intervention with women's groups on birth outcomes in Nepal: cluster-randomised controlled trial. *Lancet* 2004;364:970–9.

Chapter 13

Community interventions to reduce maternal and child mortality in low-income countries

Audrey Prost, Christina Pagel and Anthony Costello

This chapter considers progress towards maternal and child survival, the recent evidence for community health worker interventions to reduce newborn mortality and newer evidence about the effect of community mobilisation through women's groups for newborn survival. We also consider the potential for community interventions to augment health service strengthening as a way to reduce maternal mortality through family planning, financial incentives for institutional delivery and community delivery of life-saving drugs, especially in Africa. Finally, we consider the shortfall in investment for maternal and newborn health and the failure of donors and governments to provide anything close to what is required if progress is to be made towards maternal and newborn survival in the poorest countries.

Progress towards maternal and child survival

The Millennium Development Goals (MDGs) 4 and 5 expressed targets to reduce under-five mortality by two-thirds and maternal mortality by three-quarters in every country, with 1990 as the baseline year and 2015 as the endpoint.[1] In 2008, the Countdown to 2015 report described progress in 68 target countries with high baseline mortality rates.[2] Some were on track towards the under-five mortality target, namely Bangladesh, Brazil, Egypt, Indonesia, Mexico, Nepal, the Philippines, China, Haiti, Morocco and Turkmenistan. A further 28 priority countries (41%) had made insufficient progress in reducing under-five mortality, and 25 (37%) had made no progress at all. In 12 countries (Botswana, Cameroon, Central African Republic, Chad, Congo, Equatorial Guinea, Kenya, Lesotho, South Africa, Swaziland, Zambia and Zimbabwe), under-five mortality had increased. The report suggested that reliable figures for trends in newborn mortality were not available and that this gap in epidemiological information should be addressed urgently. It is important to recognise that newborn deaths now account for about half of under-five deaths in South Asia and about one-third of deaths in Africa. As under-five mortality rates fall, the proportion of deaths occurring in the neonatal period (up to 28 days after birth) rises.[3] Stillbirths do not appear in official statistics. Data on stillbirths are very limited but an estimated 3–4 million occur annually.[4]

Two countries merit special attention. India accounts for 20% of maternal deaths worldwide, 21% of all under-five deaths and 25% of all neonatal deaths.[5] Nigeria is the largest country in Africa and accounts for almost 11% of maternal[6] and 9% of under-five[7] deaths worldwide.

The most recent global review of maternal mortality trends[6] estimated that the global maternal mortality ratio (MMR) reduced from 422 per 100 000 live births (uncertainty bounds 358–505) in 1980 to 320 per 100 000 live births (uncertainty bounds 272–388) in 1990, and was 251 per 100 000 live births (uncertainty bounds 221–289) in 2008 (Table 13.1). However, the rate of decline between countries over the period 1990–2008 was very varied, with several countries having only very small reductions. More than 50% of all maternal deaths were in only six countries in 2008 (India, Nigeria, Pakistan, Afghanistan, Ethiopia and the Democratic Republic of the Congo) and only 23 countries are on track to achieve a 75% reduction in MMR by 2015. Additionally, 52% of maternal deaths in 2008 occurred in sub-Saharan Africa.[6] These latest estimates thus show progress, albeit varied, towards MDG 5. We note that substantial variation within countries can exist and the challenge in reaching women in areas with the highest maternal mortality rates remains considerable.

There is also growing evidence about inequalities in access to care across household economic quintiles, which reflects the 'inverse care law' by which families who need services most get them least and those who need them least get them most.[8,9] In part, this will contribute to the higher death rates observed in the poorest quintiles. For this reason, this chapter will later consider ways in which community approaches may augment a health systems strengthening approach.[10]

Evidence for community health worker interventions to reduce newborn mortality

In 1999, Bang and colleagues[11] published the first controlled trial of a community health worker intervention to reduce newborn mortality. The SEARCH trial intervention comprised three components: training of traditional birth attendants, health promotion and training of local village women to recognise and treat newborn sepsis with injectable gentamicin and co-trimoxazole. The study was not randomised, but reported an eventual 62% reduction in newborn mortality.[12] It demonstrated that, even in poor rural villages where access to health services was almost non-existent,

Table 13.1   Maternal mortality estimates for example regions; data from Hogan *et al.*[6]

	MMR		Change
	1990	2008	
Overall	320	251	−22%
Western Europe	10	7	−30%
East sub-Saharan Africa	690	508	−26%
Central sub-Saharan Africa	732	586	−20%
South sub-Saharan Africa	171	381	+122%
West sub-Saharan Africa	582	629	+8%
South Asia	560	323	−42%

MMR = maternal mortality ratio (maternal deaths per 100 000 live births)

substantial reductions in newborn mortality were possible. Nonetheless, there are a number of concerns about the scalability of this approach. No governments so far have approved the large-scale use of injectable antibiotics given by locally trained women to newborn infants.

More recently, three studies have looked at the impact of community health worker training on newborn mortality in India, Bangladesh and Pakistan. In Uttar Pradesh, India, the Shivgarh study[13] investigated the impact of an intensive behaviour-change programme involving community meetings and home visits by paid, non-governmental community workers. The study covered a population of around 104 000 over a 15-month period and reported a 53% reduction in neonatal mortality, with changes in home-care practices but no substantial change in care-seeking. Interpretation of this study is complicated by the fact that the control area neonatal mortality rate (NMR) rose sharply during the study, which may have distorted the true impact. In Bangladesh, the Projahnmo trial[14] evaluated two interventions: first, a home-care arm where paid non-governmental community health workers identified pregnant women, made two antenatal home visits and two postnatal home visits, and referred or treated sick neonates; and second, a 'community-care' health education arm, where birth and newborn-care preparedness as well as care-seeking from qualified providers were promoted through group sessions held once every 4 months. There were no overall differences in neonatal mortality over 30 months of intervention but a 34% reduction in the home-care arm in the final 6 months of the programme. The authors of the Projahnmo study noted that 'availability of referral services and a strong supervisory system' were essential elements of the intervention and would be required for scaling up. In Pakistan, a pilot study in Hala[15] also showed promising effects on home-care practices.

Despite these encouraging interventions, health worker home visits have rarely achieved adequate coverage, quality or effectiveness when scaled up in poor populations. Haines and colleagues[16] have described the problems in providing focused tasks, adequate remuneration, and training and supervision for large-scale community health worker programmes. They reported that only 3–12% of children born at home in five South Asian and sub-Saharan African countries received a visit from a trained health worker within 3 days of birth. An additional difficulty for large-scale commitment is that a community health worker, perhaps living in a different village, must know about a mother's pregnancy or be informed about the birth, and then be able and willing to travel for repeated postnatal visits to check for warning signs in the mother or baby, and to treat or refer promptly.

Finally, it is worth noting that two studies to evaluate the impact of the Integrated Management of Childhood Illness (IMCI) strategy, while showing encouraging improvements in health worker skills, did not show any effect on population child mortality. This is a chastening reminder that interventions largely focused on health facilities and health workers, which was the main focus of IMCI programmes, do not always produce benefit for population health outcomes.[17,18]

Community mobilisation through women's groups for newborn survival

In 2004, a cluster-randomised controlled trial in Makwanpur, Nepal,[19] showed improvements in birth outcomes in a poor rural population following a low-cost, potentially sustainable and scalable participatory intervention with women's groups. Newborn mortality rates were 30% lower in intervention areas compared with controls and the study also observed a significant fall in maternal mortality, although the numbers of maternal deaths were small and maternal mortality was not a primary outcome of the trial. The intervention involved local women who led women's groups monthly to discuss problems leading to maternal and newborn deaths, to develop practical strategies to address these problems, to link with community leaders to implement these strategies, and after two years to evaluate their outcomes. This community action cycle, adapted from a programme developed in Bolivia by Lisa Howard-Grabman and colleagues,[20] seemed to have significant health and non-health benefits. The study challenged the assumption that health outcomes, certainly for newborn infants, were primarily about use of health services. Responses to the study findings focused on questions about the generalisability and scalability of this approach in settings with different development, health and mortality indicators.[21]

New trials of a women's group approach have since been established in Nepal, urban and rural India, Bangladesh and Malawi. In India, the Ekjut study[22] of a participatory intervention with women's groups was introduced in 18 population clusters (about 7000 population per cluster) in underserved tribal communities in three districts drawn from the disadvantaged states of Jharkhand and Orissa. The baseline NMRs at nearly 60 per 1000 live births were higher than in the Nepal study. The study ran for 3 years after the introduction of the facilitated women's groups. In years 2 and 3, the NMR fell by 45% in intervention clusters compared with control clusters (Figure 13.1). What is most remarkable about this finding is that the use of antenatal care, delivery care or postnatal care showed no differences between intervention and control areas. The direct mechanism of action was probably changes in care practices in the home, especially in relation to hygiene, breastfeeding and thermal care. Women's groups, and their links with community health workers, are more than simply a vehicle for health education. They build the confidence of young mothers and have the potential to increase solidarity between women, improve relationships between women and their mothers-in-law, initiate local insurance schemes, address gender problems, assist with transport in the case of obstetric emergencies, and

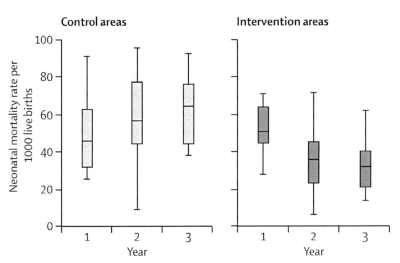

Figure 13.1 Impact of community women's groups on neonatal mortality in the Ekjut trial, India; reproduced with permission from Tripathy *et al.*[22]

provide women with a forum for respite, exchange and social support. In India, the Ekjut trial had postnatal depression as a primary outcome, and a 57% reduction was noted in moderate depression scores, which suggests that group membership has a preventive role for women at risk of depression.

In Makwanpur, Nepal, where financial support for women's groups was withdrawn in 2008 by the local research team, more than 70% of groups were self-sustaining 15 months later and network committees were being established to ensure district sustainability and expansion, without any external support.

In Bangladesh there was no significant impact of women's groups on mortality rates. The coverage of women's groups in this study was much lower than in India and Nepal, and crucially only 2% of newly pregnant women joined the groups, compared with figures ranging from 37% to 55% in the other studies. Clearly, for this intervention to succeed, there is a critical minimum coverage level, and enrolment of a sizeable proportion of newly pregnant women into the groups is necessary.

The mobilisation of women, and a focus on help for newly pregnant women, is an essential, and not costly, pre-requisite for a safer motherhood and newborn care programme. Such community mobilisation interventions can deliver substantial improvements in maternal and newborn health outcomes, especially in high-mortality settings where a high proportion of deliveries occur at home. Apart from the direct benefits of groups, mobilisation of women is also likely to increase the return on investments to strengthen essential obstetric care in hospitals and health centres through increased use and support by the local community, although further studies are needed to investigate the political influence that women's groups can produce for improvements in service delivery.

Community interventions to reduce maternal mortality

Fertility reduction

Female education and family planning have long been recognised as key components of a safer motherhood strategy. More than 50% of pregnancies are unplanned and 25% are unwanted, and complications of unsafe abortion have been estimated to cause 68 000 maternal deaths per year (13% of all maternal deaths). The unmet need for family planning services is large. Over 200 million women (one in seven women of reproductive age in developing countries) would like to use contraception but are unable to access it. Donnay[23] suggested in 2000 that meeting the existing demand for family planning services could reduce maternal deaths in developing countries by at least 20%.

Bangladesh has seen impressive gains in both female education and fertility reduction. Over the past two decades, family planning uptake has risen impressively, with concomitant reduction in fertility rates, and female literacy rates have risen greatly. However, access to maternal health services remains poor and in 2006 fewer than 15% of deliveries had a skilled attendant.[24] Nonetheless, MMR has fallen substantially from 724 per 100 000 live births in 1990 to a current estimate of 336 per 100 000 live births.

Restrictive laws that hinder the availability of safe abortion services must also be tackled, and high-quality, compassionate treatment must exist for complications resulting from unsafe abortion. Both Bangladesh and Nepal now take a progressive approach to menstrual regulation and early abortion, so that women may avoid the hazards of unsafe interventions to end pregnancy.

Financial incentives to seek care

Many countries, particularly in Latin America, have sought to raise demand for health services by providing monetary incentives to households on the condition that they engage in certain healthcare-seeking practices.[25] Nepal, Ghana, India and Bangladesh are among several countries that have introduced financial incentives to increase use of institutional deliveries or skilled birth attendants in the home. In 2005, Nepal introduced the Safe Delivery Incentive Programme (SDIP) that combines two types of incentive: a conditional cash transfer to households, along with an incentive to health staff for each delivery they attend. The SDIP was introduced to increase coverage of skilled birth attendance and to address the prohibitively high cost, particularly for travel, of trying to access professional care in childbirth.[26] Over 80% of women in Nepal continue to deliver at home and only 19% deliver with a doctor or nurse.[27] Since the launch of the SDIP, India and Bangladesh have followed suit with similar programmes of their own.

Figure 13.2, which reports data from Makwanpur, Nepal, shows that receipt of the conditional cash transfer is heavily concentrated among richer households, reflecting the fact that users of government maternity services are wealthier.[28] Inequality in the benefit incidence of the conditional cash transfer is simply illustrative of an existing inequality in the use of delivery care services, but as it is also a transfer of resources to households, it is inequitable, benefiting relatively wealthier groups within the sample of rural women. However, incentive schemes, despite early inequities, may reduce inequalities in access to hospital delivery between the richest and poorest, as has been found in later unpublished analysis of the Nepal maternity incentive scheme.

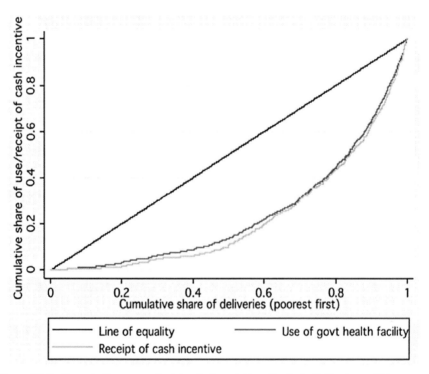

Figure 13.2 Concentration curves of uptake of a financial incentive for institutional care, Makwanpur district, Nepal; reproduced with permission from Powell-Jackson *et al.*[28]

Improving access to life-saving drugs in the community

The *Lancet* maternal health series suggested that 'a health centre intrapartum-care strategy can be justified as the best bet to bring down high rates of maternal mortality' and others have identified methods for doing this[29–31] with long-term funding and commitment from national health systems. However, as Campbell and Graham, lead authors of the maternal series, acknowledged, implementation 'cannot be achieved overnight and a legitimate question is what to do in the meantime'.

We, and others, have argued elsewhere that, by complementing a health facility strategy, it is possible to prevent and treat maternal illness at the community level.[10,32–34] The safest place for a woman to deliver is in a health facility offering essential obstetric care. However, the safest care for an individual woman and the most effective interventions for improving population outcomes are not necessarily the same thing. In populations where access to facility deliveries is beyond reach or highly inequitable, for whatever reason, and will remain so in the medium term, a facility-based approach does little to stop women dying from preventable causes following delivery at home.

The WHO review[35] of causes of death based on community surveys estimates that haemorrhage and infection cause 34% and 10% of maternal deaths, respectively, in Africa. One might argue that the estimate for infection-related deaths is far too low, because community surveys are poor at detecting symptoms or signs of infection, and experienced African obstetricians and post-mortem studies[36] suggest the true percentage may be much higher.

Prevention of deaths from haemorrhage or infection following delivery at home might be possible by the provision of drugs to mothers through antenatal clinics, community health workers, or even women volunteers at village level[37–39] in the same way that child survival has improved through community distribution of drugs.[33,40–47]

In 2009, we published a paper where we developed a mathematical model to estimate the potential impact of augmenting health facility strengthening with community drug supply on deaths from postpartum haemorrhage or sepsis following delivery.[48] Using estimates of incidence, case fatality and the effectiveness of medications derived from the literature, we evaluated several scenarios (Figure 13.3) reflecting different degrees of success in achieving the following interventions:

- improved drug supply and access to health facilities (HF)
- HF combined with antenatal care provision of prophylactic misoprostol and community health worker provision of oral antibiotics to treat infection (HF+ANC/CHW)
- HF+ANC/CHW combined with village women volunteers providing these drugs (HF+ANC/CHW+WV).

The model was applied to Malawi and sub-Saharan Africa. In all scenarios, the lowest risk deliveries were those in health facilities. The mathematical model was used to estimate the potential impact of the three strategies in reducing the number of maternal deaths from haemorrhage and sepsis. In sub-Saharan Africa, we estimated that the HF strategy could prevent 21 300, the HF+ANC/CHW strategy 43 800 and the HF+ANC/CHW+WV strategy 59 000 deaths out of a baseline estimate of 182 000 deaths from haemorrhage and sepsis annually (Figure 13.4). The estimated impact of the packages that included community interventions was greatest among poorer women.

It does seem, therefore, that community provision of misoprostol and antibiotics to reduce maternal deaths could be a highly effective addition to health facility strengthening in Africa. Community-level interventions can never address maternal

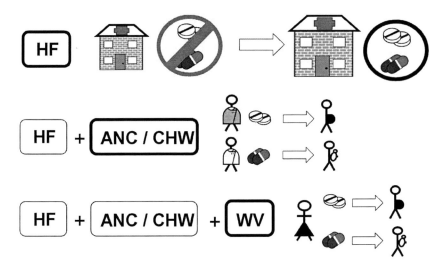

Figure 13.3 Approaches to community delivery of drugs to treat postpartum haemorrhage and sepsis; ANC = antenatal care provision of prophylactic misoprostol; CHW = community health worker provision of oral antibiotics to treat infection; HF = health facility; WV = village women volunteers providing these drugs

deaths from all causes, and access to health centre delivery remains key to reducing MMRs to below 100 per 100 000 live births. However, we do believe that modelling suggests that they can nonetheless have a significant impact in high mortality settings. We suggest that evaluation is urgently required to assess the risks, benefits and challenges of widespread implementation of such community provision. It would not, in our view, be acceptable to proceed to widespread scale-up without a controlled evaluation, because the use of misoprostol and antibiotics by unskilled providers could create risks as well as benefits. Although there is clear trial evidence that misoprostol reduces haemorrhage rates, no trial has been designed to measure its impact on maternal mortality in high mortality settings.[49] Widespread use of misoprostol at delivery could mean occasional inadvertent use before birth. Even low-dose misoprostol has been associated with uterine rupture, and inappropriate use might also increase stillbirth rates and the risks associated with twin delivery.

Investment in maternal and newborn health programmes

There is a large shortfall of investment in mother and child health in the poorest countries. Greco and colleagues[50] estimated that donor disbursements increased from US$2,119 million in 2003 to $3,482 million in 2006. Funding for child health increased by 63% and that for maternal and newborn health by 66% but from an extremely low baseline. In the 68 countries identified by the Countdown to 2015 group as a priority, child health-related disbursements increased from $4 to $7 per child between 2003 and 2006, and disbursements for maternal and neonatal health increased from $7 to $12 per live birth. But the picture is mixed. Disbursements fell in some countries, and much of the spend was directed at routine immunisation programmes. Greco and colleagues felt that aid specifically for maternal and newborn health did not seem to be well targeted towards countries with the greatest needs.

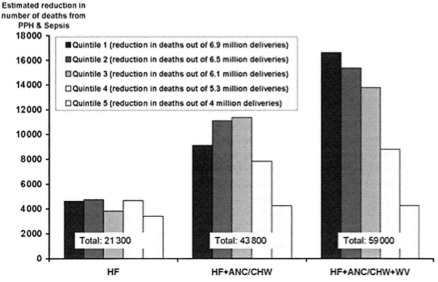

Figure 13.4 Estimated impact on deaths from sepsis and postpartum haemorrhage in sub-Saharan Africa; 182 000 deaths from postpartum haemorrhage (PPH) or sepsis from 28.8 million annual deliveries in baseline scenario

A critical issue is the lack of a coordinating mechanism for aid investment, specifically for maternal and newborn health. There have been calls for a global fund for mothers and children or alternatively to broaden the remit of the existing Global Fund for health, which currently focuses on AIDS, tuberculosis and malaria.[51,52] Health and development professionals need to advocate on behalf of mothers and children so that proper investments mean that millions of preventable deaths may be saved.

Conclusion

Health facility delivery remains the safest option for women and safer motherhood programmes must always strengthen national and district systems for facility-based obstetric care. At the same time, the reality facing millions of women is that home delivery is their only option in the foreseeable future. There is strong evidence that community interventions can have a significant impact in reducing the risk of maternal and newborn mortality in poor communities. Development programmes need much greater investment in maternal and newborn health, and an integrated approach that combines community mobilisation, access to life-saving drugs and provision of high-quality facility care.

Acknowledgements

The authors would like to acknowledge Professor Martin Utley's contribution to the section on 'Improving access to life-saving drugs in the community' as well as unpublished research findings from Tim Powell-Jackson and colleagues presented at the Department for International Development 'Towards 4+5' dissemination meeting in May 2010.

References

1.   United Nations. Millennium Development Goals [www.developmentgoals.org].

2.   Bryce, J, Daelmans B, Dwivedi A, Fauveau V, Lawn JE, Mason E, *et al.* Countdown to 2015 for maternal, newborn, and child survival: the 2008 report on tracking coverage of interventions. *Lancet* 2008;371:1247–58.

3.   Black RE, Morris SS, Bryce J. Where and why are 10 million children dying every year? *Lancet* 2003;361:2226–34.

4.   Lawn JE, Yakoob MY, Haws RA, Soomro T, Darmstadt GL, Bhutta ZA. 3.2 million stillbirths: epidemiology and overview of the evidence review. *BMC Pregnancy Childbirth* 2009;9 Suppl 1:S2.

5.   UNICEF. *The State of Asia-Pacific's Children: Child Survival.* New York: UNICEF; 2008 [www.unicef.org/publications/files/SOAPC_2008_080408.pdf].

6.   Hogan MC, Foreman KJ, Naghavi M, Ahn SY, Wang M, Makela SM, *et al.* Maternal mortality for 181 countries, 1980–2008: a systematic analysis of progress towards Millennium Development Goal 5. *Lancet* 2010;375:1609–23.

7.   UNICEF. *State of the World's Children 2009: Maternal and Newborn Health.* New York: UNICEF; 2009 [www.unicef.org/sowc/].

8.   Houweling TA, Ronsmans C, Campbell OM, Kunst AE. Huge poor–rich inequalities in maternity care: an international comparative study of maternity and childcare in developing countries. *Bull World Health Organ* 2007;85:745–54.

9.   Houweling TA, Kunst AE, Huisman M, Mackenbach JP. Using relative and absolute measures for monitoring health inequalities: experiences from cross-national analyses on maternal and child health. *Int J Equity Health* 2007;6:15.

10. Costello A, Azad K, Barnett S. An alternative strategy to reduce maternal mortality. *Lancet* 2006;368: 1477–9.

11. Bang A, Bang RA, Baitule SB, Reddy MH, Deshmukh MD. Effect of home-based neonatal care and management of sepsis on neonatal mortality: field trial in rural India. *Lancet* 1999;354:1955–61.

12. Bang AT, Reddy HM, Deshmukh MD, Baitule SB, Bang RA. Neonatal and infant mortality in the ten years (1993 to 2003) of the Gadchiroli field trial: effect of home-based neonatal care. *J Perinatol* 2005;25 Suppl 1:S92–107.

13. Kumar V, Mohanty S, Kumar A, Misra RP, Santosham M, Awasthi S, *et al;* Saksham Study Group. Effect of community-based behaviour change management on neonatal mortality in Shivgarh, Uttar Pradesh, India: a cluster-randomised controlled trial. *Lancet* 2008;372:1151–62.

14. Baqui AH, El-Arifeen S, Darmstadt GL, Ahmed S, Williams EK, Seraji HR, *et al;* Projahnmo Study Group. Effect of community-based newborn-care intervention package implemented through two service-delivery strategies in Sylhet district, Bangladesh: a cluster-randomised controlled trial. *Lancet* 2008;371:1936–44.

15. Bhutta ZA, Memon ZA, Soofi S, Salat MS, Cousens S, Martines J. Implementing community-based perinatal care: results from a pilot study in rural Pakistan. *Bull World Health Organ* 2008;86:452–9.

16. Haines A, Sanders D, Lehmann U, Rowe A, Lawn J, Jan S, *et al.* Achieving child survival goals: potential contribution of community health workers *Lancet* 2007;369:2121–31.

17. Arifeen SE, Hoque DM, Akter T, Rahman M, Hoque ME, Begum K, *et al.* Effect of the Integrated Management of Childhood Illness strategy on childhood mortality and nutrition in a rural area in Bangladesh: a cluster randomised trial. *Lancet* 2009;374:393–403.

18. Armstrong Schellenberg JR, Adam T, Mshinda H, Masanja H, Kabadi G, Mukasa O, *et al.* Effectiveness and cost of facility-based Integrated Management of Childhood Illness (IMCI) in Tanzania. *Lancet* 2004;364:1583–94.

19. Manandhar DS, Osrin D, Shrestha BP, Mesko N, Morrison J, Tumbahangphe KM, *et al.* Effect of a participatory intervention with women's groups on birth outcomes in Nepal: cluster-randomised controlled trial. *Lancet* 2004;364:970–9.

20. O'Rourke K, Howard-Grabman L, Seoane G. Impact of community organization of women on perinatal outcomes in rural Bolivia. *Rev Panam Salud Publica* 1998;3:9–14.

21. Rosato M, Laverack G, Grabman LH, Tripathy P, Nair N, Mwansambo C, *et al.* Community participation: lessons for maternal, newborn, and child health. *Lancet* 2008;372:962–71.

22. Tripathy P, Nair N, Barnett S, Mahapatra R, Borghi J, Rath S, *et al*. Effect of a participatory intervention with women's groups on birth outcomes and maternal depression in Jharkhand and Orissa, India: a cluster-randomised controlled trial. *Lancet* 2010;375:1182–92.

23. Donnay F. Maternal survival in developing countries: what has been done, what can be achieved in the next decade. *Int J Gynaecol Obstet* 2000;70:89–97.

24. Chowdhury ME, Ahmed A, Kalim N, Koblinsky M. Causes of maternal mortality decline in Matlab, Bangladesh. *J Health Popul Nutr* 2009;27:108–23.

25. Fiszbein A, Schady N. *Conditional Cash Transfers: Reducing Present and Future Poverty*. Washington, DC: World Bank; 2009.

26. Borghi J, Ensor T. Financial implications of skilled attendance at delivery in Nepal. *Trop Med Int Health* 2006;11:228–37.

27. Powell-Jackson T, Morrison J, Tiwari S, Neupane BD, Costello AM. The experiences of districts in implementing a national incentive programme to promote safe delivery in Nepal. *BMC Health Serv Res* 2009;9:97.

28. Powell-Jackson T, Neupane BD, Tiwari S, Tumbahangphe K, Manandhar D, Costello AM. The impact of Nepal's National Incentive Programme to promote safe delivery in the district of Makwanpur. *Adv Health Econ Health Serv Res* 2009;21:221–49.

29. Campbell OM, Graham WJ; Lancet Maternal Survival Series steering group. Strategies for reducing maternal mortality: getting on with what works. *Lancet* 2006;368:1284–99.

30. Koblinsky M, Matthews Z, Hussein J, Mavalankar D, Mridha MK, Anwar I, *et al*; Lancet Maternal Survival Series steering group. Going to scale with professional skilled care. *Lancet* 2006;368:1377–86. Erratum in: *Lancet* 2006;368:2210.

31. World Health Organization. *Mother–Baby Package: Implementing Safe Motherhood in Countries*. Maternal Health and Safe Motherhood Programme, WHO/FHE/MSM/94.11 Rev.1. Geneva: WHO; 1996.

32. Bhutta ZA, Darmstadt GL, Hasan BS, Haws RA. Community-based interventions for improving perinatal and neonatal health outcomes in developing countries: a review of the evidence. *Pediatrics* 2005;115(2 Suppl):519–617.

33. Kidney E, Winter HR, Khan KS, Gülmezoglu AM, Meads CA, Deeks JJ, *et al*. Systematic review of effect of community-level interventions to reduce maternal mortality. *BMC Pregnancy Childbirth* 2009;9:2.

34. Costello A, Osrin D, Manandhar D. Reducing maternal and neonatal mortality in the poorest communities. *BMJ* 2004;329:1166–8.

35. Khan KS, Wojdyla D, Say L, Gülmezoglu AM, Van Look PF. WHO analysis of causes of maternal death: a systematic review. *Lancet*. 2006 Apr 1;367(9516):1066–74.

36. Menéndez C, Romagosa C, Ismail MR, Carrilho C, Saute F, Osman N, Machungo F, *et al*. An autopsy study of maternal mortality in Mozambique: the contribution of infectious diseases. *PLoS Med* 2008;5:e44.

37. Derman RJ, Kodkany BS, Goudar SS, Geller SE, Naik VA, Bellad MB, *et al*. Oral misoprostol in preventing postpartum haemorrhage in resource-poor communities: a randomised controlled trial. *Lancet* 2006;368:1248–53.

38. Rajbhandari S, Pun A, Hodgins S, Rajendra PK. Prevention of postpartum haemorrhage at homebirth with use of misoprostol in Banke District in Nepal. *Int J Gynecol Obstet* 2006;94(Suppl 2):S143–4.

39. Sanghvi H. Preventing PPH at Homebirth: Community Based Approaches. JHPIEGO; 2007 [www.esdproj.org/site/DocServer/MAT2_Harshad_Sanghvi.pdf?docID=1003].

40. Okech BA, Mwobobia IK, Kamau A, Muiruri S, Mutiso N, Nyambura J, *et al*. Use of integrated malaria management reduces malaria in Kenya. *PLoS ONE* 2008;3:e4050.

41. Elmardi KA, Malik EM, Abdelgadir T, Ali SH, Elsyed AH, Mudather MA, *et al*. Feasibility and acceptability of home-based management of malaria strategy adapted to Sudan's conditions using artemisinin-based combination therapy and rapid diagnostic test. *Malar J* 2009;8:39.

42. Das LK, Jambulingam P, Sadanandane C. Impact of community-based presumptive chloroquine treatment of fever cases on malaria morbidity and mortality in a tribal area in Orissa State, India. *Malar J* 2008;7:75.

43.   Rasmussen Z, Pio A, Enarson P. Case management of childhood pneumonia in developing countries: recent relevant research and current initiatives. *Int J Tuberc Lung Dis* 2000;4:807–26.

44.   Bang AT, Bang RA, Sontakke PG. Management of childhood pneumonia by traditional birth attendants. The SEARCH Team. *Bull World Health Organ* 1994;72:897–905.

45.   Holloway KA, Karkee SB, Tamang A, Gurung YB, Kafle KK, Pradhan R, *et al.* Community intervention to promote rational treatment of acute respiratory infection in rural Nepal. *Trop Med Int Health* 2009;14:101–10.

46.   Hadi A. Management of acute respiratory infections by community health volunteers: experience of Bangladesh Rural Advancement Committee (BRAC). *Bull World Health Organ* 2003;81:183–9.

47.   Bryce J, Coitinho D, Darnton-Hill I, Pelletier D, Pinstrup-Andersen P; Maternal and Child Undernutrition Study Group. Maternal and child undernutrition: effective action at national level. *Lancet* 2008;371:510–26.

48.   Pagel C, Lewycka S, Colbourn T, Mwansambo C, Meguid T, Chiudzu G, *et al.* Estimation of potential effects of improved community-based drug provision, to augment health-facility strengthening, on maternal mortality due to post-partum haemorrhage and sepsis in sub-Saharan Africa: an equity-effectiveness model. *Lancet* 2009;374:1441–8. Erratum in: *Lancet* 2009;374:1422.

49.   Hofmeyr GJ, Gülmezoglu AM. Misoprostol for the prevention and treatment of postpartum haemorrhage. *Best Pract Res Clin Obstet Gynaecol* 2008;22:1025–4.

50.   Greco G, Powell-Jackson T, Borghi J, Mills A. Countdown to 2015: assessment of donor assistance to maternal, newborn, and child health between 2003 and 2006. *Lancet* 2008;371:1268–75.

51.   Costello A, Osrin D, The case for a new Global Fund for maternal, neonatal, and child survival. *Lancet* 2005;366:603–5.

52.   Brugha R. The Global Fund at three years – flying in crowded air space. *Trop Med Int Health* 2005;10: 623–6.

Section 4

Training and development

Chapter 14

Capacity development – a midwifery perspective

Frances Day-Stirk

Introduction: capacity development challenges and complexities

The lack of midwives to provide access to the worlds' 10 million women and their newborn by 2015 is well recognised and documented, with only 59% of births in the developing world attended by skilled healthcare workers – trained midwives, doctors or nurses.[1] This access deficiency aligns with countries that experience the greatest shortages. The Economic and Social Council noted in its Annual Ministerial Review that across the globe the distribution of healthcare workers is inequitable, with vast gaps between developed and developing countries, as well as within countries between urban and rural areas.[2] Capacity development and human resource shortages are interrelated: one cannot be considered independently of the other and both need to be considered as part of a system whole. While the challenge of capacity development is an issue across the globe, it is greater in developing countries and greatest in fragile states.[3] It is known that fragile states have less than one health worker for every 1000 people and one in four pregnant women gives birth alone or with a family member.[4] The lifetime risk of maternal death is one in 8000 in the Global North compared with one in 76 in the Global South. It is estimated that 75% of mothers' lives could be saved if women had access to a skilled health worker at birth and to emergency obstetric care. The case for urgent capacity development is clear. Each community, country and continent has to contend with the impact of midwife shortages: the degrees vary, as do the push–pull factors. As new cadres of worker are being introduced, so are concerns about diluted competencies, diminished quality of care and capacity development increases.

The various socio-economic determinants of capacity development – gender; women's status and education; governance (local and international); infrastructure and interdependent capacities; governmental, structural and professional – combine to create a complex picture.

This chapter explores the challenge of capacity development to achieve universal coverage, within health systems and services staffed by adequate numbers of appropriately skilled healthcare workers, which has been shown to reduce mortality among mothers and their newborn. The word 'midwife' will be used with reference to the skilled midwifery provider to mean one with essential midwifery competences as training and scope of practice defined by the International Confederation of Midwives (ICM).[5,6]

What does capacity development mean?

Capacity development at its simplest has been described as the 'how' – how a country, by it priority drivers, seeks to retain what exists in-country, to identify what requires improvement and where the gaps are and how to fill them, and to identify which human development strategies can move from aspiration to implementation[7]. It is suggested that capacity development differs from technical aid in its starting position; that is, that countries have the capacity 'at home' – endogenous capacity and the need to decide where it wants to move it and how.

This is an important redefinition of the concept, which moves away from the traditional thinking of capacity development based on technical training and foreign expertise, and captures the concept in its complexity and entirety.[8] So, while technical assistance may be part of capacity development, it should not be assumed that it is always external to the country.

Several useful definitions of capacity development are listed on the Wikipedia website:[8]

- United Nations Development Programme (UNDP) – the process through which individuals, organisations and societies obtain, strengthen and maintain the capabilities to set and achieve their own development objectives over time

- Canadian International Development Agency (CIDA) – the activities, approaches, strategies and methodologies which help organisations, groups and individuals to improve their performance, generate development benefits and achieve their objectives

- World Bank (Africa Region) – the proven ability of key actors in a society to achieve socio-economic goals on their own. ... demonstrated through the functional presence of a combination of most of the following factors: viable institutions and respective organisations; commitment and vision of leadership; financial and material resources; skilled human resources.

A number of commonalities on capacity development emerge from these definitions:

- Capacity development is a process of transformational change of capacities – people, organisations and society.

- Capacity development operates at these three different levels, which are interlinked and interdependent; therefore investment in capacity development must design and account for impact at these multiple levels.

- Capacity development results can be short term (crises and post-conflict situations) but need to be supported by a sustained resource and political commitment to yield longer term results that truly impact on existing capacities.

- Capacity development is about who and how and where the decisions are made, management takes place, services delivered, and results monitored and evaluated. Primarily an endogenous process, and while supported and facilitated by the international development community, it cannot be owned or driven from the outside.

- Leadership is essential, as is knowledge and knowledge sharing. Civil society, private sector and international development partners are all part of the capacity development equation.

- Capacity development is about capable, transformational states that enable capable and resilient societies to achieve their own development objectives over time.

UNDP provides clarity around the essentials of capacity development:[7]

- effective leadership and succession planning
- aid coordination and financial management skills
- a functioning civil service
- a skilled labour force
- a conducive environment to strengthen this foundation.

Identifying the issues

Contributors to the Global Alliance for Nursing and Midwifery (GANM) Communities of Practice online discussion[9] on the question posted by Dr Jean Yan, on the health worker shortage in Africa, identified key generic issues. A cross-section of these factors from contributors around the world can be seen to apply to capacity building:

- Trinidad and Tobago cited **education** – 'Teach the teachers' needs to be a piece of the foundation of stemming the shortage; that is, building capacity.
- The USA identified **funding** for mass training of health personnel; training is an issue – many are interested but do not have the money to pay their way.
- Jordan stated that **local strategies equal local solutions** – enlisting the support of families, government and royalty to attract female recruits. Jordan has developed a strategy that mapped the steps towards achieving the goal of building nurses' capacity and enhancing the education system. A national agenda will not be achieved without multi-sectoral collaboration and coordination.
- Papua New Guinea cited **human resource data and planning** – the biggest challenge is accessible, accurate and sound human resources information for policy direction and workforce planning.
- Cameroon suggested strategies for **stemming the brain drain** – salaries are unrealistic for the quality of work done and health workers feel unappreciated.
- Cote d'Ivoire noted **national health system review and professional regulation** – countries have to revise their national health systems, review their salary scales, reinforce the autonomy of professional boards and extend their professional control systems to positively affect all practitioners and protect the health of citizens.

When added to those mentioned earlier, these generic issues illustrate and capture a comprehensive continuum of capacity development. The urgency of capacity development of midwives and those with midwifery skills stems from the general consensus that if every birth were attended by a skilled midwifery provider the number of maternal deaths would plummet. This is further supported by the repeatedly stated position that high-quality midwifery care (and by extension good health status for women and the newborn) are more likely to occur where the role of the midwife is well articulated and they enjoy high status.[10] Hence the need to focus on midwives and human resource development, and the UK Department for International Development's support for development of training facilities, curricula and materials, particularly midwifery and pre- and in-service training, is not surprising.[11]

Gender inequities and capacity development

Capacity development cannot be achieved without consideration of the status of women. The impact of the status of women – gender discrimination experienced and lower levels of education – on maternal outcomes are well acknowledged and global efforts are being made to improve the status and education of women.[4,12] It is also acknowledged that the root cause lies in women's disadvantaged position in most countries and cultures:[13] 'In countries with similar levels of economic development, maternal mortality is inversely proportional to women's status.' That is, the worse women are treated in society, in general, the more likely they are to be in childbirth.

The World Health Organization (WHO) makes clear that the lower a woman's economic status, the less likely she is to have skilled assistance at delivery and life-saving emergency obstetric care.[14] Unsurprisingly, the converse is seen in countries where the status of women has improved. In Kerala in south India and Sri Lanka, where the maternal mortality ratio is low, there are high levels of female education. Similarly, capacity development benefits can be seen in a number of countries or states, particularly Sri Lanka, Malaysia, Tunisia, Thailand, Kerala and Tamil Nadu, that have successfully undertaken specific measures to make midwifery a respectable and attractive profession.[15]

The connection between women's status and capacity development has been made by Fauveau *et al.*[15] on the basis that efforts to strengthen midwifery are in line with UNFPA's mandate to promote gender equality, as midwives are key female members of the health workforce. It is further suggested that, as most midwives are women, there has been gross underinvestment or no investment in building or maintaining a cadre of professional midwives. With low status within their community and with little credit, midwives therefore experience the same gender-related inequalities as other women.

The place of education in capacity development

The importance of education is not simply about training to carry out specific tasks, it is about the availability of a midwife as a 'quality measure' to deliver on Millennium Development Goal (MDG) 5. There is a need to examine how people gain entry into training; they do so invariably through their level of education. Education of girls and women is critical in sustainable development, and improving the capacity and in-country resource of people to address local and national issues relating to women's and children's health is widely noted at national and international policy level.[16,17]

In the context of maternal mortality in the countries concerned, a link can be established between education and the status of women and rates of maternal and infant mortality and progress towards achieving the MDGs. Literacy and educational attainment rates among women in many of the countries affected by the highest mortality rates are low because of lack of access to education by girls and women. MDG 2, to achieve universal education for all, particularly the target on literacy rates of 15- to 24-year-olds, highlights this.[18] Article 26 of the Universal Declaration of Human Rights[19] states that everyone has the right to free education, at least in the elementary and fundamental stages, and that such education should be compulsory. However, many of the 185 mostly developing countries that have signed up to the Convention on the Elimination of All Forms of Discrimination against Women, continue to deny women this basic right.[20] To encourage the recruitment of local women to train as midwives and build capacity, they must first be educated and, in the long term, be employed and appropriately remunerated, as incentives to stay within their communities.

The status of women in countries with skills deficits needs to be urgently addressed, in terms of education and political rights, as well as the more basic right to education, which is the key to raising the status of women if capacity development is a serious consideration.

A minimum of 9 years of formal education and a minimum of 18 months of a midwifery training programme are suggested as necessary to ensure effective skilled birth attendants.[21] In terms of capacity development, a community public health approach to midwifery education in countries is ideal to ensure a balanced approach, with an emphasis on primary care. However, this needs to be country specific and appropriate midwifery education/training should have built-in continuing professional development. This forms the basis of the UNFPA/ICM Investing in Midwives programme.

Sustainable solutions – is any attendance better than no attendance?

There will be different context-specific solutions that are appropriate for different countries, as no one size fits all. However, from a capacity development perspective, local solutions should be underpinned by a common framework that would address the relevant MDGs (4 and 5) and be integrated into an overall health system funding and delivery strategy.

Many solutions have been tried in the past two decades and have been debated in the developed and developing world, with the Royal College of Midwives recommending a flexible approach to professional roles, skills mix and the development of specialist roles, provided that there are improved outcomes and women's needs are met.[22] There is concern in the midwifery world that short-term measures introduced by some countries in an effort to meet the MDG targets will become permanent solutions of questionable quality. Meanwhile, other organisations such as UNICEF have promoted midwives and other midlevel providers with shorter periods of training and requiring lower entry education qualifications forming one cadre within a spectrum of health workers, who can undertake different roles, distribute workloads and build a referrals system for women and the newborn.[4] Such examples include midwives and nurse midwives in Mozambique working alongside obstetricians providing cost-effective quality emergency obstetric care in under-serviced areas, as well as community health workers in Peru undertaking monthly visits to families at high risk.[3,23]

The ICM perspective would be midwives as primary-level providers working with other cadres of community workers, as set out in its 2008 position statement.[24] In this statement, the ICM identifies midwives as 'the professional of choice for childbearing women in all areas of the world' predicated on a universal standard of initial and continuing midwifery competency-based education. It also promotes their *Essential Competencies for Basic Midwifery Practice*[5] and *Definition of the Midwife*[6] as guides for expanding education programmes and regulatory frameworks, which will lead to an increased number of competent midwives in their country practising the full scope of midwifery, in order better to serve childbearing women and their families.

The African Medical Research Foundation (AMREF) shares this view by opposing community health workers taking on the role of professionals and instead advocating a dual strategy that provides for both the long term and the short term. The organisation calls for investment in trained community health workers who, trusted by the community, play a pivotal part in linking them with the healthcare systems. This is particularly important where health systems are weak and in pastoral communities where the majority of women give birth at home: community health workers and midwives can play an important role in preventing maternal morbidity and mortality.[25]

Open space meeting recommendations to the UK Department for International Development included:

- ensuring that links with education and empowerment MDGs are made with partner agencies
- encouraging advocacy for midwifery as a respected occupation
- strengthening professional associations as a vehicle for quality improvement.

Think global, act local

WHO estimates that the world's approximately 35 million nurses and midwives, despite making significant contributions to delivery health care within a variety of systems, are rarely involved at strategic policy level. The Global Advisory Group on Nursing and Midwifery[26] also recognises that 80% of health services in hospitals and communities are provided by nursing and midwifery personnel. Two reasons for their lack of involvement in policy and strategy are suggested, firstly the perceived status of nurses and midwives and, secondly the general level of education of the profession. Several global frameworks exist or are being developed to guide capacity development of midwives and others. This includes the WHO global education standards[27] and the ICM *Essential Competencies for Basic Midwifery Practice.*[5] The goal of the global standards is to establish educational criteria and assure outcomes that:

- are based on evidence and competency
- promote the progressive nature of education and lifelong learning
- ensure the employment of practitioners who are competent and who, by providing quality care, promote positive health outcomes in the populations they serve.

The ICM's *Essential Competencies for Basic Midwifery Practice* sets out core competencies describing a minimum requirement for midwives. Two new developments that are in progress, the Global Standards for Midwifery Education and the regulation framework, will add to the portfolio of global resources available to support midwifery capacity development.

Scaling up

> Scaling-up cost-effective interventions to achieve the MDGs requires significant increases in the supply and use of health care workers. This is an onerous task for governments and development partners that calls for innovative approaches for utilising available resources.[28]

Entry into and exit from the healthcare workforce is crucial in midwifery capacity development. Fauveau *et al.*[15] will find common support for their hypothesis that a great deal of the stagnation of maternal health programmes has been the result of confusion and careless choices in scaling up between a limited number of truly skilled birth attendants and large quantities of multi-purpose workers with short training, fewer skills, limited authority and no career pathways. It appears that this opinion has been heard and has influenced at least one major midwifery capacity development initiative – the jointly executed UNFPA and ICM Investing in Midwives programme.[29] It aims to build national capacity in low-resource countries by strengthening regulatory mechanisms, developing and strengthening education and accreditation mechanisms, and promoting the development and role of midwives' associations.

Working at the country and the global/regional levels, two key features – in-country commitment and in-country, regional and global technical advice and support – are defining factors. Scaling up the capacity of midwives includes strategies towards achieving a 'critical mass' of country midwife advisors (CMAs) working nationally and regionally to promote and enhance the role and impact of midwives and others with midwifery skills.

Another approach to capacity development involved identification of skills used in task analysis and definition of skills categories that did not correspond to jobs or cadres of health workers.[30] Skills categories included birth attendance, counselling of pregnancy-related risks and family planning, basic obstetric physical examination, monitoring of vital signs, and ordering and performing of simple tests. Estimations undertaken in Chad, Malawi and Tanzania on human resource requirements have enabled development of a healthcare package capable of achieving the MDGs.

Given the specific gender issues around midwifery, women's empowerment and gender equity will strongly influence the choice of advocacy methods, working practices and interventions for the work in each country. The Partnership for Maternal, Newborn & Child Health[31] illustrates just what is required for capacity development at country level in Box 14.1.

Scaling up of midwives has the support of WHO, UNFPA, UNICEF and the World Bank,[32] and the Health Professionals Group[31] in reaching MDGs 4 and 5, as evidenced in both statements.

Strengthening in-country professional associations

Seven hundred thousand midwives are needed in community-, primary- and secondary-level health services to dramatically reduce maternal and newborn deaths. Strengthened infrastructure and referral systems to emergency obstetric care are also key. Alongside this, changes are needed to ensure that women can access healthcare services. All of this will require political will, commitment and investment.

At country level, country-to-country twinning has achieved knowledge and skills sharing. Good practice development and bespoke in-country competency-based curriculum development has been effective in the twinning relationships between the Royal College of Midwives and the Former Yugoslav Republic of Macedonia, the Swedish Midwives Association and India, and the Royal Dutch Midwives Association and Sierra Leone.

Box 14.1 Capacity building at country level[31]

- Identifying needed competencies for all levels of maternal and child healthcare workers
- Recognising and supporting an appropriate scope of practice for each cadre of health worker to promote the best use of each group's expertise
- Influencing regulation and legislation to allow for competency-based practice by all types of health professional along the continuum of care
- Assisting with the training of professionals, upgrading of skills and provision of competency-based education as defined by the specific professional group (e.g. midwives for midwives, nurses for nurses, physicians for physicians)
- Assisting with setting standards and teaching of various levels of health worker that exist at country level
- Supporting the commitment to the ethical recruitment and retention of healthcare professionals
- Increasing capacity of professional organisations to meet the health challenges of women, newborn and children
- Increasing the visibility of health issues affecting women, newborn and children
- Assisting local agencies to have a stronger voice in women's, newborn and child health by providing support from a global level, lending credence to causes at the national level, especially where there are no established professional organisations

Accountability and governance

The UK Department for International Development is aware that making progress towards achieving MDG 5 requires long-term investment in health services and health infrastructure in the countries affected.[33]

There has been willingness by most governments and aid agencies, both in the UK and elsewhere, to fund initiatives, and other new donors have also contributed in an effort to achieve the MDG targets and, most importantly, those related to maternal and child health.[34] Nevertheless, many donors have in the past provided aid without mechanisms in place to monitor how that funding is spent or linked with specific requirements on women's rights or on accountability. There is a need for governance structures and political developments before financial donation:[25]

> Money disappears in the bureaucracy, like investment in health workers – you hardly see any change on the ground. And sometimes commitments are forgotten, especially to vulnerable groups. The UK government should push for financing mechanisms that enable funds to go to the right places.

This can be achieved through ensuring that both the donor and the recipient understand the basis for the aid and that the priority for promoting gender equality is built into the monitoring process and indicators. Leadership and involvement by women should be considered at all levels of the decision-making process in terms of how the aid would be invested and how the outcomes will be monitored against indicators. This will ensure the allocation of budgets and resources for women's health and empowerment. This position does not advocate conditionality of aid but simply ensures that aid is invested in primary healthcare, including sexual and reproductive services and the provision of free antenatal care.[35] It is critical to reiterate that it is the obligation of governments to ensure that its citizens have access to basic services such as health and education.[12] As such, governments need to develop their strategic plans, which should be realistic and costed and which can be accounted for. They must be able to demonstrate that there are systems in place for monitoring outputs. Given the fact that there has been insufficient investment in midwifery training, deployment and supervision, coupled with inadequate regulation and policies to support and protect midwives in their practice, this will take strong leadership, political will and commitment.[11]

References

1.   World Health Organization. *The World Health Report 2006 – Working Together for Health*. Geneva: WHO; 2006 [www.who.int/whr/2006/en/].
2.   United Nations Economic and Social Council (ESCOSOC). Annual Ministerial Substantive Review (AMR) 2009. e-Discussion on Global Public Health, 25 January 2009 [www.un.org/en/ecosoc/newfunct/amredis2009.shtml].
3.   Merlin. *All Mothers Matter: Investing in Health Workers to Save Lives in Fragile States*. London: Merlin; 2009.
4.   UNICEF. *State of the World's Children 2009: Maternal and Newborn Health*. New York: UNICEF; 2009.
5.   International Confederation of Midwives. *Essential Competencies for Basic Midwifery Practice 2002* [www.internationalmidwives.org/Portals/5/Documentation/Essential%20Compsenglish_2002-JF_2007%20FINAL.pdf].
6.   International Confederation of Midwives. *Definition of the Midwife 2005* [www.internationalmidwives.org/Portals/5/Documentation/ICM%20Definition%20of%20the%20Midwife%202005.pdf].
7.   United Nations Development Programme. Capacity is Development [www.undp.org/capacity/].

8. Wikipedia. Capacity Development [en.wikipedia.org/wiki/Capacity_Development].

9. Global Alliance for Nursing and Midwifery. The health worker shortage in Africa: are enough physicians and nurses being trained? Online discussion. March–April 2009.

10. Sherratt DR. Why women need midwives for safe motherhood. In: Berer M, Sundari Ravindran TK, editors. *Safe Motherhood Initiative: Critical Issues.* Reproductive Health Matters. Oxford: Blackwell Science; 1999. p. 227–37.

11. Department for International Development. Open Space Conference on Maternal and Sexual and Reproductive Health and Rights. RCOG Department for International Development, January 2009.

12. Crisp N. *Global Health Partnerships: The UK Contribution to Health in Developing Countries.* London: COI; 2007 [www.dfid.gov.uk/Documents/publications/ghp-summary.pdf].

13. Filippi V, Ronsmans C, Campbell OM, Graham WJ, Mills A, Borghi J, *et al.* Maternal health in poor countries: the broader context and a call for action. *Lancet* 2006;368:1535–41.

14. World Health Organization. *The World Health Report 2005 – Make Every Mother and Child Count.* Geneva: WHO; 2005 [www.who.int/whr/2005/en/index.html].

15. Fauveau V, Sherrat D, de Bernis L. Human resources for maternal health: multi-purpose or specialist? *Hum Resour Health* 2008;6:21 [www.human-resources-health.com/content/6/1/21].

16. UNESCO. *World Education Report 2000.* Paris: UNESCO; 2000 [www.unesco.org/education/information/wer/index.htm].

17. United Nations. *World Summit for Social Development: The Copenhagen Declaration and Programme of Action.* New York: United Nations; 1995 [www.un.org/esa/socdev/wssd/copenhagen_declaration.html].

18. United Nations Development Programme. Millennium Development Goal 2: Achieve universal primary education. [www.undp.org/mdg/goal2.shtml].

19. United Nations. The Universal Declaration of Human Rights, 1948. Article 26. Education [www.un.org/en/documents/udhr/index.shtml#a26].

20. Brazier C. The heartbreak. *New Internationalist* March 2009;420 [www.newint.org/features/2009/03/01/keynote-maternal-mortality/].

21. United Nations Population Fund. *Investing in Midwives and Others with Midwifery Skills to Save the Lives of Mothers and Newborns and Improve Their Health.* New York: UNFPA; 2007 [www.unfpa.org/webdav/site/global/shared/documents/publications/2008/midwives_eng.pdf].

22. Royal College of Midwives. *Refocusing the Role of the Midwife.* RCM Position Paper 26. London: Royal College of Midwives; 2006.

23. Pereira C, Bugalho A, Bergström S, Vas F, Cotiro M. A comparative study of cesarean deliveries by assistant medical officers and obstetricians in Mozambique. *Br J Obstet Gynaecol* 1996;103:508–12.

24. International Confederation of Midwives. *The Midwife is the First Choice Health Professional for Childbearing Women.* ICM position statement. 2008 [www.internationalmidwives.org/Documentation/PositionStatements/English/tabid/759/Default.aspx].

25. Mukasa G, African Medical Research Foundation (AMREF). The Status of Women and Global Inequalities. Presentation at the Women & Children First UK and Royal College of Midwives event, 6 May 2009.

26. World Health Organization Global Advisory Group on Nursing and Midwifery (GAGNM) [www.who.int/hrh/nursing_midwifery/networks/en/].

27. World Health Organization. *Global Standards for the Initial Education of Professional Nurses and Midwives.* Geneva: WHO; 2009 [www.who.int/hrh/documents/education/en/index.html].

28. Hongoro C, Normond C. Healthcare providers: the role of compensation and incentives. *Health Economics and Financing Exchange* Spring 2004;28:1–2 [www.hefp.lshtm.ac.uk/publications/downloads/newsletters/28.pdf].

29. United Nations Population Fund/International Confederation of Midwives. *Investing in Midwives and Others with Midwifery Skills to Accelerate Progress towards MDG5* [www.internationalmidwives.org/Partners/UNFPA/tabid/550/Default.aspx].

30. Kurowski C, Mills A. *Estimating Human Resource Requirements for Scaling up Priority Health Interventions in Low-income Countries of Sub-Saharan Africa: a Methodology Based on Service Quantity, Tasks and Productivity (THE QTP METHODOLOGY).* Health Economics & Financing Programme (HEFP) Working Paper 01/06, London School of Hygiene and Tropical Medicine (LHTM); 2006 [www.hefp.lshtm.ac.uk/publications/downloads/working_papers/01_06.pdf].

31. World Health Organization Partnership for Maternal, Newborn & Child Health. *Health Professional Groups Key to Reaching MDGs 4 & 5*. Joint statement. 2007 [www.who.int/pmnch/events/2006/HCPjointstaterev0102207.pdf].

32. World Health Organization Partnership for Maternal, Newborn & Child Health. UN Leaders' Joint Statement on Maternal and Newborn Health: Accelerating Efforts to Save the Lives of Women and Newborns. 25 September 2008 [www.who.int/pmnch/media/news/2008/20080925_jointstatement/en/].

33. Department for International Development. Millennium Development Goal Five [www.dfid.gov.uk/mdg/health.asp].

34. International Health Partnerships. Taskforce on Innovative International Financing for Health Systems [www.internationalhealthpartnership.net//CMS_files/documents/working_group_1_-_report_EN.pdf].

35. Action for Global Health. *Report Three: Health in Crisis*. 2009 [www.actionforglobalhealth.eu/uploads/media/AFGH__Health_in_Crisis__Report2009_.pdf].

Chapter 15
Increasing the capacity for essential obstetric and newborn care

Nynke van den Broek and Jan Hofman

Introduction

Each year more than 536 000 women worldwide die from complications of pregnancy and childbirth – that is one every minute.[1] Many more survive but will suffer ill health and disability as a result of these complications. Ninety-five percent of all maternal deaths occur in South Asia and sub-Saharan Africa.[2] In addition, an estimated 4 million neonatal deaths occur each year, accounting for almost 40% of all deaths under 5 years.[3] An estimated 3.2 million babies are stillborn and up to 2 million perinatal deaths are intrapartum related.[4,5] The health of the neonate is closely related to that of the mother and the majority of deaths in the first month of life could also be prevented if interventions were in place to ensure good maternal health.

The provision of skilled birth attendance and the availability of Essential (or Emergency) Obstetric Care (EOC) coupled with newborn care are key strategies that will, if implemented, reduce maternal and neonatal mortality and morbidity. A skilled birth attendant is defined as:[6]

> an accredited health professional – such as a midwife, doctor or nurse – who has been educated and trained to proficiency in the skills needed to manage normal (uncomplicated) pregnancies, childbirth and the immediate postnatal period, and in the identification, management and referral of complications in women and newborns.

The term 'skilled birth attendance' includes the person (a skilled attendant) and an 'enabling environment'. This enabling environment is less well defined but refers to a functioning health system within which the person can work and includes infrastructure, equipment, drugs and a functioning referral system. Providing skilled attendance at birth is probably the single most important strategy for preventing maternal deaths.[7,8]

Pregnancy should be a normal life event for the majority of women and yet every pregnancy carries risk. For an estimated 10–15% of all women, a potentially life-threatening complication develops during pregnancy, childbirth or the postpartum period. In most cases, this complication will be unexpected and unpredictable. It is therefore crucial that all women have access to good-quality essential (or emergency) obstetric care.[9]

At least 80% of all maternal deaths result from five complications that are well understood and can be readily treated:[10]

■ haemorrhage

■ sepsis

■ eclampsia

■ ruptured uterus as a result of obstructed labour

■ complications of abortion.

We know how to prevent these deaths – there are existing effective medical and surgical interventions that are relatively inexpensive.

In 1997, the key interventions needed were bundled into a package now known as 'Essential (or Emergency) Obstetric Care'.[11] There is unified agreement and criteria on what constitutes Essential Obstetric Care, the minimum coverage levels needed and good-quality evidence based practice.[12–14] Recent evidence, however, shows that in many setting this minimum package is not available to women and their families.

Essential obstetric and newborn care

Two levels of EOC can be distinguished: Basic Essential Obstetric Care (BEOC) and Comprehensive Essential Obstetric Care (CEOC). BEOC originally had six 'signal functions' or components (Box 15.1) but a seventh was recently added – the ability to provide basic resuscitation of a newborn baby using a bag and mask.[11,12] CEOC consists of a total of nine signal functions – those of BEOC plus the ability to provide a caesarean section and blood transfusion. In addition to agreement on the components of EOC, there are agreed specifications for the levels of coverage needed. Thus, the United Nations (UN) agencies recommend that for a population of 500 000 there should be at least one health facility that is able to provide the nine signal functions of CEOC and at least four that provide the seven signal functions of BEOC. It is important that these facilities are equitably geographically distributed with regard to distance and time needed to travel to them. Furthermore, the signal functions must be available 24 hours a day and 7 days a week for the facility to be considered fully functional.

Box 15.1   Levels of Essential Obstetric Care and their signal functions

Basic Essential Obstetric Care (BEOC):
• parenteral antibiotics
• parenteral oxytocics
• parenteral anticonvulsants
• manual removal of a retained placenta
• removal of retained products of conception (by manual vacuum aspiration [MVA])
• assisted vaginal delivery (vacuum extraction)
• basic neonatal resuscitation (with bag and mask).

Comprehensive Essential Obstetric Care (CEOC):
• all seven BEOC functions, plus:
  – caesarean section
  – blood transfusion.

For monitoring and evaluation of EOC services, six process indicators have been recommended by UN agencies. These indicators together measure the availability, accessibility, utilisation and quality of EOC for the relevant population (Box 15.2).

Measuring availability of essential obstetric and newborn care

Using a rapid assessment tool (RAT) adapted from the guidelines for assessment of availability and need for maternal and newborn health services developed by the World Health Organization (WHO),[15,16] we measured the availability of EOC and newborn care in populations in three separate sub-Saharan countries in the period 2006 to 2009.

In country 1, the surveys covered six districts with a total population of almost 2 million (conducted in two phases). In country 2, the survey was done in three adjoining districts covering a total population of over 2.8 million. In country 3, the surveys were conducted in three states with a total population of over 12 million. In each country setting, all facilities providing maternal and newborn health services were identified and visited. The level of functioning of facilities was assessed with the rapid assessment tool. The findings of these three country surveys with regard to availability of CEOC are summarised in Table 15.1. Whereas for the given population there are in principle more than sufficient hospitals in place, the functionality of these with regard to provision on the key EOC signal functions was found to be below minimum acceptable UN coverage levels for two of the three country settings. In addition, many of the hospitals that could potentially serve as fully functioning CEOC facilities were found to be unable to provide all the key signal functions.

Based on the number of caesarean sections carried out, the population-based caesarean section rate for each population covered by the survey was 0.9% in country 1, 2.7% in country 2 and 0.5% in country 3. This is well below the recommended rate of 5–15% for population coverage, thus clearly indicating a very significant unmet need for CEOC.

Lack of adequate blood transfusion when needed is an important contribution to maternal deaths and it must be noted that when the signal function 'blood transfusion' is said to be available in practice this often means that blood transfusions are given using immediate family donors even though there is in fact no functional blood bank in place at the facility.[17]

Table 15.2 presents the results of the same population-based surveys with regard to availability of BEOC. For this, all facilities below 'hospital' level that are meant to provide at least skilled birth attendance were identified and assessed. These included health centres and maternity homes. In country 3, for each state a catchment

Box 15.2	Process indicators for the availability, accessibility, utilisation and quality of Essential Obstetric Care

1. Availability of Basic Essential Obstetric Care (BEOC) and Comprehensive Essential Obstetric Care (CEOC) facilities per 500 000 population (at least one CEOC facility and four BEOC facilities)
2. Geographical distribution of EOC facilities
3. Proportion of all births conducted in EOC facilities
4. Proportion of women estimated to have major emergency obstetric complications who are treated in EOC facilities (met need for EOC)
5. Caesarean sections as a percentage of all births in the population (5–15%)
6. Case fatality rate of direct obstetric complications treated in EOC facilities (< 1%)

Table 15.1 Availability of Comprehensive Essential Obstetric Care (CEOC) in surveyed hospitals in three countries in sub-Saharan Africa

	Country 1	Country 2	Country 3
Year of survey	2006 and 2009	2006	2008
Population of survey area	1 995 034	2 812 183	12 104 109
Number of hospitals assessed (potential CEOC facilities)	24	13	51
Availability of fully functional CEOC facilities (percentage of total number of hospitals)			
Recommended number of CEOC facilities for population:	4	6	24
Actual number of fully functional CEOC facilities available	3 (12.5%)	8 (57.1%)	1 (3.9%)
Number of CEOC signal functions carried out in hospitals surveyed (percentage of total number of hospitals)			
Hospitals with 8 EOC signal functions	3 (12.5%)	8 (62%)	1 (3.9%)
Hospitals with 7 EOC signal functions	3 (12.5%)	1 (8%)	21 (41.2%)
Hospitals with 6 EOC signal functions	4 (16.6%)	0 (0%)	16 (31.4%)
Hospitals with 5 EOC signal functions	5 (20.8%)	1 (8%)	5 (9.8%)
Hospitals with 4 EOC signal functions	6 (25%)	4 (31%)	4 (7.8%)
Hospitals with 3 EOC signal functions	2 (8%)	0 (0%)	0 (0%)
Hospitals with 2 EOC signal functions	1 (4.2%)	0 (0%)	1 (2.0%)
Hospitals with 1 EOC signal function	0 (0%)	0 (0%)	2 (3.9%)
Availability of specific EOC functions in hospitals surveyed (percentage of total number of hospitals)			
Parenteral oxytocics	18 (75%)	13 (100%)	49 (94%)
Parenteral anticonvulsants	20 (83%)	13 (100%)	47 (86%)
Parenteral antibiotics	17 (71%)	13 (100%)	31 (61%)
Manual removal of retained placenta	21 (88%)	10 (77%)	46 (90%)
Evacuation of retained products of conception	16 (67%)	10 (77%)	41 (80%)
Assisted vaginal delivery	5 (21%)	10 (77%)	1 (2%)
Blood transfusion	14 (58%)	11 (85%)	46 (90%)
Caesarean section	11 (46%)	10 (77%)	43 (84%)

Table 15.2   Availability of Basic Essential Obstetric Care (BEOC) in surveyed health facilities in three countries in sub-Saharan Africa

	Country 1	Country 2	Country 3
Year of survey	2006 and 2009	2006	2009
Population of survey area	1 995 034	2 812 183	1 631 556
Health facilities with maternity services surveyed	76	60	49
Availability of fully functional BEOC facilities			
Recommended number of BEOC facilities for population	16	24	13
Actual number of fully functional BEOC facilities	0	0	1
Number of BEOC signal functions carried out in health facilities with maternity services (percentage of total number of facilities)			
Maternity services with 6 BEOC signal functions	0 (0%)	0 (0%)	1 (2%)
Maternity services with 5 BEOC signal functions	12 (16%)	2 (3%)	6 (12%)
Maternity services with 4 BEOC signal functions	17 (22%)	13 (22%)	6 (12%)
Maternity services with 3 BEOC signal functions	21 (28%)	33 (55%)	5 (10%)
Maternity services with 2 BEOC signal functions	11 (14%)	9 (15%)	11 (22%)
Maternity services with 1 BEOC signal function	7 (9%)	2 (3%)	8 (16%)
Maternity services with 0 BEOC signal functions	8 (11%)	0 (0%)	11 (22%)
Availability of specific EOC functions in health facilities with maternity services (percentage of total number of facilities)			
Parenteral oxytocics	52 (68%)	55 (92%)	29 (59%)
Parenteral anticonvulsants	46 (61%)	49 (82%)	17 (35%)
Parenteral antibiotics	55 (72%)	54 (90%)	30 (61%)
Manual removal of retained placenta	39 (51%)	20 (33%)	22 (45%)
Evacuation of retained products of conception	18 (24%)	3 (5%)	8 (16%)
Assisted vaginal delivery	5 (7%)	1 (2%)	1 (2%)

population of 500000 was identified and all relevant facilities in each catchment population assessed. The results illustrate that, in most cases, the minimum need for BEOC services is not currently being met and, with one exception, of a total of 185 health facilities surveyed none could be considered a fully functioning BEOC facility.

A number of other surveys have assessed the availability, accessibility and quality of EOC in countries with high maternal mortality. These surveys consistently find that coverage of EOC facilities is inadequate and minimum UN agreed standards are not yet in place.[18–22]

In addition, these surveys show that in many cases there are relatively large numbers of health facilities but these are often not providing the full complement of signal functions for either BEOC or CEOC. Furthermore, the geographical distribution of facilities is such that these tend to be clustered in urban areas, with poor coverage particularly in more rural areas.

Basic newborn care is also frequently not in place, with a lack of simple equipment (bag and mask) or an identified area for newborn resuscitation, a source of heat unavailable and methods such as kangaroo mother care not yet adopted.

The reasons for the non-availability of EOC facilities and signal functions are a lack of skilled professional staff, a lack of knowledge and skills to perform the signal functions among the existing healthcare providers and failures in the enabling environment.

One of the signal functions that is least well carried out is that of assisted vaginal delivery.[23,24] This may be because this skill is no longer or rarely taught or because the cadre of staff allowed to carry out assisted delivery is not available at the facility. Many of the health facilities that should provide BEOC are not staffed by medical doctors, who are in many cases still the 'lowest' cadre of staff allowed to carry out assisted deliveries. However, it has been shown that this task, as well as manual removal of the placenta and manual vacuum aspiration, can be effectively delegated to clinical officers or nurse-midwives trained in life-saving skills for EOC.[25,26] Many developing countries are currently facing a severe shortage of skilled healthcare providers. There are many reasons for this, including poor planning and management of available human resources, lack of incentives to work in rural areas and external migration.[27] The quality of services provided is often substandard owing to lack of knowledge and skills of existing staff, who are frequently poorly supervised and demotivated.

Training for essential obstetric and newborn care

It has been well documented that suboptimal care in many cases contributes to maternal and neonatal deaths and that this includes inability of available staff to recognise and manage complications of pregnancy and childbirth in a timely and effective manner.[28,29] Similarly, in-depth assessments of availability and coverage of EOC have shown that in many cases structures are in place and equipment and consumables are available but the existing staff lack competency and skills and for this reason are unable to provide all the signal functions of EOC and essential newborn care.[19–23]

Healthcare professionals as well as health service managers have a crucial role in implementing these interventions and ensuring they are available to all pregnant women and newborns. The combination of lack of knowledge and of skills is a key reason why many beneficial evidence-based practices are still not used in many resource-poor settings.[14]

In 2006, a new Life Saving Skills: Essential Obstetric Care and Newborn Care (LSS-EOC&NC) training package was designed and developed specifically for the developing country setting by the Liverpool School of Tropical Medicine (LSTM) and the Royal College of Obstetricians and Gynaecologists (RCOG). It is based on the WHO manual on integrated management of pregnancy and childbirth[30] and has been developed in collaboration with the Department of Making Pregnancy Safer at WHO and in consultation with a wide range of experts with multidisciplinary backgrounds (including midwives, obstetricians, public health specialists and anaesthetists) and extensive practical experience of maternal and newborn health in resource-poor areas as well as educational methods. The training package was piloted extensively in 2007 and is now used in a variety of settings in both Africa and Asia.

The purpose of the LSS-EOC&NC training package is to develop capacity of existing health systems in developing or resource-poor countries to meet demand and provide a standard of care that will improve women's health.

The course is designed to cover the five major causes of maternal death – haemorrhage, sepsis, eclampsia, obstructed labour and complications of abortion. The focus is on the signal functions of CEOC and BEOC and is inclusive of early newborn care. There are a number of core modules, which include the following:

- communication, triage and referral
- resuscitation of mother and newborn
- shock and the unconscious patient
- severe pre-eclampsia and eclampsia
- haemorrhage
- obstructed labour
- sepsis
- assisted delivery (vacuum extraction)
- common obstetric emergencies (shoulder dystocia, breech delivery, cord prolapse)
- complications of abortion
- early newborn care.

The training package includes a section on surgical skills (caesarean section, B-Lynch suture, venous cutdown) and on normal delivery (skilled birth attendance).

There are pre-designed materials for delivery of the training package, which include a simple manual[31] and a set of accompanying teaching aids (manikins, models and DVDs).

Lectures and content of breakout sessions, discussions and demonstrations are standard and documented in the Facilitator Guide. This also contains practical details of the course infrastructure. Both the manual and course content were designed with an awareness of the very real barriers to accessing care that women in resource-poor countries have, as well as with the realisation that many healthcare providers trying to provide skilled attendance at birth and EOC for women with complications work in difficult circumstances with limited resources. All case scenarios are based on actual everyday scenarios that would be encountered in a BEOC or CEOC facility in sub-Saharan Africa or Asia.

A multidisciplinary approach has been seen by many as the basis for effective delivery of LSS-EOC&NC training, thus all cadres of staff involved in obstetric and newborn care are targeted and preferably trained as a team.

To ensure maximum effectiveness, the LSS-EOC&NC training package is designed to be deliverable (generally 3 days' duration), educationally sound and adhering to the principles of adult learning (that is, it includes various methods of learning – lectures, skills teaching, scenarios, discussions, workshops, demonstrations, videos, etc.), supportive (mentoring, small-group constructive feedback sessions), evidence based, relevant and adaptable to the local in-country conditions, and strongly supportive of national essential drugs lists, policies and practices.

In each country setting it is important to identify which cadres of staff are involved in delivering skilled birth attendance and EOC. Depending on the country setting, this may include doctors, nurse-midwives, clinical officers and medical assistants. Representation from the ministry of health, training institutions (medical and midwifery), professional associations and healthcare providers in management positions is encouraged.

Sustainability is ensured via a process of training of trainers. At the time of the first LSS-EOC&NC training, future facilitators will be identified from among the participants. These participants will be offered a 1- to 2-day theoretical training of trainers (TOT) course and then will work alongside external faculty to help deliver the immediate next LSS-EOC&NC courses. A model for scale-up and subsequent quality assurance has been developed and is being piloted in a number of countries. All equipment and demonstration material is left in the host facility (health facility or training institution) for use in further courses or regular follow-up 'skills and drills' practice in the facility or training institution.

Retention of learned interventions is promoted via a series of wall charts and posters that complement the training and can be posted in the workplace to guide an approach to clinical management of specific emergencies. These cover, for example, the ABC approach used for resuscitation, management of an eclamptic fit, and postpartum haemorrhage, and can easily be adapted to reflect specific protocols. Where these are not yet available, protocols and standards for skilled birth attendance and EOC can be developed.

Monitoring and evaluation of training in essential obstetric and newborn care

A systematic review by Black and Brocklehurst[32] identified six papers describing LSS-EOC&NC training programmes and only four papers documenting an evaluation of such programmes. All evaluations involved the use of questionnaires completed by course participants. No studies comparing one form of training with another were found. Descriptions of training in developing countries were excluded from this review. Training courses were between 1 and 3 days long and all resulted in a significant increase in confidence in handling obstetric emergencies. Although these studies were not yet able to assess clinical outcome measures, a more recent study from the UK was able to document improved clinical outcome with a reduction in the number of babies born with low Apgar scores (less than 7) and a reduction in incidence of neonatal encephalopathy following a series of pre-designed 1-day training sessions for all midwifery and obstetric staff to be attended annually.[33]

Where training in developing countries has been evaluated, this has so far generally taken the form of evaluation via simple questionnaires, with or without observation of skills on, for example, dummies. In these settings, short-term structured skills training has been shown to result in significantly improved scores for knowledge and scenario-based practice among participants.[34,35] Uptake of new practice concepts introduced as part of the training was anecdotally reported as having occurred, for example the use of a new technique (balloon tamponade for haemorrhage) and the development of protocols for use of magnesium sulphate.

In Kenya, to improve EOC in eight health facilities in Nyanza, mid-level staff were given 2 weeks' training in life-saving skills followed by a 1-week course on post-abortion care. This was followed by supportive supervision visits at 6 weeks, 2 months and then quarterly intervals. Using facility records, observation, focus-group discussion and in-depth interviews with both providers and clients, improved outcomes included an increased number of deliveries in the facilities, an improved system for referral of cases for surgery (caesarean section) with presumed improved earlier recognition of complications requiring referral, increased use of infection prevention practices and recognition of the importance of effective client–provider communication.[36]

In general, however, there is relatively poor documentation of the effect of training in EOC and there is currently no accepted published international framework available for monitoring and evaluation of the effect of LSS-EOC&NC training on the delivery of skilled birth attendance and EOC. Recent publications have highlighted the need for development of such a framework and have suggested examples of frameworks for evaluating other areas of capacity development such as health research capacity development, a framework for dissemination and implementation of evidence-based medicine and a model for institutionalising quality assurance.[37–39]

To complement the EOC and newborn care training package developed by the RCOG, LSTM and WHO, a generic framework for evaluation of the effect of training was designed that includes measurement of the effect on competency and motivation of the healthcare provider, utilisation (or uptake) of skilled birth attendance and EOC services, and effect on health outcomes. Both quantitative and qualitative research methodologies are used when implementing this framework.

The monitoring and evaluation framework makes use of and assesses the four key levels of learning as described by Kirkpatrick[40] and is adapted to incorporate the UN process indicators (Box 15.2). These include:

1. participants' reaction to training
2. improvement in knowledge and skills
3. change in behaviour (clinical practice)
4. societal outcomes (UN process indicators).

To complement assessments made as part of the evaluation framework, careful documentation of concurrent activities involving improved quality of care and/or the system of healthcare delivery is important as these are likely to have a 'multiplier' effect and may facilitate the effectiveness of the training package per se.

To date, programmes have generally assessed only the immediate effects of training; whether and how training can have a longer lasting effect on care delivery requires further study, as does the optimum frequency of training.

During the pilot phase, the standardised 3-day LSTM/RCOG training package in LSS-EOC&NC was delivered to 380 participants in six sub-Saharan African countries (Tanzania, Kenya, Zimbabwe, Malawi, Somaliland and Swaziland).

Using the generic monitoring and evaluation framework, an evaluation of levels 1 and 2 was carried out. Anonymous standardised questionnaires were used to assess pre- and post-course knowledge. The assessment was via a series of true or false questions for each of eight modules:

1. airway, breathing and circulation (ABC) and maternal and newborn resuscitation
2. shock and the unconscious patient
3. eclampsia and severe pre-eclampsia

4. communication and triage

5. obstetric emergencies

6. haemorrhage

7. obstructed labour

8. sepsis and abortion complications.

The maximum score for each section was 5 and the minimum was 0.

Using a separate questionnaire, participants were also asked to score how useful each of the sessions was (on a scale of 1–10, with 1 being not useful and 10 being extremely useful) and level of enjoyment (also on a scale of 1–10, with 1 being not enjoyable and 10 being extremely enjoyable). In addition, direct subjective feedback was received either through small-group discussions or by anonymous written responses.

Among all levels of healthcare providers (nurse-midwives, doctors, clinical officers and specialists), knowledge about the diagnosis and management of complications of pregnancy and childbirth as well as newborn care significantly increased ($P < 0.001$). The median scores for enjoyment of learning and usefulness were between 8 and 9 out of 10 in all countries. Participants expressed a high level of satisfaction and a need for scale-up of this form of capacity development. The training resulted in increased enthusiasm and motivation among participants to provide a better quality of care, and increased awareness of the need for evidence-based care. It also encouraged team work.

Longer term studies are needed to address the contribution of this form of capacity development to retention of staff, sustained improvement in clinical services and improved maternal and newborn outcomes. A programme is currently under way in five countries, three African and two Asian, to evaluate the longer term effects of training in EOC and newborn care on the availability of signal functions and quality of care at facility level, as well as the effect on healthcare provider competencies.

References

1. Hill K, Thomas K, AbouZahr C, Walker N, Say L, Inoue M, *et al*. Estimates of maternal mortality worldwide between 1990 and 2005: an assessment of available data. *Lancet* 2007;370:1311–19.

2. World Health Organization. *Maternal Mortality in 2005. Estimates Developed by WHO, UNICEF, UNFPA and the World Bank.* Geneva: WHO; 2007.

3. Lawn JE, Cousens S, Bhutta ZA, Darmstadt GL, Martinez J , Paul V. Why are 4 million newborn babies dying each year? *Lancet* 2004;364:399–401.

4. Lawn JE, Yakoob MY, Haws RA, Soomro T, Darmstadt GL, Bhutta ZA. 3.2 million stillbirth: epidemiology and overview of the evidence review. *BMC Pregnancy Childbirth* 2009;9(Suppl 1):1–17.

5. Lawn JE, Lee AC, Kinney M, Sibley L, Carlo WA, Paul VK, *et al*. Two million intrapartum-related stillbirths and neonatal deaths: Where, why, and what can be done? *Int J Gynecol Obstet* 2009;107:S5–19 [www.ijgo.org/issues/contents?issue_key=S0020-7292%2809%29X0010-X].

6. World Health Organization. *Making Pregnancy Safer: the Critical Role of the Skilled Attendant.* A joint statement by WHO, ICM and FIGO. Geneva: WHO; 2004 [www.who.int/making_pregnancy_safer/topics/skilled_birth/en/index.html].

7. World Health Organization. *Making a Difference in Countries – Strategic Approach to Improving Maternal and Newborn Survival and Health. Ensuring Skilled Care for Every Birth.* Geneva: WHO; 2006.

8. World Health Organization. *Reduction of Maternal Mortality.* A joint WHO/UNFPA/World Bank statement. Geneva: WHO; 1999.

9. World Health Organization. *The World Health Report 2005: Make Every Mother and Child Count.* Geneva: WHO; 2005.

10. Khan KS, Wojdyla D, Say L, Gülmezoglu AM, Van Look PF. WHO analysis of causes of maternal deaths: a systematic review. *Lancet* 2006;367:1066–74.

11. UNICEF, World Health Organization, United Nations Population Fund. *Guidelines for Monitoring the Availability and Use of Obstetric Services.* 2nd edition. New York: UNICEF; 1997 [www.who.int/making_pregnancy_safer/documents/9280631985/en/index.html].

12. World Health Organization, UNFPA, UNICEF, AMDD. *Monitoring Emergency Obstetric Care: a Handbook.* Geneva: WHO; 2009 [www.who.int/reproductivehealth/publications/monitoring/9789241547734/en/index.html].

13. Enkin M, Keirse M, Neilson J, Crowther C, Duley L, Hodnett E, *et al. A Guide to Effective Care in Pregnancy and Childbirth.* 3rd edition. Oxford: Oxford University Press; 2000.

14. Fauveau V, de Bernis L. "Good obstetrics" revisited: too many evidence-based practices and devices are not used. *Int J Gynaecol Obstet* 2006;94:179–84.

15. World Health Organization. *Safe Motherhood Needs Assessment.* Geneva: WHO; 2001.

16. World Health Organization. *Making Pregnancy Safer: a Planning Guide for Districts.* Geneva: WHO; 2005.

17. Bates I, Chapotera GK, McKew S, van den Broek N. Maternal mortality in sub-Saharan Africa: the contribution of ineffective blood transfusion services. *BJOG* 2008;115:1331–9.

18. Paxton A, Bailey P, Lobis S, Fry D. Global paterns in availability of emergency obstetric care. *Int J Gynaecol Obstet* 2006;93:300–7.

19. Pearson L, Shoo R. Availability and use of emergency obstetric services: Kenya, Rwanda, Southern Sudan, and Uganda. *Int J Gynaecol Obstet* 2005;88:208–15.

20. Olsen OE, Ndeki S, Norheim EF. Availability, distribution and use of emergency obstetric care in northern Tanzania. *Heath Policy Plan* 2005;20:167–75.

21. Islam MH, Hossain M, Islam MA. Improvement of coverage and utilisation of EmOC services in south western Bangladesh. *Int J Gynaecol Obstet* 2005;91:298–305.

22. Kongnyuy E, Hofman J, Mlava G, Mhango C, Van den Broek N. Availability, utilisation and quality of Basic and Comprehensive Emergency Obstetric Care services in Malawi. *Matern Child Health J* 2009;13:687–94.

23. Bailey P. The disappearing art of instrumental delivery: time to reverse the trend. *Int J Gynaecol Obstet* 2005;91:89–96.

24. Ameh CA, Weeks AD. The role of instrumental delivery in low resource settings. *BJOG* 2009;116:22–5.

25. De Luz Vaz M, Bergström S. Mozambique – delegation of responsibility in the area of maternal care. *Int J Gynaecol Obstet* 1992;38:S37–9.

26. Duale S. Delegation of responsibility in maternity care in Karawa rural health zone, Zaire. *Int J Gynaecol Obstet* 1992;38:S33–5.

27. Moyo NT, Liljestrand J. Emergency obstetric care: impact on emerging issues. *Int J Gynaecol Obstet* 2007;98:175–7.

28. Drife J, Lewis G, editors. *Why Mothers Die. Report on Confidential Enquiries into Maternal Deaths in the United Kingdom 1994–96.* London: The Stationery Office; 1998.

29. Pattinson RC. *Saving Mothers – Third Report on Confidential Enquiries into Maternal Deaths in South Africa 2002–2004.* Pretoria: Department of Health; 2006.

30. World Health Organization. *Managing Complications in Pregnancy and Childbirth: a Guide for Midwives and Doctors.* Integrated Management of Pregnancy and Childbirth. Geneva: WHO; 2005.

31. van den Broek NR. *Life Saving Skills Manual: Essential Obstetric and Newborn Care.* London: RCOG Press; 2007.

32. Black RS, Brocklehurst P. A systematic review of training in acute obstetric emergencies. *BJOG* 2003;110:837–41.

33. Draycott T, Sibanda T, Owen L, Akande V, Winter C, Reading S, *et al.* Does training in obstetric emergencies improve neonatal outcome? *BJOG* 2006;113:177–82.

34. Johanson B, Akhtar S, Edwards C, Dewan F, Haque Y, Jones P. MOET: Bangladesh – an initial experience. *J Obstet Gynaecol Res* 2002;28:217–23.

35. Johanson BR, Menon V, Burns E, Kargramanya E, Osipov V, Israelyan M, *et al.* Managing Obstetric Emergencies and Trauma (MOET) structured skills training in Armenia, utilising models and reality based scenarios. *BMC Med Educ* 2002;2:5.

36. Orero S, Oguttu M, Omondi E, Oyoo C, Ambrose M, Ombaka C. The importance of Life Saving Skills Training for mid-level providers of Emergency Obstetric Care in a low resource

setting, Averting Maternal Death and Disability (AMDD) Program Network Conference, 2003, Kuala Lumpur, Malaysia. Abstract 62.

37.   Bates I, Akoto AY, Ansong D, Karikari P, Bedu-Addo G, Critchley J, *et al.* Evaluating health research capacity building: an evidence-based tool. *PLoS Med* 2006;3:e299.

38.   Garner P, Meremikwu M, Volmink J, Xu Q, Smith H. Putting evidence into practice: how middle- and low-income countries 'get it together'. *BMJ* 2001:329:1036–9.

39.   Silimperi DR, Franco LM, Veldhuyzen T, MacAulay C. A framework for institutionalizing quality assurance. *Int J Qual Health Care* 2002;14(Suppl 1);67–73.

40.   Kirkpatrick DL, Kirkpatrick JD. *Evaluating Training Programs: the Four Levels.* 3rd edition. San Francisco: Berrett-Koehler Publishers; 2006.

Chapter 16

The role of the Royal Colleges in training and development

Anthony Falconer (RCOG), Kate Grady (RCoA), Frances Day-Stirk (RCM) and Stephen Allen (RCPCH)

Royal College of Obstetricians and Gynaecologists (RCOG)

Setting standards to improve women's health is the core philosophy of the Royal College of Obstetricians and Gynaecologists. This theme is central to our principal functions of training and standard setting in obstetrics and gynaecology. The organisation has almost 12 000 Members and Fellows and just under 50% work outside the UK. Members work in 90 separate countries and the potential network of influence is considerable. This article will focus on issues of training and development delivered under the auspices of the RCOG but developed specifically for the under-resourced areas where Millennium Development Goals 4 and 5 present major challenges.

UK-based training

Historically, many postgraduate doctors came to the UK to work and train within the NHS. Such an experience was not time limited and often provided the trainee with a skewed experience of the discipline. Successful trainees would return home with new clinical and management skills and a postgraduate examination certificate. Membership of the RCOG would enable such doctors to develop a lifelong relationship with the facilities of the college.

However, recently such opportunities have decreased owing to a rapid expansion of British medical graduates. Opportunities, coordinated by the RCOG, now allow a limited number of overseas doctors to work under supervision for up to 2 years. It is anticipated that shortly some more senior doctors will come to the UK for exposure to subspecialty and special interest work. Such experiences allow the trainers to become part of a competency-based training assessment process.

MRCOG

Overseas doctors would submit for the MRCOG, which is an examination aimed at assessing knowledge rather than clinical competence and which is passed by British trainees between their intermediate and their advanced training. Currently, 90% of doctors writing the examination come from outside the UK, although many of them are working within the UK. The examination is structured around principles of UK medicine but nevertheless many of those sitting the examination from overseas desire a certificate from a UK institution. Many doctors with this certificate will never work in the UK but will continue to receive the educational and standards products of the RCOG.

Distance learning

StratOG, a distance learning resource produced by the RCOG and pitched at a level commensurate with the MRCOG, is available internationally. Sadly, its wide distribution has been curtailed by economic factors. This modular programme covers the whole extent of obstetrics and gynaecology.

More recently, learning resources have been developed with the intention of assisting medical staff in-country in more defined functions and incorporating elements of competency into the programme. The obstetric fistula programme is a modular course, developed jointly by the RCOG, the International Federation of Gynecology and Obstetrics (FIGO) and the International Obstetric Fistula Surgeons Group. The course includes a curriculum, core knowledge principles, clinical competencies including objective structured assessment of technical skills (OSATS) and suggested further study. This project is currently undergoing field testing in certain fistula institutions within Africa. It is hoped that, through training the trainers, a group of trainees will be created in these hospitals who will be able to incorporate our contemporary educational methods into this vital area of women's health. Such modelling may be extended to other areas of maternity care.

The potential for developments in e-learning are wide and represent a challenge and a creative and 'green' way to provide learning.

Direct interaction learning

Postgraduate courses, including courses franchised to other obstetric and gynaecological organisations, will continue to provide a focus for academic advancement. Such courses include basic surgical skills and a variety of intrapartum care learning.

Scientific courses are an effective medium for knowledge transfer. Currently, the RCOG attempts to sponsor and organise one course per year overseas.

Multiprofessional learning

More recently, the need to break down professional barriers has been central to the learning philosophy of the RCOG. It is widely accepted that most clinical care is provided by multiprofessional teams rather than by individuals and therefore learning should logically occur in a similar manner.

The evolution of the Life Saving Skills: Essential Obstetric Care and Newborn Care (LSS-EOC&NC) courses has attempted to address this concept in intrapartum care in under-resourced communities. This method has provided evidence of improvement in knowledge acquired and skills leant in all cadres of staff.

Within some communities, much health care is provided by clinical staff who have no formal medical qualification. Providing training and learning opportunities for mid-level providers presents a fresh challenge.

The RCOG is involved with the World Health Organization (WHO) Reproductive Health Library to define a modular training package for those involved in providing women's health care within Africa. Intrapartum care, obstetric fistula, family planning, unsafe abortion, sepsis and cervical cancer will form some components of the course.

Standards

Through a large and comprehensive library of guidelines, the RCOG has the ability to connect with many different communities with regard to investigation and management of common conditions. Methodologies have been developed to allow alterations of guidelines for local use. The current quoted standards are those that are appropriate for UK practice.

Challenges

Quality assurance of learning is an imperative. Evaluation of some of the methods described above is challenging. The process for reproducibility and reliability for the MRCOG is now a standard component of conducting the examination. In comparison, quality assurance for the fistula training package may be far more unreliable and will be described following the piloting of the technical aspects of the resource.

Sustainability of progress needs to be defined. Decay of information and the development of new knowledge has stimulated the development of continuous professional development. Ideally, such structures should be fundamental to any development. The progress that has occurred in e-technology should facilitate these processes.

New knowledge requires reinforcement and this can be very difficult to guarantee in resource-poor and busy healthcare facilities.

Summary

The medical Royal Colleges have a central role to play in the development, delivery, assessment and quality assurance of new learning technologies that can be applied to under-resourced health facilities. However, such developments should occur in liaison with local practitioners familiar with the local needs.

Royal College of Anaesthetists (RCoA)

The perspective of the RCoA

The RCoA has significant expertise in training, education and assessment in clinical anaesthesia, including critical care and pain medicine:

- it addresses the status of anaesthesia worldwide
- it embraces the issues of perioperative care, the non-doctor role and maternal mortality
- it has a key role in the setting of standards internationally
- it promotes the highest standards of anaesthetic practice worldwide
- it is a recognised expert in the provision of learning resources, in particular its e-learning project.

The AAGBI

The RCoA has close professional links with the Association of Anaesthetists of Great Britain and Ireland (AAGBI). The AAGBI, through its International

Relations Committee (IRC), coordinates likeminded specialists to contribute to the development of anaesthesia in the resource-poor world through:

- learning materials
- website discussion groups
- local support
- support for those anaesthetists undertaking overseas work.

The IRC of the AAGBI has brought together a group of anaesthetists and others keen to improve anaesthesia in the developing world. The group comprises representation from the RCoA, the RCOG, the Obstetric Anaesthetists' Association (OAA) and individuals working on projects and endeavours to train anaesthetists and develop anaesthesia.

   This group has been proactive in linking to the WHO Department of Making Pregnancy Safer and, as a partnership, they have linked to the World Federation of Societies of Anaesthesiologists (WFSA). These organisations together have designed a short course designed to improve standards of the practice of anaesthesia, to a level where safe obstetric anaesthesia can be delivered. The course template, a 3-day in-country course, has been designed and interactive learning materials are currently being written. The RCoA has donated access to some of its e-learning material to the course. The course will be complemented by a training the trainers course for local faculty in-country and it will have integrated monitoring, evaluation and quality assurance. The course will be piloted in Bangladesh in October 2010.

Other anaesthesia projects

Many individual and groups of UK anaesthetists are involved in training and teaching initiatives, mentoring and advocacy in widespread areas of sub-Saharan Africa and South Asia, including:

- Bangladesh
- Ethiopia
- Liberia
- Malawi
- Tanzania
- Uganda
- Nepal.

Potential future roles

Further roles of the specialty of anaesthesia could include:

- support and continuing development of the above and other training programmes
- advocacy, recognition and support through visiting and distance mentoring
- addressing deficiencies in equipment and drug provision, engaging with partners at government and international level
- campaign for assistance for the anaesthetist (including the non-doctor anaesthetist) intraoperatively and in recovery

- creation of a culture and introduce methods of professional reflection and move away from immediate blame
- international senior, large-scale advocacy and support for training and status.

Royal College of Midwives (RCM)

Introduction

The Royal College of Midwives has an international history and has sought to work with and support midwives from all over the world, through international organisations, committees and networks and by fostering links with individual midwives and associations. Since President Edith Pye was honoured with the French Chevalier of Cross of the Legion of Honour in recognition of valuable services rendered during World War I, the Medal of the City of Rheims for services to mothers also during World War I and the Greek Red Cross Medal for services during 1940–41, the RCM has established its international credentials.

Subsequently its activities have focused primarily on supporting in-country capacity development of midwifery education (in Botswana, Spain, Tanzania, Zimbabwe and the Former Yugoslav Republic of Macedonia), regulation (in British Columbia and Ontario) and association development (in Bulgaria, Romania, Sierre Leone and FYR Macedonia).

In 1999, the RCM set out its commitment in a position paper entitled *Supporting World Midwifery.*[1] This position paper outlines the RCM's mission, values and principles underpinning this activity, which seeks continual improvements to the care provided for women and babies throughout the world (Figure 16.1).

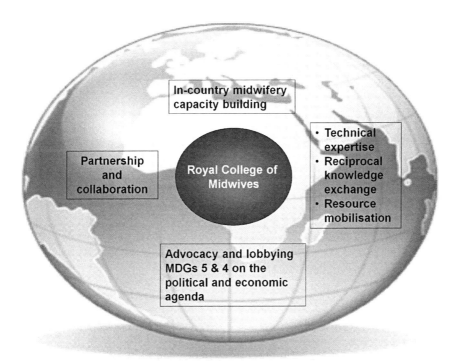

Figure 16.1 The Royal College of Midwives' global commitments

Mission, values and guiding principles

The RCM's mission is to promote the art and science of midwifery at a worldwide level, to exchange information and to improve international understanding. This is in the belief that midwives collectively are empowered through unity at international level and that cooperation and collaboration among nations will further the goal of all midwives. The RCM's international activities are underpinned by the following central values:

- midwifery focus
- objective orientated
- reciprocal value
- resource neutral
- establishing networks
- international credibility.

This role is directed by a number of guiding principles:

- the development of strategies that support and empower midwives to achieve professional autonomy
- midwives in-country should develop projects themselves with our assistance
- provision of technical expertise in the form of service reviews, education and practice study tours, curriculum development and fundraising activities
- maintaining mutually beneficial relationships with colleagues, other agencies and governments
- above all, being clear about the value of an international project/activity in the UK.

International networks

The RCM is engaged in a wide range of midwifery and other international networks, non-governmental and civil society organisations, and is also designated a WHO Collaborating Centre for Midwifery (Figure 16.2). In terms of interprofessional

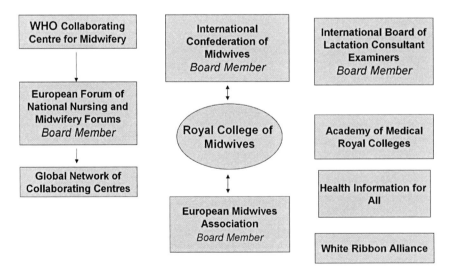

Figure 16.2 The Royal College of Midwives' international networks

partnerships and capacity building, the RCM has a Memorandum of Understanding with RCOG and the White Ribbon Alliance to guide joint activities.

International Day of the Midwife

On 5 May each year, the International Day of the Midwife[2,3] is the focal point to profile safe motherhood issues and highlight the pivotal role of the midwife.

International Confederation of Midwives

The RCM is an active member of the International Confederation of Midwives (ICM),[4] an accredited non-governmental organisation with over 90 member associations in 85 countries in four regions of the world: Africa, the Americas, Asia-Pacific and Europe. The RCM hosted the ICM 28th Triennial Congress in Glasgow, June 2008, which was attended by more than 3000 midwives from all regions of the world. The UK prime minister, Gordon Brown, delivered a video address to the opening ceremony and his wife, Sarah, was a guest plenary speaker. The RCM has enjoyed several board positions and currently holds the vice-presidency.

European Midwives Association

The RCM is a full member of the European Midwives Association (EMA),[5] an international non-profit and non-governmental organisation of midwives representing midwifery organisations from the member states of the European Union (EU), the European Economic Area (EEA) and EU applicant countries. Its aims and objectives are to:

- lobby for minimum educational standard for European midwifery
- promote women's reproductive health
- support midwifery associations
- develop EU-wide legislation on midwifery education and practice.

European Forum of National Nursing and Midwifery Associations and WHO

The RCM is a full member of the European Forum of National Nursing and Midwifery Associations (EFNNMA),[6] which was founded in November 1996 as a joint initiative of European national nursing and midwifery associations and WHO. The RCM, as a full member association and steering committee member, participates in the remit to:

- inform debate on improving health in Europe
- promote exchange of information between midwifery and nursing associations and WHO
- form consensus on policy issues relating to midwifery and nursing.

WHO Collaborating Centre for Midwifery

RCM was designated a WHO Collaborating Centre in March 1993 and received re-designation in February 1998 and April 2009, renewing its commitment to interagency collaboration on international midwifery. As a WHO Collaborating Centre, the RCM forms part of a global network of over 30 designated, primarily nursing, collaborating centres. Each collaborating centre has a plan or terms of reference with WHO that is consistent with WHO's programme goals. Every 4 years, RCM priorities are set with WHO Europe around:

- education, research and developing standards
- capacity building in-country
- assisting with developing midwifery associations.

An example of this is a 2-year capacity-building Safe Motherhood project in FYR Macedonia, Educating the Educators.

Ad hoc activities

The RCM also participates in *ad hoc* activities such as the intercollegiate Kenya Safe Motherhood standard setting in partnership with the RCOG, the Royal College of Nursing and the UK Department for International Development (DFID). It holds an annual event, 'Working Overseas', in collaboration with the Royal College of Nursing, VSO and Médecins Sans Frontières (MSF), and is also actively engaged with the Maternal Mortality Campaign and Healthcare Information for All (HIFA2015) campaign.[7] The RCM also facilitates international exchanges and study visits, undertakes accreditation of international learning programmes that involve midwives and engages in inter-agency collaboration with non-governmental organisations such as Maternity Worldwide and Merlin.

Summary

The RCM's four main international roles in supporting midwifery and safe motherhood are:

- role modelling
- capacity building through twinning and providing technical expertise, information and resources
- inter-agency collaboration on international midwifery and safe motherhood
- interprofessional partnerships.

Royal College of Paediatrics and Child Health (RCPCH)

Background

Paediatricians based in the UK have a long tradition of contributing to improving the health of children in poorer countries through a wide range of activities, including clinical service, education of health professionals, medical aid and disaster relief. In 1997, the RCPCH membership mandated the College to have a specific role in international child health. The RCPCH International Board was established in 2000 and acts as the reference point for the numerous College activities outside the UK.

A key event was the establishment of the David Baum International Foundation (DBIF) in 2001.[8] This followed the untimely death of Professor Baum, the then College President, and, in recognition of his great contribution to international child health, sought to improve the health of children in disadvantaged areas of the world by improving standards of paediatric education.

The international programme was expanded in May 2006 when Overseas Directors for Africa, Asia and the Middle East were appointed to support the David Baum International Fellow in the organisation of events and activities. There followed a series of discussions both within the College and with key overseas partners. The College sought to extend its influence beyond the UK, where it can make a significant impact on specific problems in child health by:

- working through paediatric associations in other countries to find sustainable solutions to specific problems in areas in which we have particular expertise, such as education and training
- running our examinations overseas where there is a demand and a need for them
- aiming to give *Archives of Disease in Childhood* a higher international profile, particularly through collaboration with the European Academy of Paediatrics.

RCPCH International Strategy

The International Strategy was adopted in July 2006 to act as a framework to guide international activities.[9] This reaffirmed the primary aim of supporting paediatricians outwith the UK through education programmes. A number of key partnerships and a network of postgraduate events across the world to promote appropriate best practice in health for children and adolescents were further developed according to specific criteria:

1. The main aim is to deliver the support in the country of origin. It is appreciated that some training or expertise may require visits to the UK and it is likely that this may be accommodated in the first instance through the various award schemes of the College, managed by the Academic Board.

2. Each training and education programme should be based on a 'Memorandum of Understanding' between a local organisation and the RCPCH, through the International Board. Where there is not a strong local or national body representing paediatricians, consideration should be given either to the appropriateness of establishing a training programme or directing the programme towards supporting the establishment of a local body involved in the governance of paediatric and child health care practice.

3. Consideration must be given when designing any programme to its sustainability. This has to be discussed with the RCPCH and potential funding bodies such as DBIF in detail. All programmes must include a detailed business plan. Programmes should be developed initially for a reasonable duration (ideally 3–5 years), although it is accepted that short-term projects may occasionally be appropriate.

4. Training and education programmes should be delivered through established medical education approaches and use methodology considered to be effective. The use of e-learning methods is considered to be a major way forward, even in areas currently under-resourced for this form of learning.

5. Two themes have emerged as priority projects for the International Board: 'training the trainers' and 'evidence-based practice'. However, other education programmes will need to be considered if and when appropriate.

6. All programmes must be delivered with appropriate consideration to the cultural context.

7. While accepting that many RCPCH members are involved in medical aid and disaster relief work, and while it is accepted that on occasions RCPCH,

through the International Board, may work closely with organisations involved in this area (for example, WHO, DFID and UNICEF), the priority is for the delivery of training and education to paediatricians and other appropriate health professionals involved in the care of children and adolescents. The International Board activities must be governed by UK Government advice on the specific countries involved in relation to medical and personal safety.

8. The International Board has the remit to establish links with other international paediatric bodies, outside of Europe. The International Board is the College reference point for the International Paediatric Association (IPA).

Funding

Core funding for international activities is derived from:

- ▨ a top slice from membership fees (£45,000 per year)
- ▨ additional support from general funds (£45,000 per year)
- ▨ DBIF funds.

Programmes

The activities of the International Board are grouped into three broad programmes:

1. **International Policy Programme:** The International Board links with the Academic Board, the International Child Health Group and the RCPCH Advocacy Committee to advise and comment on international events and activities. It is the forum, when appropriate, to consider specific links with other international bodies, such as the International Paediatric Association.

2. **International Training Programme:** The International Board advises from an international perspective and receives requests from several groups involved with education and training, such as the Education and Training Board, the International Paediatric Training Scheme, VSO, the Nutrition Committee and the Overseas Examinations Committee.

3. **International Development Programme:** Postgraduate activities ('training the trainer' courses, evidence-based medicine workshops and advanced paediatric life support [APLS] courses) with memoranda of understanding between RCPCH and a variety of international organisations since 2000 in the following areas:

   - Middle East: Occupied Palestinian territories, Iraq/Jordan
   - Africa: West African College of Physicians, Tanzania, South Africa, Kenya
   - Asia: India, Pakistan, Bangladesh
   - other areas: Brazil, West Indies.

International Development Programme current activities

Africa

Current projects in Africa are the following:

1. **West African College of Physicians (WACP):** A Memorandum of Understanding was signed with the Faculty of Paediatrics, West African College of Physicians in 2006. This has led to collaboration on sharing materials and

experience in assessments and examinations between the two institutions. To assist the WACP Faculty of Paediatrics in evaluating submitted dissertations, the RCPCH supported an evidence-based medicine workshop at the WACP Annual General and Scientific Meeting in Abuja, Nigeria, in November 2008, and discussions are under way regarding further developments of this initiative.

2. **Emergency Triage Assessment and Treatment and post-admission care (ETAT+), East Africa:** The ETAT+ course was developed from WHO's ETAT course by KEMRI/Wellcome Programme researchers with the Kenyan Ministry of Health and the University of Nairobi. It focuses on identifying and managing seriously ill children and newborns and is linked to a set of evidence-based clinical practice guidelines for common causes of child mortality. Since 2006, training has been delivered to large numbers of Kenyan health workers, the undergraduate paediatric curriculum and the postgraduate course in paediatrics at the University of Nairobi, Kenya. The DBIF has selected this programme as their main flagship project and, in January 2009, approved over £100,000 to support the training over the following 8 years. This will include establishing a critical mass of trainees and rolling out the training in Kenya and also consideration of extending the training throughout the sub-region. Two of the Kenyan ETAT+ trainers were supported by the College to attend the RCPCH Annual Meeting in York in April 2009 and presented summaries of their work at the joint RCPCH International/International Child Health Group session. Working with the Paediatric Association of Tanzania and the Kenya team, the College also supported a training workshop on the evidence behind the current WHO management guidelines of the sick child in Dar es Salaam, Tanzania, in 2007.

3. **Tanzania Art Project:** DBIF has supported Mrs Angela Baum and a colleague to deliver workshops in art therapy for children at Moshi Deaf School.

4. **International Health Training Project:** In a collaboration with the Royal Society of Tropical Medicine and Hygiene and the Wellcome Trust, the DBIF provided funding to develop an online information resource for lecturers in Africa. The College supported an extensive evaluation of the resource at the College of Medicine, University of Ibadan, Nigeria.

5. **Child protection:** Following on from the programme in India (see below), a training workshop in child protection was held in Addis Ababa in May 2009 in association with the Ethiopian Paediatric Society. Means of establishing the programme in Ethiopia and possibly extending within East Africa is being considered.

South Asia

Current projects in South Asia are the following:

1. **Evidence-based medicine:** Under a Memorandum of Understanding with the Indian Academy of Pediatrics (IAP), the main emphasis of training has been in evidence-based child health. With support from the College and funding through the DBIF, the Centre for Evidence-Based Child Health (CEBCH) has run three courses in Chandigarh. Over 70 clinicians from across India attended the courses and six Indian tutors were also trained. A further evidence-based medicine workshop was held at a neonatal meeting in Pune and, through collaboration with the *Archives of Disease in Childhood*, one of the Indian tutors

is now editing a new evidence-based medicine synopsis series for the journal *Indian Pediatrics*. Support for continuation of this programme has been awarded by the DBIF, with the emphasis over the next 2 years being to train a full Indian faculty under the auspices of the IAP by running four 'training the trainers' courses alongside two further 'provider' courses.

2. **Child protection:** Training courses in child protection in association with IAP were delivered in Mumbai and Chennai early in 2007. Following this, at the request of IAP, the RCPCH donated to the IAP a number of full copies of all child protection training materials (readers, DVDs, etc.) with which the IAP developed its own training package and subsequently rolled out eight complete training courses across India.

Middle East

Current projects in the Middle East are the following:

1. **Palestine Child Health Diploma:** This programme is the longest running overseas education course supported by the College and remains its flagship programme. It was initiated by Professor David Baum in 1998. Teaching in primary healthcare is provided for paediatric residents (Makassed group) and for GPs and nurses (Ramallah group) and is organised into 11 modules covering acute paediatrics, chronic illness, clinical skills, disability, nutrition and growth, mental health, child protection, health promotion and children's rights. Training is delivered in Makassed Hospital and Ramallah and each course lasts 18 months. Successful candidates are awarded the RCPCH Palestinian Child Health Diploma. The key partners are MAP-UK (currently funding the Palestinian part of the course), Juzoor (the main training, organisational and community mobilisation partner), the Palestinian Paediatric Association (links with local paediatricians), Al Quds University Medical School (local accreditation), the Ministry of Health (oversight and regulation to ensure compatibility with the National Health Plan), and the United Nations Relief and Works Agency (oversight and support in regulation, standardisation and integration of emergency services). RCPCH International provides technical training and support, and has prepared all the materials, which are now being further developed in collaboration with Palestinian paediatricians. A summary of the programme was published in the *Lancet*[10] and the College was pleased to host a meeting in March 2009 to launch the *Lancet* Palestinian health series.

2. **Postgraduate education course – training trainers in teaching paediatrics and child health and emergency care:** This programme is undertaken with the Jordanian Paediatric Society. Seven teaching paediatrics courses and nine resuscitation courses have been delivered in Amman and attended by over 200 trainees from Jordan, Iraq and Palestine.

3. **Child mental health in Gaza:** This course is being developed with MAP-UK and is currently in the planning stage.

4. **Postgraduate paediatric course, Iraq:** In association with the Iraq Paediatric Association, the College delivered a 5-day course focusing on paediatric life-support and evidence-based medicine at the Hawler Medical University, Erbil, Kurdistan, in September 2009.

Other activities

The RCPCH and VSO Fellowship Scheme offers UK Specialist Trainees 1-year placements working to improve child health in developing countries. Fellowship placements are out of programme experience, with structured support from the College to provide evidence of their personal and professional learning. There are currently 12 volunteers allocated to eight placements in six developing countries.

The RCPCH International Paediatric Training Scheme supports both junior and senior paediatric trainees from overseas to undertake fixed-term posts within the NHS. Doctors enter the UK under Tier V of the immigration regulations. There are currently 30 trainees in post and many more applications being processed.

The College has an important role in advocacy for children living in developing countries and works with several organisations, including the IPA, the International Malnutrition Task Force and the UK Government, to this effect.

Summary

Paediatricians based in the UK have a long-standing tradition of contributing to improving the health of children living in poor countries. In recent years, RCPCH International and the DBIF have focused their activities on a number of strategic partnerships in Africa, South Asia and the Middle East. We are confident that these working partnerships are sustainable and are already making a significant contribution to children's health. We look forward to extending our activities where appropriate in the future.

References

1.   Royal College of Midwives. *The RCM: Supporting World Midwifery*. Position Paper 7a. London: RCM; 1999 [www.rcm.org.uk/college/standards-and-practice/position-papers/].
2.   Royal College of Midwives. International Day of the Midwife [www.rcm.org.uk/college/international/international-day-of-the-midwife/].
3.   International Confederation of Midwives. International Day of the Midwife [www.internationalmidwives.org/CongressesEvents/InternationalDayoftheMidwife/tabid/327/Default.aspx].
4.   International Confederation of Midwives. [www.internationalmidwives.org/AboutICM/tabid/225/Default.aspx].
5.   European Midwives Association [www.europeanmidwives.eu/ema/].
6.   European Forum of National Nursing and Midwifery Associations [www.euro.who.int/efnnma].
7.   Healthcare Information for All [www.hifa2015.org/].
8.   Royal College of Paediatrics and Child Health. David Baum International Foundation [www.rcpch.ac.uk/About-the-College/RCPCH-International/David-Baum-International-Foundation/].
9.   Royal College of Paediatrics and Child Health. RCPCH International [www.rcpch.ac.uk/About-the-College/RCPCH-International].
10. Waterston T, Halileh S, Odeh J, Rudolf M, Hamilton P. Teaching child health in the occupied Palestinian territory. *Lancet* 2009;373:878–80. Erratum in: *Lancet* 2009;373:1174.

Section 5

Specific challenges in specific countries

Chapter 17
Challenges faced in Afghanistan

Jacqueline Hill and Eric Sinclair

Introduction

In 2002, a report by UNICEF and the Centers for Disease Control and Prevention (CDC) concluded that 'Afghanistan is among the worst places on the globe in which to be pregnant'. This conclusion was reached following review of preliminary data from a large well-designed maternal mortality study conducted from 1999 to 2002 that was subsequently published in the *Lancet* and that reported an overall maternal mortality ratio () of 1600 maternal deaths per 100 000 live births (95% CI 1100–2000).[1] Maternal death was the leading cause of death in women of reproductive age (15–49 years) and the MMRs were among the highest in the world. In the district of Ragh in Badakhshan province, the MMR was the highest ever recorded at 6507 per 100 000 live births. The study concluded that 87% of these deaths were 'preventable' and that maternal death was intimately linked to neonatal death (74% of babies born alive to mothers who died also died).

In 2003, my husband and I left the UK for Kabul, Afghanistan, to work with Medair (www.medair.org), a Swiss-based humanitarian relief and rehabilitation organisation. Eric took up the position of country director and I, after a short language course, moved to Ragh to begin developing Essential Obstetric Care (EOC) services in four Medair clinics as part of their Primary Health Care programme. In the ensuing months, I experienced first-hand what life was like for women in these remote villages.[2] Every kind of obstetric emergency came my way and I began to realise that sustainability would only be possible by training and capacity building national medical staff who would commit to improving the health care of their own people. With this in mind, in 2005 I moved to Kabul to work with another humanitarian organisation, Cure International (www.cureinternational.org). Their mandate was to develop and manage a hospital that would be a training centre for Afghan doctors. Training programmes would concentrate on family medicine together with obstetrics and gynaecology. The long-term goal was to send these trained doctors out into the provinces on a rotational basis. In the following 3 years, we saw the vision become reality.

Country background

Afghanistan is struggling to recover from nearly 30 years of conflict, displacement and destruction of its infrastructure. Its health status and human development indicators are among the worst in the world (Table 17.1). The country is approximately 2.5 times the size of the UK (Figure 17.1) but with 30% of its population (24.5 million), 78% of whom live in rural areas. At least 5 million people live in Kabul, 3 million refugees live outside the country (mainly in Pakistan) and around 1.5 million are internally displaced. Afghanistan is an Islamic state with 84% Sunni and 15% Shiite Muslims. The main ethnic groups are the Pashtuns (44%), the Tajiks (25%), the Uzbeks (8%), the Turkmen (5%) and the Hazaras (10%). Other minorities include Baluchis, Nuristanis and Kuchi nomads (8%). Natural resources include gas, petroleum, coal, copper, talc, sulphur, lead, zinc, iron, salt and (semi-) precious stones but, sadly, Afghanistan is better known as the largest producer of illicit opiate products.

The country was founded in 1747 by Ahmad Shah Durrani and it served as a buffer between the British and Russian empires until it won independence from notional British control in 1919. A brief democracy ended in a 1973 coup. In 1978, a Communist counter-coup made way for the Soviet Union invasion in 1979, beginning a long, destructive war with the internationally supported anti-Communist mujahedin rebels. A series of subsequent civil wars, which left very little infrastructure in place, saw Kabul fall in 1996 to the Taliban, a hardline Pakistani-sponsored movement that emerged in 1994 to end the country's civil war and anarchy. The rule of the Taliban had particularly devastating effects on health, especially maternal health, summed up in the title of a letter in the *Lancet*: 'The Taliban's war on women'.[3]

Following the terrorist attacks in New York City on 11 September 2001, a US, Allied and anti-Taliban Northern Alliance military action defeated the Taliban, who were sheltering Osama Bin Laden. The UN-sponsored Bonn Conference in 2001 established a process for political reconstruction that included the adoption of a new constitution, a presidential election in 2004 and National Assembly elections in 2005. Hamid Karzai became the first democratically elected president of Afghanistan. In the post-Taliban era, the Ministry of Health in the Islamic Republic of Afghanistan committed itself to improving health and placed strong emphasis on improving reproductive health.[4] Despite gains towards building a stable central government, corruption, the resurgent Taliban and continuing provincial instability – particularly in the south and east – remain serious challenges for the Government.

Maternal health in Afghanistan

Mortality and morbidity

The best-known indicator of maternal health is the maternal mortality ratio (MMR). High MMRs are indicators of poor health and status of women and point to deeper issues of underdevelopment of social, political and economic processes as well as to women's human rights issues.[5] Two published studies have been conducted in Afghanistan. One was in Herat by Physicians for Human Rights[5] using the indirect sisterhood method (MMR estimated at 593 per 100 000 live births [95% CI 557–630]). The other, the UNICEF/CDC survey,[1] identified deaths by verbal autopsy (MMR estimated at 1600 per 100 000 live births [95% CI 1100–2000]). Vast differences were noted between urban and rural areas: the MMR in Kabul was 400 whereas in Badakshan it was 6507.

Table 17.1 Human development indicators; data from Afghanistan Health Survey (AHS),[15] UNDP,[28] CIA[29] and UNICEF[27]

Indicator	Value
Infant mortality rate (2008)	165 per 1000 live births
Under-five mortality rate (2008)	257 per 1000 live births
Life expectancy at birth (2007)	43.6 years (males: 43.6 years; females: 43.5 years)
Total fertility rate (2005–10)	6.6 births per woman
Literacy rate (age 15+; 1997–2007)	28% (males: 43.1%; females: 12.6%)
Access to basic health care	29–35%
Access to safe water	6–13%
Gross domestic product (2008 estimate)	US$23.1 billion
Gross domestic product per capita (2008 estimate)	US$800

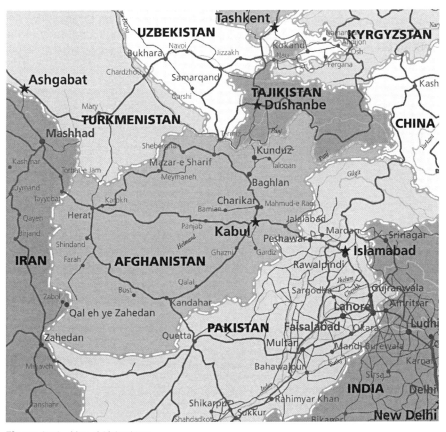

Figure 17.1 Map of Afghanistan

As in other global reports,[6] the most common cause of maternal death was haemorrhage (30%). However, obstructed labour was the second leading cause overall (23%) and the first in Ragh, Badakshan (Figure 17.2), suggesting that many women died undelivered and that obstetric fistula would be a likely outcome for those who survived.

Mortality statistics are the tip of the iceberg. The number of women suffering illness and disability associated with pregnancy and childbirth is far greater than the number who die.[7] Measuring morbidity may better assess programme impact but, with no internationally agreed definitions and the difficulty in identifying and classifying morbidity, few studies have attempted this. However, an assessment of obstetric fistula or severe hypotension leading to renal failure or brain damage would be very relevant in Afghanistan.

Despite the fact that the prevalence of obstetric fistula in Afghanistan is unknown, Cure International Hospital (CIH), with funding from Women's Hope International (www.whi.org) began a programme of repair for women with fistula. In 2 years, 78 women from all over the country have been operated on. More resources are needed to educate and inform the population about obstetric fistula and the fact that help is available.

Why obstructed labour should be the leading cause of maternal death in Badakhshan is an interesting question. Obvious answers include the remoteness of the area, the lack of access to health facilities and the fact that girls are often married before puberty. However these factors are present in other areas around the world where death due to obstructed labour is not so prevalent. A potential exacerbating factor in Badakhshan may be that of vitamin D deficiency and the effects of vitamin D myopathy and osteomalacia on the labour and delivery process. An interesting recent study in the USA found an inverse association between caesarean section and maternal serum

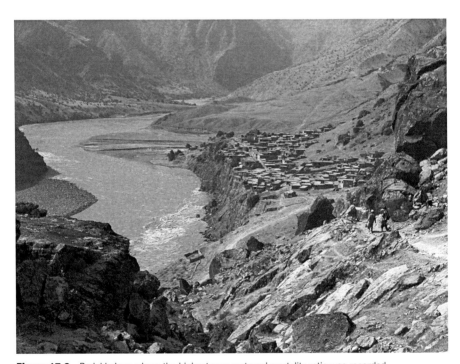

Figure 17.2 Badakhshan, where the highest ever maternal mortality ratio was recorded

vitamin D concentrations.[8] A pilot study, carried out in CIH in Kabul, found a high prevalence of vitamin D deficiency among newly delivered mothers. Only 2.8% of the study population had vitamin D levels within the 'normal' range.[9] In Badakhshan, I witnessed many women brought to the health clinics who were no longer able to walk owing to pain and weakness in their legs and many of the women we operated on with obstructed labour had signs and symptoms of osteomalacia. Further research in this field is certainly warranted.

Other reproductive and maternal health indicators

The World Health Organization (WHO) in 1996 selected 15 global indicators and two complementary indicators for monitoring reproductive health targets set at the International Conference on Population and Development (ICPD) in Cairo in 1994. Table 17.2 overleaf presents data for seven of these indicators for Afghanistan, together with estimates from other countries for comparison.

UNICEF, WHO and UNFPA also developed a series of process indicators to measure availability, use and quality of obstetric care by providing information on EOC coverage and performance (Table 17.3).[10] Analysis of these indicators has been used successfully in developing countries to identify problems with under-use of obstetric services and to stimulate national policy discussions leading to programme design, implementation and evaluation.[11]

Compared with 2002, when only 11 of Afghanistan's 32 provinces had the capacity to provide comprehensive EOC and only 17 of the country's 174 hospitals could perform caesarean sections,[12] there have been significant improvements. The province of Nuristan is now reportedly the only one without the availability of caesarean section.

Table 17.3 Essential Obstetric Care (EOC) process indicators and minimum acceptable level

Indicator	Minimum acceptable level
Number of EOC facilities per 500 000 people:	
Basic[a]	At least 4
Comprehensive[b]	At least 1
Geographic distribution	Minimum levels met in sub-national areas
Percentage of births in EOC facilities	At least 15% of all births in the population
Met need for EOC (percentage of women treated in EOC facilities)	All women with obstetric complications treated in EOC facilities (estimated at 15% of all births)
Caesarean section rate	Not less than 5% and not more than 15% as a proportion of all births in the population
Case fatality rate	Not more than 1%

[a] Basic EOC can:
  1. administer parenteral antibiotics
  2. administer parenteral oxytocic drugs
  3. administer parenteral anticonvulsants for pre-eclampsia and eclampsia
  4. perform manual removal of placenta
  5. perform removal of retained products (via manual vacuum aspiration)
  6. perform assisted vaginal delivery.

[b] Comprehensive EOC can provide all the basic services, i.e. 1–6 above, plus:
  1. perform surgery (i.e. caesarean section)
  2. perform blood transfusions.

Table 17.2 Reproductive health indicators; data for Afghanistan from the Ministry of Public Health[31]

Indicator	Existing Afghanistan data			Other country estimates		
	Source	Date	Afghanistan	More developed	Less developed	Least developed
1 Total fertility rate (per woman)	UNICEF[27]	2008	6.6	1.5–1.6	2.9–3.2	5.2
2 Contraceptive prevalence (percentage of women aged 15–49 years)	AHS[15]	2006	15.4%	75%	55%	<23%
3 Maternal mortality ratio (per 100 000 live births)	WHO[30]	2002	1600	21	440	1000
4 Antenatal care coverage (percentage of women attended)	AHS[15]	2006	32.3%	97%	65%	
5 Births attended by skilled health personnel (percentage of births attended)	AHS[15]	2006	18.9%	99%	54%	26–30%
6 Perinatal mortality ratio (per 1000 total births)	WHO[30]	2000	96	8–11	>30	
7 Low birth weight prevalence (percentage of live births)	WHO[30]	2000	20%	6%	18%	22%

Maternal and child health services

In 2002, only 17% of all health facilities could provide basic reproductive health services.[13] Only 25% of primary care facilities could provide all the basic mother and child services.[12] The availability and quality of maternal and child health services varied considerably between provinces, even in the same region. In Herat province, 11% of women accessed antenatal care and 12% used family planning services.[5] The situation appeared to be better in Kabul, where 79% of the women interviewed in a knowledge, attitudes and practices (KAP) survey had attended antenatal clinics in their last pregnancy and 23% were using a family planning method.[14]

The Afghanistan Health Survey (AHS)[15] has shown some improvement over the past 6 years in both access and utilisation of healthcare services by women in rural and urban areas (Figure 17.3): the contraceptive prevalence rate increased from 5.1% to 15.5%, skilled antenatal care contacts increased from 4.6% to 18.9% and skilled attendants at delivery increased from 6% to 18.9%.

Skilled attendance at delivery

Having a skilled attendant at delivery has been shown to reduce maternal mortality.[16] A 'skilled attendant' is defined by WHO as a trained midwife, nurse, nurse/midwife or doctor who has completed a set course of study and is registered or legally licensed. There is, however, another, slightly broader definition from WHO/UNFPA that defines skilled attendants as 'people with midwifery skills necessary to manage normal deliveries and diagnose, stabilise and refer obstetric complications'. Trained traditional birth attendants (TBAs) could fit into this definition.

In a review by Sibley *et al.*,[17] it was shown that training TBAs did not, in the absence of back-up from a functioning referral system or support from professionally

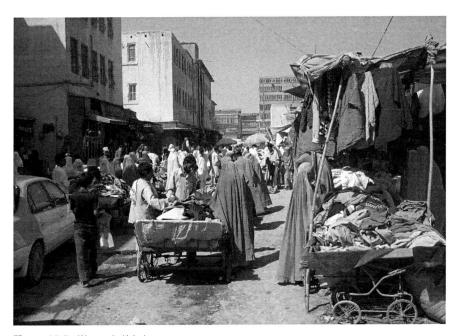

Figure 17.3 Women in Kabul

trained health workers, decrease women's risk of dying in childbirth: this has been used by some to argue that training TBAs is of no value. However, in Badakhshan, where obstructed labour is the number one killer, it could be argued that even well-trained midwives will be unable to make a significant impact on maternal mortality, as the main requirement in these cases is for a functioning referral system and access to caesarean section.

Another concern regarding training of TBAs is that it may be viewed as a cheaper alternative to training midwives or doctors. In 2003, there were only 3500 doctors in Afghanistan, with a doctor-to-nurse/midwife ratio of 1 : 1. There were 11 000 medical students in eight medical schools but only 2500 students in intermediate schools for nurses/midwives.[18] Since 2003, there has been a big drive to develop programmes to train midwives and nurses across the country. Despite these efforts, it will take many years to provide enough trained doctors and midwives to ensure attendance by them at all deliveries and, even as the numbers increase, the challenge of getting trained female healthcare workers out into the rural areas remains. The AHS[15] showed that TBAs conduct the majority of antenatal visits and are the main birth attendants in Afghanistan.

Access to and quality of maternal health services

In 2002, there were just 756 health facilities in the country (over 80% of which provided only basic primary health services). The population-to-health facility ratio was an average of 27 243 : 1. Now there are 1701 health facilities (25% of which can provide comprehensive primary health services).[15]

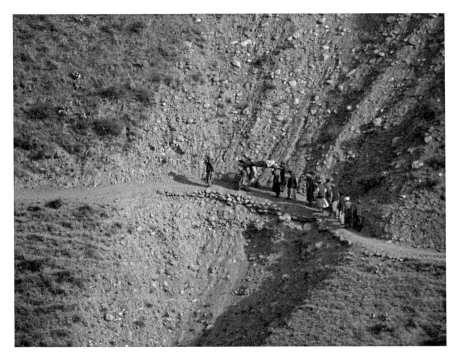

Figure 17.4 A woman in labour being carried by stretcher to the clinic

In rural Afghanistan, access is limited by geographical terrain: there are high mountains to overcome and rivers to cross. Winters are severe and summers harsh. Few roads are functional and there are significant security issues. Most travel outside Kabul is on foot or by donkey or horseback (Figure 17.4). Poverty is such that few families own any form of transport. There are still areas where next to nothing is known about the health situation except to say that, with no access in or out of the area, it must be very poor.

Lack of finance restricts access. In Afghanistan, the constitution requires healthcare provision by the government to be free of charge. In practice, there are costs involved in obtaining each and every service[19] and families may feel they cannot afford the costs of travel or of treatment. Projects that provide emergency loan funds or health insurance can increase access to health services and reduce maternal mortality.[20,21]

Poor-quality care, which includes substandard clinical care due to lack of knowledge or training, lack of drugs and supplies, delays in referral, and poor interaction between the women and the healthcare providers, prevents women and their families accessing health services.

Factors contributing to poor maternal health in Afghanistan

Conflict

Security remains a major issue and the lack of it prevents both UN agencies and non-governmental organisations (NGOs) from working in many parts of the country. The International Security Assistance Forces (ISAF) police Kabul and its immediate surroundings but, beyond that, local warlords and militia groups remain in control. Unexploded landmines remain a major problem within the country. There are estimated to be around 10 million landmines in Afghanistan, covering an area of 725 km^2.[22]

Although violence against women occurs during peacetime as well as during war, it tends to take a more extreme form during war. In Afghanistan, Amnesty International have said that 'a multitude of women have undergone war-related trauma',[23] that is, multiple rape, forced prostitution, slavery, and other forms of gender-related violence. Women suffer abuse through neglect during wars. Food and medical resources are taken from women and given to male soldiers, resulting in high levels of malnutrition and hunger-related diseases that affect the society for generations to come.[23]

The pressures of war and of brutal regimes such as the Taliban also result in mental health problems. In one study of 160 Afghan women during the Taliban regime, 42% reported symptoms that met diagnostic criteria for post-traumatic stress disorder, 97% demonstrated evidence of major depression and 86% had significant anxiety symptoms.[22]

Another important war-related problem that affects the healthcare system is that of emigration of educated people, including teachers and health professionals.

Politics, religion and culture

Each of politics, religion and culture has an effect on maternal health but they are often interrelated and difficult to separate. Politics has contributed to the poor health situation in that, until recently, health services were not the priority of the governing factions. Political cultures marked by corruption and inefficiency take their toll on maternal health.[23] Women and their families will use health facilities as a last resort if they know that they will have to pay bribes for each service required (Figure 17.5). Political will is crucial if health systems are to function effectively.

In relation to religion, it is argued that the teachings of Islam do not inherently affect women's rights but that those in power manipulate these teachings for their own ends.[24] Extreme Islamic fundamentalist views do little to protect women and children. On the contrary, the Taliban actively persecute women, ignoring their basic human rights.[3] Maternal mortality ratios remain high in cultures that undervalue women and allow men to control women's reproductive capacities, and where the practice of purdah (wife seclusion) restricts women's access to medical care.[25]

Cultural and religious beliefs can promote or discourage female education. Where female illiteracy is common, harmful cultural or religious beliefs and practices are more likely to occur.[1] Cultural views regarding gender roles are also relevant both to the provision of health care and its uptake. Of particular concern in Afghanistan is the lack of availability of female health workers in health facilities. During the rule of the Taliban, female children were prohibited from attending school and women were prohibited from working in public places. If then women are only permitted to seek health care from other women, women will inevitably suffer. The value of female health workers cannot be underestimated, but it is also important to remember that the underlying issue is one of trust. In the clinic in Ragh, there was initially only one male doctor who at first was permitted to see only male patients and children. During the year he lived and worked in the surrounding villages, he built up relationships of trust. When the wife of the village leader became sick, the village leader eventually permitted this doctor to see and examine her. Following her recovery, more women started to come to the clinic and by the time I came to join this Afghan doctor, he was seeing more women than men. The same has been true for a number of male doctors I have worked with in Afghanistan and this should not be forgotten.

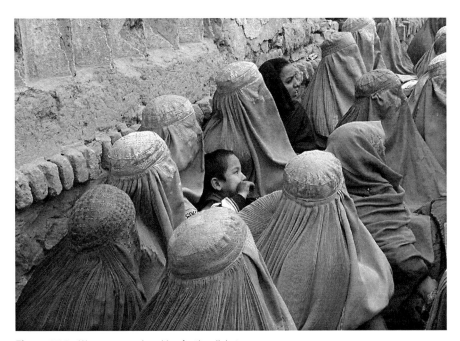

Figure 17.5 Women covered, waiting for the clinic to open

Since 2002 girls have been attending school and women have been allowed to go back to work but the extent to which they have done so has been less than hoped for. Many have been beaten, insulted or killed and take significant risks every day of their lives.

For women to use the health facilities in this culture, the majority still have to ask for permission from their husbands or fathers. This can lead to significant delay in seeking help when problems occur. Many women are still not free to leave their homes unless in the company of a male family member. In Ragh I met women who had never stepped out of their compound since the day they were married.

Education – general and medical

'If you think education is expensive, try illiteracy' – Nigerian saying

'There is, in our time, no well-educated literate population that is poor; there is no illiterate population that is other than poor' – JK Galbraith, 1994

Education, especially among girls, is an important factor in improving maternal health. It has been associated with several healthy outcomes and better care of the children.[16,26] World Bank experts judge it as 'the most influential investment', with high financial returns. It is possible, though, that it is not just the education *per se* that is important, but that the society places enough value on women to want to educate them.

Education for both boys and girls in Afghanistan has been limited over the past 20 years and for girls during the Taliban regime it was almost non-existent. The education of boys suffered as 70% of teachers were female. The literacy rates in the country are low, at 46–51% for males and 15–21% for females.[27] According to the AHS,[15] school attendance remains low, with only 28% of girls currently in school (Figure 17.6) and 49% of boys.

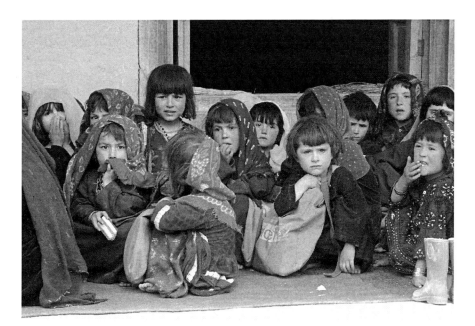

Figure 17.6 Girls outside school

The impact of lack of educational resources, both personnel and material, is felt not just in schools but also in colleges and universities. Medical students graduate with knowledge and experience levels far below standard and are then expected to function as independent 'general' practitioners. Patients are oftentimes harmed rather than helped by the medical profession and distrust between patient and doctor results in patients' 'shopping' around from doctor to doctor. There is an urgent need to channel medical graduates, many of whom sincerely want to help and care for their own people, into well-run postgraduate medical education programmes.

Cure International Hospital (Figure 17.7) developed a 3-year 'residency' programme for young doctors to specialise in family medicine. This has been a tremendously successful programme. For every trainee post, 100 applications are received. The programme was modelled on the US system and produces 'generalist' doctors of a far higher calibre than are otherwise available in Afghanistan. Emphasis is placed on maternal and child health and we ensure that each resident is able to safely perform caesarean section as well as being able to administer both spinal and general anaesthesia using ketamine. Alongside this residency programme, we developed a 1-year obstetrics and gynaecology Fellowship programme that focused on training national doctors already specialised according to current Ministry of Public Health criteria. During the 1-year programme, we modified and used RCOG material such as assessment and appraisal forms and log books in order to improve not only knowledge and skills but also attitudes. Emphasis was placed on mentoring, a method that appeared to pay dividends. In CIH we could control who was appointed and could hold our trainees accountable. Although this sounds obvious, it is not the case in government hospitals, where it is almost impossible to discipline anyone and where the disorder is such that no one takes any responsibility and no one is ever accountable when things go wrong. Graduates from both training programmes, in their graduation speeches, expressed in their own words what their training meant to them. An extract from the speech of one of the first graduates in the Fellowship programme is shown in Box 17.1. The challenges remain to convince the Ministry of Public Health and the Ministry of Higher Education of the value of these programmes and to continue to find resources not only to sustain but to expand them.

Government policies regarding maternal health and other agency involvement

The Ministry of Public Health is responsible for rebuilding health services in the country. In early 2002, it produced a national health policy document that listed reproductive health among the health sector priorities for saving and improving lives. Working in coordination with partner agencies (including the European Commission, UNICEF, USAID, the World Bank, WHO and others), the policy has

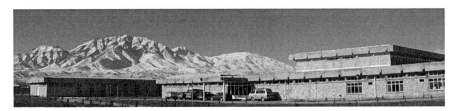

Figure 17.7 Cure International Hospital, Kabul

Box 17.1	Graduation speech, 31 January 2007

I am proud of being one of the fellow doctors graduating from Cure OBGYN fellowship programme. Being a trainee on this program gave me the true understanding of what is the standard level of medical care for a patient. It is obvious that the three decades of war has damaged our medicine badly. The war has pushed our medicine decades back and I am sad to say that our medicine is far away from standard levels. Three decades of war has made our smart brains to leave the country, destroyed our resources and cut our contact with the outside modern world. During the war, our medicine was trapped in a well and from the whole sky of knowledge it could only see the circle which was above it. It couldn't hear, see or feel the new discoveries. Cure OBGYN Fellowship programme is a model step to help Afghan medicine to get out of this well, to give it real prestige and to make it a part of new modern medicine.

been to develop the 'Basic Package of Health Services' (BPHS) and contract out the delivery of the BPHS to NGOs in performance-based partnership agreements (PPAs) where NGOs provide the services on behalf of, and monitored by, the Ministry, with payment dependent on the meeting of predetermined performance indicators.[18] The AHS[15] was carried out in 2006 to quantify the impact of this policy. The results were tentatively encouraging.

The situation in Afghanistan is far from settled. With corruption increasingly prevalent and widespread, it is not clear what the best course of action is: invest more funding into central government on top of the many hundreds of millions of dollars already donated as part of the international community's commitment to 'rebuild' the healthcare services, or reappraise the contribution made by international NGOs in various health sectors since the early part of this century and continue to fund them directly? My vote would be with the latter.

Conclusion

The present situation in Afghanistan with regard to maternal health remains awful. The country has one of the highest maternal mortality ratios in the world[1] and, despite the removal of the Taliban, women continue to daily experience violations of their human rights.[3,21] There is, however, relatively little published work on the maternal health situation in Afghanistan and many of the figures quoted are taken from reports written for donor agencies and governments and therefore not entirely without bias.

As has been said before, political will is crucial if maternal health is to be improved. It was encouraging that the Government of Afghanistan, in its National Health Policy document, made maternal health a priority, but words are meaningless unless translated into action. From our own experience in the country, three areas that are worth focusing on are:

1. **Postgraduate medical training programmes, particularly in family medicine and in obstetrics and gynaecology:** Training doctors is essential. Increasing not just the number but the quality has to be a priority in order to save mothers' lives. Nurse/midwifery programmes are currently being run throughout the country but, in the rural areas, where most deaths occur, the healthcare workers are generally young male doctors who have graduated from a deficient medical school training programme and have practically no knowledge or experience of women's health issues. The Government has recently recognised family medicine as a specialisation but so far the training programme

is only being run at CIH. This programme needs to be expanded so that more doctors can be trained and deployed throughout the country. Doctors trained as family medicine practitioners are able to provide comprehensive EOC. They can perform caesarean section, administer anaesthesia, resuscitate the newborn and manage a wide range of medical and surgical problems, while knowing when to refer onwards. It is far more cost-effective, not to mention realistic, to place two family medicine practitioners in a rural hospital than to try to find an internist, a surgeon, a paediatrician and an obstetrician for the same hospital. There is a need also for further training for obstetricians and gynaecologists, already specialised according to Ministry of Public Health criteria. The Government needs to improve its system whereby professional qualifications and training are regulated (such as through continuing medical education) andx workers should be better supervised. At present, there is a great deal of corruption and nepotism within the healthcare system, thus disheartening and demotivating those who genuinely want to bring improvement and accountability. Better-trained and better-qualified specialists in the provincial hospitals can more effectively manage the complications referred to them as well as being able to function as teachers and pass on their skills to junior trainees and family medicine residents.

2. **Research:** As discussed previously, morbidity is not easy to define or measure, but a study looking at chronic obstetric morbidity, especially obstetric fistula, would be valuable in this country, where prevalence is expected to be high. The information obtained from such a study could help to stimulate national policy discussions, leading to changes in programme design, implementation and evaluation of obstetric services and practice. The possible link between vitamin D deficiency and obstructed labour is also interesting and should be investigated further as it may be that preventing vitamin D deficiency through supplementation could reduce the prevalence of obstructed labour and that of obstetric fistula.

3. **EOC facilities:** There is no doubt that EOC facilities should be established in geographically strategic areas and more work needs to be done to ensure supplies of drugs, equipment and personnel, especially female personnel. As an example, at LAMB hospital (a rural hospital) in Bangladesh, a primary school was established and free education offered to the children of the hospital workers to attract staff away from the cities. Better salaries may also have to be offered to recruit health workers to remote areas.

Projects that focus on reducing maternal mortality can indeed be successful, as shown by a large number of studies from around the world.[16] The focus has to be on providing good-quality EOC facilities with skilled personnel attending births and with a good referral system in place. There are organisations in Afghanistan working on these very issues but so much more needs to be done.

References

1. Bartlett LA, Mawji S, Whitehead S, Crouse C, Dalil S, Ionete D, *et al*; Afghan Maternal Mortality Study Team. Where giving birth is a forecast of death: maternal mortality in four districts of Afghanistan, 1999–2002. *Lancet* 2005;365:864–70. Erratum in: *Lancet* 2005;365:2006.
2. Hill JC. Dying to give birth: obstructed labour in the Hindu Kush. *Obstet Gynaecol* 2005;7:267–70.
3. Palmer C. The Taliban's war on women. *Lancet* 1998;352:734.

4. General Directorate of Health Care and Promotion, Women's and Reproductive Health Directorate, Reproductive Health Task Force. *National Reproductive Health Strategy for Afghanistan.* Kabul: Ministry of Health; 2003.

5. Amowitz LL, Reis CJ, Iacopino V. Maternal mortality in Herat Province, Afghanistan, in 2002: an indicator of women's human rights. *JAMA* 2002;288:1284–91.

6. Family Care International. *The Safe Motherhood Action Agenda: Priorities for the Next Decade – Report on the Safe Motherhood Technical Consultation. 18–23 October 1997, Colombo, Sri Lanka.* New York; Family Care International in Collaboration with the Inter-Agency Group for Safe Motherhood; 1998.

7. Mantel GD, Eckhart B, Rees H, Pattinson RC. Severe acute maternal morbidity: a pilot study of a definition for a near-miss. *BJOG* 1998;105:985–90.

8. Merewood A, Mehta SD, Chen TC, Bauchner H, Holick MF. Association between vitamin D deficiency and primary cesarean section. *J Clin Endocrin Metab* 2009;94:940–5.

9. Hill JC, Holman MJ, Reading I, Boucher B. Ionised calcium and vitamin D status in mothers and their newborn in Kabul, Afghanistan: a pilot study. *BJOG* 2008;115(Suppl 1):249–50.

10. UNICEF/WHO/UNFPA. *Guidelines for Monitoring the Availability and Use of Obstetric Services.* New York: UNICEF; 1997.

11. Pathak LR, Kwast BE, Malla DS, Pradhan AS, Rajlawat R, Campbell BB. Process indicators for safe motherhood programmes: their application and implications as derived from hospital data in Nepal. *Trop Med Int Health* 2000;5:882–90.

12. MSH/HANDS. *Afghanistan National Health Resources Assessment: Preliminary Results.* MSH, HANDS and MSH/Europe; 2002.

13. Central Statistics Office, Afghanistan Transitional Authority. *Afghanistan Multiple Indicator Cluster Survey 2003: Moving Beyond 2 Decades of War: Progress of Provinces.* Central Statistics Office and UNICEF; 2004 [www.childinfo.org/files/AfghanistanMICS2003.pdf].

14. IbnSina/ICRH. *KAP Survey Regarding Reproductive Health.* Kabul; 2002 [www.icrh.org/files/KAPsurveyKabulICRHIbnSina.pdf].

15. Ministry of Public Health. *Estimates of Priority Health Indicators.* The Afghanistan Health Survey. Ministry of Public Health; 2006.

16. POLICY Project. *What Works: a Policy and Programme Guide to the Evidence on Family Planning, Safe Motherhood and STI/HIV/AIDS Interventions.* Module 1: Safe Motherhood. Washington, DC: Futures Group; 2003 [www.policyproject.com/pubs/generalreport/SM_WhatWorksps2.pdf].

17. Sibley LM, Sipe TA, Brown CM, Diallo MM, McNatt K, Habarta N. Traditional birth attendant training for improving health behaviours and pregnancy outcomes. *Cochrane Database Syst Rev* 2007;(3):CD005460.

18. Cook J, Reeve G. *Reconstruction of the Health System in Afghanistan – Capacity Building in Primary Care and Public Health.* Report on the workshop at the London School of Hygiene & Tropical Medicine, April 2003 [www.medact.org/content/wmd_and_conflict/ACF5B94.doc].

19. Nahar S, Costello A. The hidden cost of free maternity care in Dhaka, Bangladesh. *Health Policy Plan* 1998;13:417–22.

20. Maine D. Lessons for programme design from the PMM projects. *Int J Gynaecol Obstet* 1997;59;S259–65.

21. Celik Y, Hotchkiss D. The socio-economic determinants of maternal health care utilisation in Turkey. *Soc Sci Med* 2000;50:1797–806.

22. Rasekh D, Bauer HM, Manos MM, Iacopino V. Women's health and human rights in Afghanistan. *JAMA* 1998;280:449–55.

23. Wali S, Gould E, Fitzgerald P. The impact of political conflict on women: the case of Afghanistan. *Am J Pub Health* 1999;89:1474–6.

24. Obermeyer CM. Reproductive choice in Islam: gender and state in Iran and Tunisia. *Stud Fam Plann* 1994;25:41–51.

25. Wall LL, Dead mothers and injured wives: the social context of maternal morbidity and mortality among the Hausa of northern Nigeria. *Stud Fam Plann* 1998;29:341–59.

26. Harrison KA. The importance of the educated healthy woman in Africa. *Lancet* 1997;349:644–7.

27. UNICEF. The State of the World's Children [www.unicef.org/rightsite/sowc/].

28. United Nations Development Programme. *Human Development Report 2009* [hdrstats.undp.org/en/countries/data_sheets/cty_ds_AFG.html].

29. Central Intelligence Agency. *The World Factbook 2009.* Washington, DC: CIA; 2009.

30. World Health Organization Department of Measurement and Health Information Systems (MHI). *Evidence and Information for Policy (EIP). WHO Under-five Mortality. Unpublished Country Estimates Computed for the World Health Report 2005.* Geneva: World Health Organization; 2004.

31. Ministry of Public Health. *Afghanistan Health Indicators, Fact Sheet - August 2008* [www.moph.gov.af/en/reports/Afg-Health-Indicators-Factsheet-August2008.pdf].

Chapter 18
Challenges faced in Zimbabwe

Stephen Munjanja

Introduction

Zimbabwe faces enormous challenges in meeting the Millennium Development Goals (MDGs) 4 and 5. Some of the problems the country faces are similar to those affecting other sub-Saharan African countries but others are unique to Zimbabwe. There was a relatively stable environment for about 15 years after the country gained its independence from Britain in 1980. However, the past 10 years have been characterised by political instability and a rapidly deteriorating socio-economic environment. This has severely affected the health of women and children, who are the first to suffer under such circumstances. In this chapter, the challenges Zimbabwe has faced in the past three decades, and attempts to overcome them, will be described.

Profile of MDG indicators in Zimbabwe

The indicators for the MDGs show very slow progress or worsening since 1990 (Table 18.1).[1] There has been a decrease in the gross national income (GNI) per capita from US$810 in 1990 to US$360 in 2005. The goal to eradicate extreme poverty and hunger is not on track and there is an increasing prevalence of malnutrition in children under 5 years. There has either been no change or there has been a worsening in the following indicators since 1990: primary school completion rate, births attended to by skilled attendants, condom use among females aged 15–24 years, incidence of tuberculosis, and life expectancy.

Maternal mortality

The maternal mortality ratio (MMR) for Zimbabwe in 1990 is not known. Although there have been six national estimates reported since 1987, three from Demographic and Health Surveys[2–4] and three from the World Health Organization (WHO),[5–7] their imprecision precludes the monitoring required by the MDGs. Other estimates from Zimbabwe were facility based and cannot be used to establish trends.

Population–based estimates in an urban area (Harare) were first done in 1983, when the MMR was found to be 56 per 100000 live births.[8] In 1987, it was similar at 53 per 100000 live births,[9] but by 1990 it had risen to 85 per 100000.[10] This was then followed by a rapid increase in the MMR to 224 per 100000 live births by 1997.[11] These urban reports, which were done using the same methodology and on the same

Table 18.1   Millennium Development Goal indicators for Zimbabwe; data from the World Bank[1]

Goal	1990	1995	2000	2005	2008
Goal 1: Eradicate extreme poverty and hunger					
Malnutrition prevalence, weight for age (percentage of children under 5 years)	8.0%	11.7%	11.5%	14.0%	14.0%
Goal 2: Achieve universal primary education					
Primary completion rate, total (percentage of relevant age group)	93%	96%	89%	81%	–
Goal 3: Promote gender equality and empower women					
Proportion of seats held by women in national parliaments	11%	15%	14%	17%	15%
Ratio of female to male primary enrolment	99%	97%	97%	99%	99%
Goal 4: Reduce child mortality					
Measles immunisation (percentage of children aged 12–23 months)	87%	87%	75%	66%	66%
Infant mortality rate (per 1000 live births)	62	77	77	65	59
Under-five mortality rate (per 1000)	95	122	122	101	90
Goal 5: Improve maternal health					
Adolescent fertility rate (births per 1000 women aged 15–19 years)	–	106	88	69	65
Births attended by skilled health staff (percentage of total)	70%	69%	73%	69%	69%
Contraceptive prevalence (percentage of women aged 15–49 years)	43%	48%	54%	60%	60%
Proportion of pregnant women receiving prenatal care	91%	93%	93%	94%	94%
Goal 6: Combat HIV/AIDS, malaria and other diseases					
Condom use, female (percentage of females aged 15–24 years)	–	12%	11%	9%	9%
Condom use, male (percentage of males aged 15–24 years)	–	48%	56%	52%	52%
Incidence of tuberculosis (per 100 000 people)	329	474	685	824	782
Prevalence of HIV, total (percentage of population aged 15–49 years)	14.2%	27.3%	27.3%	19.0%	15.3%
Other					
Fertility rate, total (births per woman)	5.1	4.3	3.9	3.6	3.5
Gross national income per capita, Atlas method (current US$)	US$810	US$600	US$460	US$360	–
Life expectancy at birth, total	60 years	52 years	44 years	43 years	45 years
Population, total (millions)	10.5	11.7	12.5	12.5	12.5

population, clearly show an increase in maternal mortality in Harare between 1987 and 1997. Part of the increase was attributed to indirect deaths from complications of HIV/AIDS such as meningitis, tuberculosis and pneumonia, but there had also been a decline in the quality of care.[11] There were no periodic reports from any rural areas of Zimbabwe, so a similar analysis is not possible. There has been only one population–based report from a rural area of Zimbabwe and the MMR was 168 per 100 000 live births in 1990.[10] However, it is reasonable to infer that the same trend of an increase in MMR detected in urban Harare was also occurring in the rural areas.

The first population-based national study of maternal mortality levels was done in 2007.[12] This reported an MMR of 725 per 100 000 live births (95% CI 648–810). The settings and methodology of the previous studies were not comparable to the latest one, so it cannot be assumed that the MMR has risen further since 1997, although this is quite likely. What is clear, however, is that it will not be possible in 2015 to establish whether the MDG 5 target has been reached or not since a precise estimate for 1990 does not exist and the first population-based national study was only conducted in 2007.

The leading causes of maternal mortality in 2007 were HIV/AIDS (26%), postpartum haemorrhage (14%), eclampsia/hypertensive disorders (13%), puerperal sepsis (8%), abortion complications (6%), malaria (6%) and obstructed labour (3%). Postpartum haemorrhage, eclampsia/hypertensive disorders, obstructed labour and malaria are still causing the same proportions of deaths that they did in 1990,[10] showing that the health system has made no progress in addressing these problems (Table 18.2). HIV/AIDS is now the leading cause of maternal death, and this is due to the large number of women who fall pregnant without knowing their HIV status, the low rate of testing in pregnancy and the small proportion of HIV-positive women who receive effective anti-retroviral (ARV) drugs during pregnancy.[12] HIV/AIDS also contributes indirectly to the deaths due to malaria by making women more susceptible to the infection.[13] As a result, despite widespread availability of prophylaxis, malaria still contributes significantly to maternal mortality in Zimbabwe.

The other MDG indicators related to maternal health show a mixed picture (Table 18.1). Adolescent fertility has fallen since 1995 by more than one-third and contraceptive prevalence has increased but there has been little change in the percentage of women receiving antenatal care or being attended to by skilled attendants at delivery. The national caesarean section rate, which was 4.8% in 2005–6[4] had fallen in a period of less than 2 years to 4.4% in 2007.[12]

Table 18.2   Causes of maternal deaths in Zimbabwe; data for 1990 from Mbizvo et al.[10] and for 2007 from Ministry of Health and Child Welfare[12]

Cause	Proportion of maternal deaths	
	1990	2007
Haemorrhage	18%	19%
Abortion complications	17%	6%
Puerperal sepsis	13%	8%
Hypertension/eclampsia	12%	13%
Obstructed labour	3%	3%
HIV/AIDS	5%	26%
Malaria	5%	6%
Unknown	9%	10%

Perinatal mortality

It is widely accepted that to achieve MDG 4, which is a reduction by two-thirds in child mortality, major efforts need to be made to reduce newborn mortality.[14] At the international level, the number and causes of newborn deaths are now known[15] but, at country level, the information is frequently lacking. This lack of information is worse for perinatal mortality, as stillbirths are more difficult to identify in settings where a large proportion of women deliver at home.

In Zimbabwe, there have been no population-based perinatal data until recently. The published reports have been from isolated urban and rural districts. Urban population-based perinatal audits were conducted in Harare and Bulawayo in the 1980s and 1990s. These reported a perinatal mortality rate (PNMR) of 39 per 1000 births for Harare in 1983[16] and 36 oer 1000 births in Bulawayo in 1991.[17] A study to determine various PNMRs for the period 1980–89 in Harare showed that all rates fell at the beginning of the 1980s: neonatal mortality rate (NNMR) from 17 to 15 (1980–85), PNMR from 40 to 35 (1980–85) and fetal death rate from 21 to 20 (1983–85). Between 1986 and 89, however, all rates increased: NNMR from 19 to 23, PNMR from 41 to 47 and fetal death rate from 24 to 26.[18] The reasons proposed for the increases from 1986 included demographic changes in mothers, the rising prevalence of HIV and deterioration in the quality of care. Maternal HIV infection has now been shown to be associated with a higher risk of perinatal mortality,[19,20] and this is worse in settings where it coexists with malaria.[13,21,22]

In rural areas of Zimbabwe, there have been very few population-based estimates of the PNMR. In Gutu, a district with a population of 200 000, the PNMR was 23 per 1000 births in 1992–93.[23] By 1998, it had risen to 28 per 1000 births.[24]

In 2007, a population-based national study was conducted and this reported a PNMR of 29 per 1000 births (95% CI 27.3–30.4).[12] The main causes of death were preterm birth (33.6%), intrapartum birth asphyxia and birth trauma (26%), unexplained intrauterine death (17.4%), multiple pregnancy (4.6%), maternal hypertension (3.6%) and infection (3.3%). Syphilis infection was no longer a significant cause of perinatal mortality because the prevalence in pregnant women has declined from levels of 11% in Bulawayo in 1992[17] and 4.8% in Harare in 2005[25] to 1% in both cities currently.[12] At the national level, 0.3% of women received treatment for syphilis and there was only one death from congenital syphilis out of 1296 perinatal deaths.

Child mortality

Infant and under-five mortality rose during the 1990s but has been declining since. This is illustrated in Figure 18.1, which shows data from Demographic and Health Surveys done in 1988, 1994, 1999 and 2005–06.[2–4,26] The same trend is shown in Table 18.1, with data from the World Bank. This table also shows that a simple but important service delivery intervention, immunisation of measles, is being conducted very poorly. The indicators for child mortality are back to the same level they were in 1990, having initially risen. There is no prospect of MDG 4 targets being achieved by 2015.

The increase in child mortality was due to a variety of factors. The failure to eradicate poverty and hunger has exposed more children to malnutrition. The decrease in GNI per capita from US$810 to US$360 means that the whole population is surviving on less than a dollar a day, a situation of extreme poverty. Maternal and infant malnutrition is inevitable under these circumstances and 14% of children were underweight for age in 2008.[1] A significant proportion of the population is surviving on food relief from international donors.

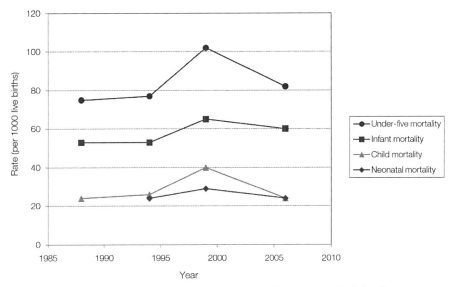

Figure 18.1 Trends in early childhood mortality in Zimbabwe from 1988 to 2006; data from Zimbabwe Demographic and Health Surveys 1988, 1994, 1999 and 2006[2–4.26]

The HIV/AIDS epidemic, which has had its epicentre in southern Africa for a decade, has had a huge impact in increasing childhood morbidity and mortality. Mother-to-child transmission (MTCT) of the virus has resulted in a large number of infants dying in childhood because of the lack of capacity within the health system to deal with the huge problem. The rate of transmission of the virus through this route was found to be as high as 31.9% in one study in Zimbabwe, in the absence of prevention of mother-to-child transmission (PMTCT) interventions.[27] Between 1980 and 2005, of approximately 10 million children born in Zimbabwe, a cumulative 504 000 (range 362 000–665 000) were vertically infected with HIV. MTCT of HIV decreased from 8.2% (range 6.0–10.7%) in 2000 to 6.2% (range 4.9–8.9%) in 2005. The decline in MTCT during 2000–2005 was attributed more to the concurrent decrease in HIV prevalence in pregnant women than to the PMTCT interventions because the levels of coverage (50%) and acceptance (42%) remain low.[28]

A range of interventions are available to reduce the risk of MTCT of HIV, including:

- testing of all women for HIV status before pregnancy
- reducing unwanted pregnancies among HIV-positive women
- testing of couples during pregnancy
- ARV drugs for HIV-positive pregnant women and newborns
- safe intrapartum practices
- optimal feeding practices.

Zimbabwe has opted for exclusive breastfeeding as a policy because of the evidence that this improves infant outcomes for both HIV-exposed and non-exposed infants,[29,30] and also because of the limited availability of alternative feeding options. All the above interventions are part of the PMTCT programme for Zimbabwe but the national maternal mortality study showed that only 34% of pregnant women were being offered the test. The percentage of women known to be HIV positive in pregnancy was 5.4%, instead of 17.5% as was expected from the latest survey.[4] The number of women who took ARVs was 1.8%.[12] The number of HIV-positive women detected was therefore only one-third and those prescribed ARV drugs one-tenth of the expected number. This indicates how much work needs to be done to meet the challenge of MTCT of HIV.

HIV/AIDS

The changes that have occurred in the prevalence of HIV infection in Zimbabwe since 1981 are shown in Figure 18.2. The data show that the prevalence increased in men and women aged 15–49 years from 0.85% in 1981 to a peak of 29.3% in 1997 before falling to 13.7% in 2009. An estimated 1 320 739 Zimbabweans were living with HIV and AIDS at the end of 2007. The decline from 1997 is thought to be due to an increase in adult mortality in the early 1990s and a decline in HIV incidence in the mid-1990s. Survey data also showed that there was an improvement in the adoption of protective behavioural measures, especially in decreasing the number of sexual partners and increasing condom use.[31]

While the decline is encouraging, it is only partly due to interventions within the health system. One in seven Zimbabweans is infected with the virus so the effect on maternal and newborn health will be felt for a long time. Reducing the maternal and perinatal mortality from HIV/AIDS is more complicated since this requires an array of interventions throughout the life cycle from the fetal stage of an individual to the end of his/her reproductive life. Effective ARV drug treatment will also increase the number of HIV-positive women who fall pregnant with wanted or unwanted pregnancies, meaning that the interventions that are put in place have to be sustained over a long period.

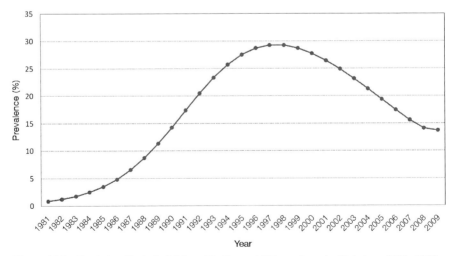

Figure 18.2 Trends in estimated adult (age 15–49 years) HIV prevalence in Zimbabwe, 1981–2009; data from Ministry of Health and Child Welfare[31]

Main challenges faced in Zimbabwe

Political

The political challenges that Zimbabwe faces are well known. At one level are the problems of credibility that the current government faces domestically and internationally. These have an impact on the next level, which is that of creating a vision for maternal and newborn health for the country, and translating political will into action. The administration is sapped by the political problems of trying to stay in power and has no time or energy to devote to the important issues in health.

Officially, the government is committed to the goals of the declarations and conventions that it has signed. After signing up to the programme of action at the International Conference on Population and Development in Cairo in 1994,[32] the Ministry of Health and Child Welfare developed guidelines that recognised the sexual and reproductive health rights (SRHR) agreed to in Cairo.[33] However, there has been little real advocacy for SRHR and policy changes that were needed to implement the guidelines did not occur. At other times, there was even resistance to change. The attempts by health professionals to make termination of pregnancy more easily available legally were stopped at the political level and have not yet succeeded. The intolerant speeches that some leaders make about homosexuality show that, at the political level, SRHR have not been accepted as a package.

The same failures of political commitment have occurred with the actions that followed Zimbabwe's signing of the Millennium Declaration.[34] The agricultural policies that have been implemented have severely reduced food production, increasing poverty and hunger. The governance problems in Zimbabwe make it difficult to create a national vision for the MDGs.

In 2001, the African Union recommended that member countries should allocate at least 15% of government expenditure to health.[35] The health budget has never reached 15% of expenditure and has ranged between 8% and 12% since Zimbabwe signed the declaration.[1,36]

Policy-level challenges

The challenges at the policy level occur at formulation, dissemination and implementation. The process of policy formulation within the Ministry of Health and Child Welfare is not clear and there is often little technical consultation. Local experts are sometimes ignored in preference to international consultants. The background data required to develop policies is often inaccessible, which results in policies based on inadequate information.

The final policy documents are rarely widely disseminated to the public or to health workers. The Ministry does not have a library or website of policy documents that can be accessed or referenced. Sometimes there are two opposing policies on one issue in the public domain at the same time. The 'user fee' issue is a case in point. The Ministry says publicly that maternal and newborn care is free up to district level in rural areas. However, all rural district hospitals charge pregnant women 'user fees' at the point of service delivery because they are required by their local authorities to recover costs. The confusion caused by these two policies has reduced access to women with complications and has doubtless led to many maternal and newborn deaths.

Another issue which has not been articulated well is the policy on feeding options for PMTCT. The official policy is that all women should practise exclusive breastfeeding to reduce the risk of HIV transmission, but it is not mentioned that this is because it carries a lesser risk than mixed breastfeeding. The result is that many women think that exclusive breastfeeding prevents MTCT and are not aware that it actually does carry a risk of transmission. Other women stop exclusive breastfeeding early to avoid transmission even though it is the incorrect thing to do.[37]

The implementation of policies is not monitored and evaluated. A policy can only become effective if it is backed up by budgetary allocation. Within the health budget, maternal and newborn health is not prioritised, in the face of major problems such as HIV/AIDS, tuberculosis, malaria and childhood diseases.

There is no laid-down process to review policies regularly or in the light of new evidence. Policies can even be changed without good reason or evidence of the need to do so. For example, the training of clinical officers (non-physicians) was stopped in the 1990s without collecting information about their contribution to the management of obstetric emergencies at rural district hospitals. The Ministry was forced to resume that training in 2007 because doctors were not accepting deployment to district hospitals, which were functioning very poorly as a result.

Challenges at the health–system level

The three major challenges at health-system level are the shortage of resources, the skills shortage and HIV/AIDS.

The financial resources available to Government were affected by the reduced income from taxation as a result of the economic deterioration and there has been little assistance from the international community owing to political problems. The allocation for health per capita in 2009 was US$7, which is far below the US$60 that WHO has recommended for health systems in developing countries.[38] The underfunding led to a policy of cost recovery and 'user fees' were introduced. The fees are demanded at the point of service delivery at district and tertiary hospitals, the only institutions that manage complications. Furthermore, women are asked to pay more for the treatment of complications. The result is that the very women who need emergency care are denied access, and this barrier has contributed to the high MMR of the country. In some cases, the fee demands have been made so vigorously that women are 'detained' in hospital after delivery until they have paid. Apart from the differences in fees between complicated and uncomplicated pregnancies, local authorities, church-related institutions and private hospitals are also allowed to charge their own fees, resulting in a complete 'free for all'. The national maternal mortality study has highlighted the barrier of 'user fees' and has recommended a review of the policy.[12] There are lessons from reviews and the experiences of other countries that Zimbabwe can draw upon.[39–42]

The second major challenge that the health system faces is the shortage of skills caused by the emigration of health workers and the reduction in the capacity of training institutions due to loss of staff. Although doctors continue to be trained in the same numbers as before, midwifery, nurse anaesthesia and clinical officer training have been severely affected by the loss of tutors. Retention of health workers in the system is very poor owing to bad conditions of service. In 2007, doctors earned the equivalent of US$36 per month and midwives US$18. The transport to get to work costs more than the salaries. Health workers subsidised the service less if they stayed at home, and in 2008 many did, which forced the closure of most of the tertiary hospitals in the country for 3 months. This was the lowest point in the deterioration of the health service. Women in labour arrived at the doors of maternity units to find them locked because there had been no public warning. Those who failed to deliver at home had to travel up to 100 km away to rural faith-based hospitals that continued to offer a service throughout the crisis. Many must have died during this time but there has been no documentation of the numbers.

Emigration of health workers has contributed the most to the loss of skilled attendants. In the early 1990s, Zimbabwe had 6000 trained midwives but only 1500 were left in the country by the end of 2009. Similarly, of an estimated 18 000 nurses, many of whom carried out midwifery functions, only 11 000 are still in the service. A survey of Comprehensive Emergency Obstetric Care (CEOC) carried out in 2007–8 found out that only 35% of midwifery posts and 30% of medical officer posts were filled in district hospitals. Only 26% of district hospitals met the criteria for providing CEOC.[12] With emigration, the most highly skilled workers leave first, leaving the service short of trainers and this worsens the skills shortage. The fewer health workers who are left are also less well trained.

The third major challenge for the health system is HIV/AIDS, which is like an elephant in the room. The pandemic has caused major distortions in resource allocation and for many years maternal and newborn health 'fell off the radar'. Despite the availability of substantial amounts of money for HIV/AIDS programmes in Zimbabwe, there has been little benefit for mothers and children, as shown by the indicators mentioned above. A lot of the money has been disbursed to non-governmental organisations (NGOs), which are seen as being transparent with its use. The problem is that the NGOs run vertical programmes in selected sites, with little potential for scale-up. Failure to prioritise women's health in HIV/AIDS programmes has led to the limited success of PMTCT.

HIV/AIDS has also contributed to the skills flight. There is a very high risk of occupational exposure in obstetric and neonatal care and health facilities do not always have post-exposure prophylaxis available. There have been documented cases of health workers acquiring the infection from accidents at work and this has contributed to the emigration to countries with a lower prevalence of HIV. Health workers have also acquired the virus sexually and thousands have died from AIDS.

Apart from the three major challenges mentioned above there is also the lack of reliable information within the health system about the magnitudes of the various problems, the inputs into programmes and the process or impact outcomes. This is due to two problems. Firstly, the information may not exist because no monitoring or evaluation has been put in place. Secondly, the information may exist but not be published, usually owing to lack of appreciation of the need for dissemination, but occasionally owing to deliberate suppression.

Challenges at the population level

The mass emigration of skilled people has inevitably led to demographic changes at the population level. Zimbabwe has lost two and a half million people, most of them highly educated and skilled. Those remaining have been disempowered by the socio-economic changes and by the political atmosphere of intimidation and violence. There is less demand for good-quality services and for accountability. The health service is the source of many reports of impunity: care denied without explanation, arrogant behaviour by administrators, rudeness of health workers, etc. The root cause, as with the problem at the larger political stage, is the loss of the 'middle class'.

Meeting some of the challenges

Prioritising maternal and newborn health

Among certain stakeholders and partners there was already acknowledgement that maternal and newborn health was not getting enough attention, but there was no information on the true magnitude. The Ministry of Health and Child Welfare proposed a study to estimate the MMR and this was conducted by a team from the University of Zimbabwe.[12] The UK Department for International Development (DFID) funded the study. The study has led to raised awareness of the extent of the problems and it is being used in many forums for advocacy. The report will be used to sensitise ministers of government responsible for youth, education and gender affairs about maternal and newborn health and a meeting with parliamentarians with the same aim has been scheduled for the first half of 2010.

Dissemination of the 'road map' for maternal and newborn health

At the same time that the study was being conducted, the Ministry produced a programme document for maternal and newborn health entitled *Zimbabwe Maternal and Neonatal Health Roadmap*.[43] This document sets out a framework for the maternal and newborn health programme, and, importantly, emphasises monitoring and evaluation. The document had never been properly disseminated but the national process started in November 2009. Provincial workshops are planned for 2010 so that, by the end of the year, all the 62 districts will have been covered.

Implementation of the recommendations of the maternal and perinatal mortality study

Five key recommendations are already being acted upon: increasing skilled attendance by greater use of maternity waiting homes (MWHs), training health workers in life-saving skills, expanding the training of clinical officers and nurse anaesthetists, a review of the 'user fee' policy, and scaling-up of facility-based audit nationally.

Zimbabwe's rural hospitals have always used MWHs to house primigravidae and women with complications, but this has never been recommended for all rural women. Observational studies have already demonstrated some benefits[44,45] and, because Zimbabwe has the potential to admit all rural women to await delivery, a randomised controlled trial is being planned on MWHs. If their use is linked to the availability of a cheaper form of transport, it opens up the possibility of eliminating the first and second delays. A pilot of the use of such a cheaper form of transport, the motorbike ambulance, also funded by DFID, has started.

The training of health workers in Life Saving Skills, using a course developed by the International Office of the Royal College of Obstetricians and Gynaecologists (RCOG) in conjunction with the Liverpool School of Tropical Medicine started in 2008 and 165 senior midwives and district medical officers have gone through the course. A two-pronged strategy has now been adopted: in-service training for those already working in facilities, and imparting the skills to those still undergoing professional training.

The training of mid-level cadres will be stepped up as a result of the inadequacies noted at district hospitals, especially in rural areas. Nurse anaesthetists have always provided more than 80% of the service for obstetric complications but their training and supervision had become compromised by lack of funds and tutors. Clinical officers have resumed training after a gap of more than 15 years. Both courses need strengthening, and the conditions of service of these cadres need improvement. Discussions with stakeholders have started to improve the resources for their training.

Lastly, there is an initiative to expand maternal and perinatal audit, which has been recommended internationally as a way of improving quality of care.[46] Facility-based audit is already done in certain districts and provinces but there is no national coordination.[47] Facility-based audit misses the deaths in the community (49% in Zimbabwe[12]), so the report[12] recommended district-based audit. However, finding deaths at home and conducting verbal autopsies on all of them would be difficult with the available resources, and thus good facility-based audit should be the aim initially. Maternal and perinatal audit has resumed in several tertiary hospitals and a seminar is planned to create a national committee.

All these initiatives require funding; some of it will be found internally but a significant amount will have to come from elsewhere. For the sake of women and children, the government needs to arrange a political dispensation that allows potential partners to assist Zimbabwe.

Summary

Zimbabwe will not reach the MDGs for child and maternal health. The indicators for child health worsened in the late 1990s and are now improving but not rapidly enough to reach the target in 2015. The indicators for maternal health are still deteriorating. There have been challenges at the political, policy-making and health-system levels. The HIV/AIDS pandemic caused a diversion of resources that reduced maternal and newborn health to a lesser priority. The disempowerment at population level has reduced the demand for good-quality care.

The health system is experiencing a slow recovery in which maternal and newborn health is being prioritised, partly as a result of a recent national maternal and perinatal mortality study. Some recommendations from the study are being implemented, although their sustainability depends on funding being available. Ultimately, this will depend on whether a new political dispensation occurs.

Acknowledgements

Many thanks to the UK Department for International Development who were the main funders of the Zimbabwe Maternal and Perinatal Mortality Study that is referred to in the chapter. Thanks also to the country offices of the World Health Organization (WHO), the United Nations Children's Fund (UNICEF) and the United Nations Population Fund (UNFPA) for the technical assistance during the study. I am grateful to Gladys Dube, Eunice Tahuringana and Maxwell Chirehwa for the assistance with data retrieval and the tables and graphs.

References

1.   World Bank. *World Development Indicators 2009*. Washington, DC: World Bank; 2009.
2.   Central Statistical Office (Zimbabwe), Macro International. *Zimbabwe Demographic and Health Survey 1994*. Calverton, MD: Central Statistical Office and Macro International; 1995.
3.   Central Statistical Office (Zimbabwe), Macro International. *Zimbabwe Demographic and Health Survey 1999*. Calverton, MD: Central Statistical Office and Macro International; 2000.
4.   Central Statistical Office (Zimbabwe), Macro International. *Zimbabwe Demographic and Health Survey 2005–6*. Calverton, MD: Central Statistical Office and Macro International; 2007.

5.   World Health Organization/UNICEF/UNFPA. *Maternal Mortality in 1995*. Estimates developed by WHO, UNICEF, UNFPA. Geneva: WHO; 2001.

6.   World Health Organization/UNICEF/UNFPA. *Maternal Mortality in 2000*. Estimates developed by WHO, UNICEF, UNFPA. Geneva: WHO; 2004.

7.   World Health Organization/UNICEF/UNFPA, World Bank. *Maternal mortality in 2005*. Estimates developed by WHO, UNICEF, UNFPA and the World Bank. Geneva: WHO; 2007.

8.   Crowther CA. Maternal deaths at Harare Maternity Hospital during 1983. *S Afr Med J* 1986;69:180–2.

9.   Ashworth MF. Harare Hospital maternal mortality report for 1987 and a comparison with previous reports. *Cent Afr J Med* 1990;36:209–12.

10.   Mbizvo MT, Fawcus S, Lindmark G, Nystrom L. Maternal mortality in rural and urban Zimbabwe: social and reproductive factors in an incident case-referent study. *Soc Sci Med* 1993;36:1197–205.

11.   Majoko F, Chipato T, Iliff V. Trends in maternal mortality for the Greater Harare Maternity Unit: 1976 to 1997. *Cent Afr J Med* 2001;47:199–203.

12.   Ministry of Health and Child Welfare. *Maternal and Perinatal Mortality Study 2007*. Harare: Government of Zimbabwe; 2009.

13.   Ticconi C, Mapfumo M, Dorrucci M, Naha N, Tarira E, Pietropolli A, *et al.* Effect of maternal HIV and malaria infection on pregnancy and perinatal outcome in Zimbabwe. *J Acquir Immune Defic Syndr* 2003;34:289–94.

14.   Darmstadt GL, Bhutta ZA, Cousens S, Adam T, Walker N, de Bernis L. Evidence-based, cost-effective interventions: how many newborn babies can we save? *Lancet* 2005;365:977–88.

15.   Lawn JE, Cousens S, Zupan J; Lancet Neonatal Survival Steering Team. 4 million neonatal deaths: when? Where? Why? *Lancet* 2005;365:891–900.

16.   Crowther CA, Brown IM. A review of perinatal mortality in an urban situation in a developing country. *J Perinat Med* 1986;14:325–30.

17.   Aiken CG. The causes of perinatal mortality in Bulawayo, Zimbabwe. *Cent Afr J Med* 1992;38:263–81.

18.   Iliff PJ, Kenyon N. Perinatal mortality statistics in Harare 1980–1989. *Cent Afr J Med* 1991;37:133–6.

19.   Aiken CG. HIV-1 infection and perinatal mortality in Zimbabwe. *Arch Dis Child* 1992;67:595–9.

20.   Brocklehurst P, French R. The association between maternal HIV infection and perinatal outcome: a systematic review of the literature and meta-analysis. *Br J Obstet Gynaecol* 1998;105:836–48.

21.   Noble A, Ning Y, Woelk GB, Mahomed K, Williams MA. Preterm delivery risk in relation to maternal HIV infection, history of malaria and other infections among urban Zimbabwean women. *Cent Afr J Med* 2005;51:53–8.

22.   Bloland PB, Wirima JJ, Steketee RW, Chilima B, Hightower A, Breman JG. Maternal HIV infection and infant mortality in Malawi: evidence for increased mortality due to placental malaria infection. *AIDS* 1995;9:721–6.

23.   Nilses C, Nystrom L, Munjanja S, Lindmark G. Self-reported reproductive outcome and implications in relation to use of care in women in rural Zimbabwe. *Acta Obstet Gynecol Scand* 2002;81:508–15.

24.   Majoko F, Munjanja SP, Nystrom L, Mason E, Lindmark G. Randomised controlled trial of two antenatal care models in rural Zimbabwe. *BJOG* 2007;114:802–11.

25.   Pham L, Woelk GB, Ning Y, Madzime S, Mudzamiri S, Mahomed K, *et al.* Seroprevalence and risk factors of syphilis infection in pregnant women delivering at Harare Maternity Hospital, Zimbabwe. *Cent Afr J Med* 2005;51:24–30.

26.   Central Statistical Office (Zimbabwe), Macro International. *Zimbabwe Demographic and Health Survey 1988*. Calverton, MD: Central Statistical Office and Macro International; 1990.

27.   Nathoo K, Rusakaniko S, Zijenah LS, Kasule J, Mahomed K, Mashu A, *et al.* Survival pattern among infants born to human immunodeficiency virus type-1 infected mothers and uninfected mothers in Harare, Zimbabwe. *Cent Afr J Med* 2004;50:1–6.

28.   Dube S, Boily MC, Mugurungi O, Mahomva A, Chikhata F, Gregson S. Estimating vertically acquired HIV infections and the impact of the prevention of mother-to-child transmission

program in Zimbabwe: insights from decision analysis models. *J Acquir Immune Defic Syndr* 2008;48:72–81.

29. Piwoz EG, Humphrey JH, Tavengwa NV, Iliff PJ, Marinda ET, Zunguza CD, *et al.* The impact of safer breastfeeding practices on postnatal HIV-1 transmission in Zimbabwe. *Am J Public Health* 2007;97:1249–54.

30. Koyanagi A, Humphrey JH, Moulton LH, Ntozini R, Mutasa K, Iliff P, *et al.* Effect of early exclusive breastfeeding on morbidity among infants born to HIV-negative mothers in Zimbabwe. *Am J Clin Nutr* 2009;89:1375–82.

31. Ministry of Health and Child Welfare. *Zimbabwe National HIV and AIDS Estimates 2008.* Harare: Ministry of Health and Child Welfare; 2009.

32. United Nations. Action for the 21st Century: Reproductive Health and Rights for All. Program of Action. International Conference for Population and Development, 1994, Cairo.

33. Ministry of Health and Child Welfare. *Reproductive Health Guidelines.* Harare: Government of Zimbabwe; 2003.

34. United Nations. *Millenium Development Goals.* New York: United Nations; 2000.

35. Economic Commission of Africa. *Abuja Declaration.* Abuja: Organisation of African Unity; 2001.

36. World Bank. *World Development Indicators.* Washington, DC: World Bank; 2005.

37. Lunney KM, Jenkins AL, Tavengwa NV, Majo F, Chidhanguro D, Iliff P, *et al.* HIV-positive poor women may stop breastfeeding early to protect their infants from HIV infection although available replacement diets are grossly inadequate. *J Nutr* 2008;138:351–7.

38. World Health Organization. *World Health Report 2000 – Health Systems: Improving Performance.* Geneva: WHO; 2000.

39. Gilson L. The lessons of user fee experience in Africa. *Health Policy Plan* 1997;12:273–85.

40. Weissman E, Sentumbwe-Mugisa O, Mbonye A. Costing safe motherhood in Uganda. In: Berer M, Sundari Ravindran TK, editors. *Safe Motherhood Initiatives: Critical Issues.* Oxford: Blackwell Science; 1999.

41. World Bank. *World Development Report 2004. Making Services Work for Poor People.* Washington, DC: World Bank; 2004.

42. James CD, Hanson K, McPake B, Balabanova D, Gwatkin D, Hopwood I, *et al.* To retain or remove user fees?: reflections on the current debate in low- and middle-income countries. *Appl Health Econ Health Policy* 2006;5:137–53.

43. Ministry of Health and Child Welfare. *Zimbabwe Maternal and Neonatal Health Roadmap 2007–2015.* Harare: Ministry of Health and Child Welfare; 2007.

44. Millard P, Bailey J, Hanson J. Antenatal village stay and pregnancy outcome in rural Zimbabwe. *Cent Afr J Med* 1991;37:1–4.

45. Tumwine JK, Dungare PS. Maternity waiting shelters and pregnancy outcome: experience from a rural area in Zimbabwe. *Ann Trop Paediatr* 1996;16:55–9.

46. World Health Organization. *Beyond the Numbers: Reviewing Maternal Deaths and Complications to Make Pregnancy Safer.* Geneva: WHO; 2004.

47. Pearson L, deBernis L, Shoo R. Maternal death review in Africa. *Int J Gynaecol Obstet* 2009;106:89–94.

Chapter 19

How Egypt has overcome the challenges

Oona Campbell, Lauren Foster Mustardé, Nevine Hassanein and Karima Khalil

Introduction

Discussion of the Millennium Development Goal to improve maternal health (MDG 5) is often pessimistic, yet some low-income countries are well under way to achieving this goal and have lowered maternal mortality. Egypt is one such case. Since 1992, maternal mortality has been reduced by 68%, and the absolute level of 55 per 100 000 live births reported in 2008 is low by many standards, although it remains 5–10 times higher than those countries with the lowest mortality. This chapter addresses three questions:

▦ Has maternal mortality in Egypt actually declined?

▦ What else was happening at the same time?

▦ What interventions and policies made these changes come about?

Has maternal mortality in Egypt actually declined?

Maternal mortality levels

Maternal mortality has declined in Egypt over the past 30 years (Table 19.1, Figure 19.1). Two comprehensive National Maternal Mortality Studies (NMMS) in 1992–93[1] and in 2000[2] showed a dramatic decline in the maternal mortality ratio (MMR) from 174 to 84 per 100 000 live births. Although all methods are likely to miss some maternal deaths, the similar approach used in both of these studies means the degree of underestimation is probably similar. Subsequently, Egypt adopted a Maternal Mortality Surveillance System (MMSS) that has reported maternal mortality annually since 2002. Considerable effort seems to have gone into implementing the MMSS. For example, requests for free formula to feed infants whose mothers have died during delivery are collated centrally and checked against maternal deaths identified through the MMSS. These do not provide a systematic assessment of the quality of the data yielded by the MMSS but, if correct, they suggest maternal mortality continues to decline and was 55 per 100 000 live births in 2008.

Table 19.1   Population-based studies of maternal mortality in Egypt

	Period	No. of maternal deaths	MMR	Reference
Lower Egypt				
Alexandria	1963–82	183	163	El Ghamry *et al.* (1984)[47]
Menoufia (RAMOS)	1981–83	385	190	Fortney *et al.* (1984)[48] (1986)[49]
Giza study	1985–86	153	150	El Kady *et al.* (1989)[50]
Upper Egypt				
Assiut (Kausaih)	1984–85	16	178	Abdullah *et al.* (1985)[51]
Sohag	1984–85	23	471	Abdullah *et al.* (1985)[51]
Quena	1984–85	34	323	Abdullah *et al.* (1985)[51]
Quena	1989–90	185	207	Saleh (1992)[52]
Assiut and three villages	1987–88	29	368	Abdullah *et al.* (1992)[53]
National				
National Sisterhood method estimate[a]	~1976	150	170	Stanton *et al.* (1997)[54]
National Sisterhood method estimate[a]	~1979	87	177	Abdel-Azeem *et al.* (1993)[55]
Urban[a]	~1979	NS	150	Abdel-Azeem *et al.* (1993)[55]
Rural[a]	~1979	NS	193	Abdel-Azeem *et al.* (1993)[55]
National Maternal Mortality Study (NMMS)[a]	1992–93	772	174	MOHP (1994)[1]
Rapid Assessment Survey	1997	NS	96	MOHP (1997)[56]
National Maternal Mortality Study (NMMS)	2000	585	84	MOHP (2001)[2]
National Maternal Mortality Surveillance System (MMSS)				
	2002	NS	75	IDSC Egypt (2009)[57]
	2003	NS	68	IDSC Egypt (2009)[57]
	2004	1251	68	Roushdy (2007)[10]
	2005	NS	63	IDSC Egypt (2009)[57]
	2006	1143	59	Roushdy (2007)[10]
	2007	NS	55	IDSC Egypt (2009)[57]
	2008	NS	55	IDSC Egypt (2009)[57]

IDSC = Information Decision Support Center; MOHP = Ministry of Health and Population; MMR = maternal mortality ratio (per 100 000 live births); NS = not stated; RAMOS = reproductive age mortality survey

[a] Excluding frontier governorates

Stillbirth and neonatal mortality levels

It is expected that improvements in maternal health care should also reduce neonatal mortality and stillbirth rates. Figure 19.2, using data from population-based surveys, shows that declines have indeed occurred in neonatal mortality, albeit not as substantially as those seen in infant mortality. The most recent estimate of neonatal mortality from the Egypt Demographic and Health Survey in 2008 (EDHS2008)[3] is 16 per 1000 live births, down from over 60 per 1000 live births seen 40 years

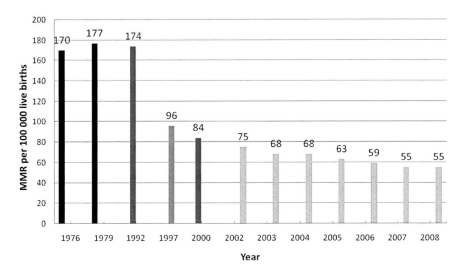

■ Sisterhood Method ■ RAMOS study ■ Rapid study ▨ RAMOS surveillance

Figure 19.1 National population-based maternal mortality ratios in Egypt; RAMOS = reproductive age mortality survey; data from Stanton *et al*,[54] Abdel-Azeem *et al*,[55] Ministry of Health and Population,[1,2,56] Roushdy[10] and IDSC Egypt[57]

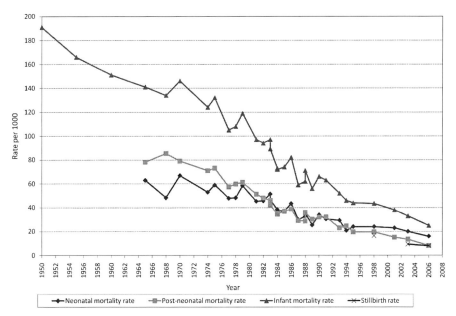

Figure 19.2 Stillbirth and neonatal, post-neonatal and infant mortality rates in Egypt; data from Stanton *et al*,[58] Abdel-Azeem *et al*,[55] Ministry of Health and Population,[1,2,59] Roushdy[10] and IDSC Egypt[57]

previously. There is a paucity of population-based data on stillbirth rates (Table 19.2), making it problematic to look at trends confidently, but the most recent estimate in EDHS2008 is 8 stillbirths per 1000 births, down from 16 in EDHS2000,[6] while the perinatal mortality rate is 19 per 1000 births, down from 33 in EDHS2000.

What else was happening at the same time?

Availability of normal delivery services and emergency care

Egypt has more resources than some of the world's poorest countries. In 2005, it spent 6.1% of its gross domestic product on health. Most (62%) was private expenditure, of which 95% was out of pocket. The per capita government expenditure on health (purchasing-power-parity [PPP] international) was $106 while the per capita total expenditure on health (PPP int.) was $279.[4]

Egypt's infrastructure of facilities and roads is well developed. Communication systems are also good, with nearly two-thirds (63%) of households in possession of a telephone and 41% with a mobile phone.[3] These features facilitate access to obstetric care in case of emergency and for normal delivery. Its high population density also means that most women, except for the 1% living in the Frontier Governorates, live within close reach of medical facilities. Data as far back as 1989 on the availability of services[5] suggest that even in rural areas 99% of women lived within 30 km of at least one government hospital.[6] Since then, there have been improvements in roads and it is now estimated that 95% of the population is within 5 km of a medical facility.[5] Ambulance services have also been upgraded in recent years, potentially contributing to better access to health care in emergencies of all causes, including pregnancy-related complications.[7]

Egypt also has many medical doctors.[6] In 2005, 24 physicians and 34 nursing/midwifery personnel per 10 000 population – a total of 58 per 10 000[*] – were recorded.[6] There is a dearth of nationally representative data on facility preparedness. A 2004 Service Provision Assessment (SPA2004) survey[5] looked at service preparedness in a random sample of government facilities and large non-governmental organisation (NGO) services but excluded private sector services, which cover 62% of deliveries in facilities. It found that 26% of 645 facilities did normal deliveries, with 6% offering caesarean section. Among the 167 facilities offering delivery services, 80% had all the necessary delivery infrastructure and furnishings (beds, examination lights, and visual and auditory privacy), 58% had capacity for sterilisation (knowledge of time needed and automatic timing devices) and 2% had other elements for supporting quality (service guidelines or protocols, partographs, and a 24-hour provider on site or on call with a duty schedule observed). Only 18% had all items needed for infection control, with hand-washing soap most often missed (missed in 51% of facilities), followed by latex gloves (missed in 48% of facilities) and a sharps box (missed in 30% of facilities). In terms of supplies, 33% had all essential supplies for delivery, 18% had supplies for common complications and 3% had supplies for serious complications. Among the 39 general hospitals offering delivery services, 45% and 41%, respectively, could assist labour with forceps or vacuum. Blood transfusion capability was 62%, while caesarean section capability was 67%.

Nevertheless, the 2000 NMMS[2] found that, with the exception of blood, the lack of appropriate facilities does not prevent many women from obtaining care. The

---

[*] The World Health Organization[4] reported in 2006 that countries with fewer than 25 physicians, nurses and midwives per 10 000 population failed to achieve adequate coverage rates for selected primary healthcare interventions as prioritised by the MDG framework.

Table 19.2 Estimates of stillbirth and early neonatal and perinatal mortality rates in Egypt; based on Arafa[60]

Source of data	Period	Sample size	SBR	ENMR	PNMR	Reference
Population-based studies						
Vital registration						
National	1917–60		12.1–7			Sarhan et al. (1967)[61]
National	1992	>1 700 000 births				United Nations (1998)[62]
Stillbirths from 20 weeks or later			3.4	5.0	8.4	
Stillbirths from 28 weeks or later			1.7	5.0	6.7	
Retrospective surveys						
National	1980	11 371 births	26	–	–	CAPMAS (1987)[63]
National EDHS92	1987–92		16	27	43	El-Zanaty et al. (1993)[64]
National EDHS95	1990–95		14	19	34	El-Zanaty et al. (1996)[65]
Menoufiya	1990–95	4315 births	10	–	–	EFCS (1995)[66]
Assiut, Sohag and Quena	1994–96	1 232 births	21	–	–	EFCS (1996)[67]
Minya and Qalyoubia	1995–97	2 128 pregnancies	16–18[a]	14	30–31[a]	Stanton and Langsten (1999)[68]
Prospective studies						
Minya[b]	1996–97	596 pregnancies	–	–	30	Stanton and Langsten (1999)[68]
Qalyoubia[b]	1996–97	380 pregnancies	–	–	39	Stanton and Langsten (1999)[68]
Hospital-based studies						
Public hospitals	1972–77		–	–	88	Aboulghar and Hussein (1984)[69]
Public hospitals	1978–82		–	–	83	Aboulghar and Hussein (1984)[69]
Private hospitals	1972–77		–	–	16	Aboulghar and Hussein (1984)[69]
Private hospitals	1978–82		–	–	14	Aboulghar and Hussein (1984)[69]
Al-Azhar/AlGalaa Hospital	1977–78	6 990 births	73.3	11.8	83	Hefnawy et al. (1983),[70] Serour et al. (1981),[71] Younis et al. (1981)[72]

SBR = stillbirth rate (per 1000 live and stillbirths); ENMR = early neonatal mortality rate (deaths in the first week of life per 1000 live births); PNMR = perinatal mortality rate (per 1000 live and stillbirths)

[a] A range is given because the report quotes 32 and 35 stillbirths at different points

[b] A combined stillbirth rate at 65 months of 16.7 per 1000 live and stillbirths and an early neonatal mortality rate of 16.6 per 1000 live births could be calculated using Langsten et al.[73]

lack of blood banks was the leading contributor (16%) to maternal death, followed by distance (4%) and/or lack of transportation (5%), or both together (7%). Lack of drugs (2%) supplies (2%) and equipment (5%) in health facilities contributed to 6% of maternal deaths. Lack of available operating theatre, back-up facilities and anaesthetist/ anaesthetic facilities contributed to 2%, 2% and 4% of maternal deaths, respectively.

Use of delivery care: where women deliver and who delivers them

Most deaths occur during delivery or on the first day postpartum. Figure 19.3 shows that the percentage of births attended by a skilled attendant (doctor or midwife/ nurse) increased from 11% in 1977 to 79% in 2006. These skilled attendants are largely doctors (94% of skilled attendants), mainly obstetricians, with one of several degrees: the Diploma; the MS, the MD, the MRCOG and the Egyptian Board degree for Obstetrics and Gynaecology.[8,9] Midwives/nurses are the remaining 6% of skilled attendants. Births by traditional birth attendants (dayas) and by relatives have decreased to 20% and 1% of deliveries, respectively. Figure 19.3 also shows that the proportion of births occurring in health facilities increased from 6% in 1976 to 72% in 2006. Unusually for many countries, doctors and midwives attend just over one-quarter of the 28% of births that occur at home (11% of deliveries in the home are by doctors and 15% by midwives).

In EDHS2000,[9] health facility births in the private sector (26%) overtook births in the public sector (22%). For the most recent period,[3] these figures were 45% and 27%, respectively, meaning that nearly two-thirds (62%) of facility deliveries were in the private sector. It is very likely that home deliveries by doctors were also private. Women delivering with dayas and relatives were rural, of higher parity, with less education and not working for cash. Fifty-five percent of women in the lowest wealth quintile had a skilled attendant compared with 97% of the wealthiest fifth of the population.

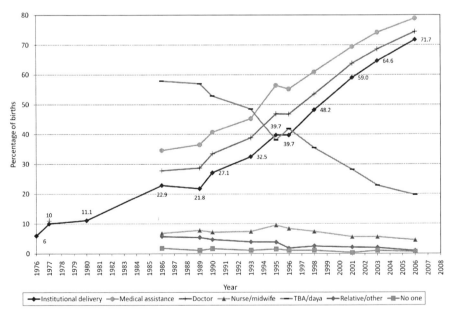

Figure 19.3 Percentage of births in health facilities and by type of attendant in Egypt; data from CAPMAS,[63] World Health Organization[74] and El-Zanaty and Way[3,9,12,75]

Use of emergency care and referral

Population-based data on emergency care use by women with complications could not be found. However, caesarean section rates reached 28% in EDHS2008,[3] well beyond the 5–15% recommended as indicating met need for caesarean sections (Figure 19.4). Even among the poorest fifth of the population, rates of 14% (compared with 45% among the richest) were seen, suggesting that even poor women needing the procedure are likely to get it.

There is other evidence that most women with complications appear to access emergency care. The 2000 NMMS[2] showed that, of maternal deaths, 62% were in medical facilities, 29% occurred at home and 9% occurred during transportation, and that 93% of these women accessed medical care at some point during the events leading to their deaths. The 2006 Maternal Mortality Surveillance System (MMSS)[10] showed that 73% died in medical facilities, with 27% still dying outside. This indicates that most maternal deaths had some sort of care and suggests an improvement in access over time.

Similarly, no population-based survey data were found on referral. It is known from SPA2004[5] that only 10% of government facilities had emergency transport support for maternity emergencies. The 2000 NMMS review of maternal deaths[2] revealed that there was no proper referral system in place, with problems occurring in both where and when to refer cases. The first medical provider's failure to refer correctly was associated with 13% of deaths. In a disproportionately large number of cases, private practitioners delayed referring women on to hospital facilities. A worrying feature is that around one-quarter of women delivering in facilities died at home or during transportation (27% for those delivering in private facilities and 23% for those delivering in public sector facilities), suggesting possible problems with referrals or premature discharge.

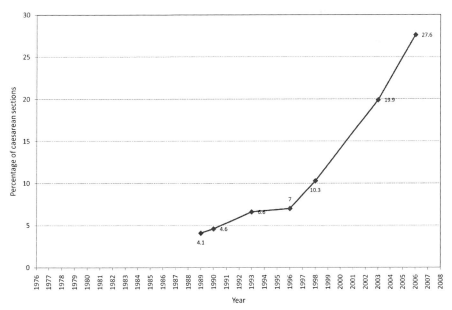

Figure 19.4 Percentage of caesarean section births in Egypt; data from El-Zanaty and Way[3,9,12,75] and Sayed et al.[23]

Quality of delivery care

There are limited national data on the quality of normal delivery care but insights can be gleaned from SPA2004[5] and EDHS2008.[3] Evidence reported above suggests many government facilities do not have equipment and supplies to manage normal deliveries adequately. Moreover, given that over one-quarter of births occur at home, the population-based caesarean section rate of 28% seen in EDHS2008 suggests overly interventionist and poorly regulated services that risk mimicking the 'caesarean section epidemics' seen in Latin America.[11] Indeed, among women delivering in private health facilities the caesarean section rate is 42%, while in the public sector it is 33%. This suggests caesarean section indications are probably not strictly adhered to.

Moreover, women in EDHS2008 were able to report birth weights for only 42% of births. Furthermore, the reporting of weights has not improved over time – it was 47% in EDHS2005.[12] Although being unable to report a weight this does not necessarily mean a baby was not weighed, earlier audits of facility deliveries suggest this basic element is not routine. If babies whose mothers could not report a weight were not weighed, then 37% of all babies were delivered by a skilled birth attendant but were not weighed.

Finally, among women having a facility delivery, 55% stayed less than 24 hours in the facility, with 40% staying less than 6 hours. A further 34% stayed 1–2 days and 11% stayed 3 or more days. This did not improve much from 2005 when these data were first collected and suggests a lost opportunity to check on the health of both the woman and the neonate.

There are other small-scale investigations that suggest deficits in quality. A 2001 study[13] in an Egyptian teaching hospital documented practices for 176 normal births by directly observing women for their entire labour and delivery. Although the facility's preparedness was acceptable, high levels of inappropriate practice were documented. Among the most clinically significant were inadequate assessment procedures, routine labour augmentation and inappropriate third-stage management. For example, third-stage active management was correct for only 15% of women observed. High caseload, absence of written protocols for normal labour, and providers' relative focus on high-risk obstetric cases were felt to contribute to the poor practices documented. Others have also documented various aspects of poor quality of care.[14–16]

In the 2000 NMMS,[2] poor care by obstetricians played a major role in the avoidable factors contributing to maternal death, with failure of early diagnosis and poor management contributing to 19% and 42% of all deaths, respectively. The MMSS have not reported on substandard care but smaller studies in the Damietta Governorate in 2004[17] and the Dakahlia Governorate in 2004–05[18] indicate that substandard care by health providers, in particular obstetricians and GPs, remains the most important avoidable factor contributing to 54% of maternal deaths in Damietta and 51% in Dakahlia.

Barriers to use of normal delivery services and emergency care

Early studies suggested that women's perceptions of poor-quality services and financial cost were barriers to using antenatal and delivery services, respectively.[19] SPA2004[5] indicated that 25% of government services charged user fees for antenatal care and 41% charged for delivery care. Cost is the second most common reason given for not delivering in a health facility (23%), with the most common being stating that it was 'not customary' (63%).[3] Length of stay following delivery increases with increasing wealth, suggesting again that cost is a consideration.[3]

Data on whether cost is a financial barrier to emergency care were not identified. In 1996, a cost-recovery programme was introduced to all hospitals but services were meant to be provided free when needed.[20]

When asked about their ability to seek care when they were sick (general illness not related to pregnancy), 80% of women reported having at least one problem accessing health care. In order of frequency, 64% were concerned that drugs would not be available, 63% that there would be no provider, 44% that they needed money to be treated, 40% that there would be no female providers, 26% did not want to go alone, 20% because of having to take transport, 17% because of distance from the facility and 7% because of needing permission.

Family factors also play a role. To achieve relatively low mortality with one-fifth of births occurring at home with traditional birth attendants or relatives, families need to be able to access emergency care rapidly when complications arise. Both the 1992/93[1] and 2000 NMMS[2] showed that maternal deaths occurred because of a delay in seeking care on the part of the woman and her family. These in turn complicated the management of the obstetric emergencies presenting at health facilities. However, distance and lack of transport were rarely avoidable factors, suggesting the reasons for delay or non-adherence with referral were probably because families and women did not recognise danger signs and complications in pregnancy, because those attending the birth did not have decision-making capacities regarding transfer, because health facilities were not judged to be of good quality or because complying with recommendations was costly (either financially or socially). There is also evidence that delay is still caused by the intermediate steps of women seeking care at private practitioners who are incapable of dealing with the medical emergency involved, or who delay transfer to higher level facilities.

EDHS2000[9] showed that only 18% of women attending antenatal care were told about danger signs in pregnancy and only 14% were told where to go should they have a complication. In EDHS2008,[3] this increased to 34% and 31%, respectively. Moreover, in EDHS2008, 21% of ever-married women aged 15–49 years had received information about danger signs. Of these, 56% heard them from television and 33% from a service provider.

Studies in Egypt have highlighted that many women cannot take autonomous decisions concerning their own health and must persuade other decision makers (the husband or mother-in-law) of the importance of their illness.[21,22] EDHS2000[9] indicated that 36% of women made decisions regarding their own health care on their own, 24% made it jointly with the husband or someone else, while for 38% of women it was the husband alone who took the decision and in 2% it was someone else. In EDHS2008,[3] 27% of women made decisions regarding their own health care on their own, 61% made them jointly with the husband, while for 12% of women it was the husband alone who took the decision and in 1% it was someone else.

Availability of antenatal care tetanus toxoid and postnatal care

Most antenatal care is delivered in the private sector (74%) and no information on these services was identified. SPA2004[5] looked at service preparedness in a random sample of government facilities and large NGO services. It found that 87% could provide antenatal care, 70% postnatal care and 68% tetanus toxoid. Eighteen percent of facilities had all essential supplies for antenatal care (iron and folic acid tablets, tetanus toxoid vaccine, blood pressure apparatus and fetoscope (Pinard), 52% for physical examination (visual and auditory privacy [private room], examination table and examination light), 10% for infection control (soap and water, clean latex gloves, disinfecting solution and sharps box) and 5% for counselling (visual aids for health education, guidelines or protocols for antenatal care, and individual client card or record). The percentage with capacity to conduct diagnostic tests was 66% for anaemia, 66% for urine protein, 59% for urine glucose, 29% for blood grouping and 29% for ultrasound. Only 3% could give antihypertensives.

Use of antenatal care, tetanus toxoid and postnatal care

The most recent EDHS2008 data[3] suggest that 74% of women seek antenatal care (19% in the public sector and 55% in the private sector) (Figure 19.5). Most care (99.5%) is given by doctors and 90% of those getting antenatal care have four or more visits. Most of those getting antenatal care (82%) do so within the first 3 months of pregnancy and 94% get their last visit at 8 months of pregnancy or later. Maternal mortality nearly halved in Egypt between 1992 and 2000 without a substantial increase in the percentage of women having antenatal care.

There has also been a tremendous increase in tetanus toxoid coverage, with 81% of women getting tetanus toxoid (40% one immunisation, 41% two or more immunisations). This is almost exclusively provided in the public sector (94%), with women going to a different provider for antenatal care. This increase is unlikely to have a major contribution to maternal mortality decline but may well have reduced neonatal mortality (Figure 19.6).

One-third of women (34%) had no postnatal care. Among the 66% with postnatal care, the vast majority received it from doctors, mostly early, and nearly all within the first 24 hours after delivery. However, 18% of women delivered by a doctor or midwife had no postnatal care.

Antenatal care quality

EDHS2008[3] found that 94% of women had some sort of medical care during pregnancy or birth. Of these, 88% were weighed and 87% had blood pressure measured, and 69% gave a urine sample and 71% a blood sample. forty-four percent bought or received iron tablets or syrup. This is an improvement over earlier years: in EDHS2000,[9] when 85% sought medical care during pregnancy, the respective percentages were 60%, 58%,

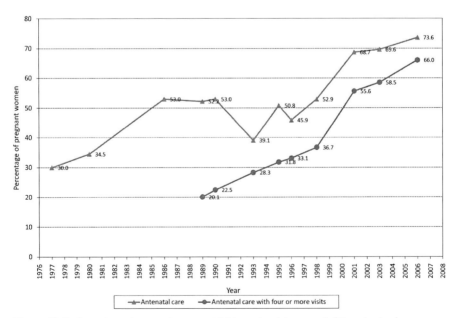

Figure 19.5 Percentage of pregnant women obtaining antenatal care and of those having four or more visits in Egypt; data from El-Zanaty and Way[3,9,12,75] and Sayed *et al.*[23]

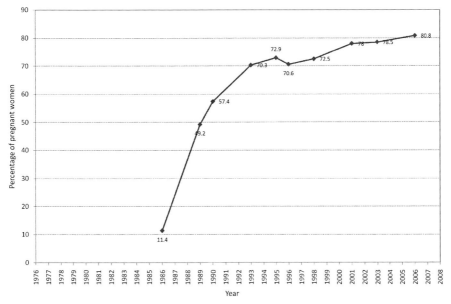

Figure 19.6 Percentage of women receiving one or more tetanus toxoid immunisation during pregnancy in Egypt; data from El-Zanaty and Way[3,9,12,75] and Sayed *et al.*[23]

46%, 47% and 28%. Observations in the SPA2004[5] government facilities concur with these findings but also note poor interpersonal communication skills of providers.

The Ministry of Health has also asked tetanus toxoid providers to recommend antenatal care checks.[5] Twenty percent of women had tetanus toxoid but no antenatal care, 14% had antenatal care but no tetanus toxoid and 77% of those obtaining tetanus toxoid said they were not advised to seek antenatal care, suggesting poor compliance with these protocols.

In 2000, nearly one-fifth of maternal deaths were in women who had attended antenatal care but received poor-quality care.[2] The percentage of deceased women without antenatal care reduced slightly from 35% in 1992/93[1] to 32% in 2000, whereas the percentage with ten or more visits increased from 13% to 24%, suggesting the possibility of greater care-seeking among women with complications. The MMSS has not reported comparable data to date.

Fertility patterns, contraceptive use and abortion

Egypt has made sustained efforts to reduce its fertility rate and prevent unwanted births. Figure 19.7 shows national estimates of the contraceptive prevalence rate. The use of modern contraception increased from 23% in 1980 to 58% in 2008; the total fertility rate reduced from 5.3 births in 1980 to 3.0 births in 2008.[3,23]

In 1984–88, 24% of births were not wanted at all and 16% were wanted later[23] but, by 2004–08, only 9% of births were not wanted at all and 5% wanted later,[3] suggesting a substantial improvement in contraceptive access (Figure 19.8). There is scope for improvement, though: in EDHS2008,[3] 9% of women had an unmet need for family planning (3% in need of spacing and 6% in need of limiting).

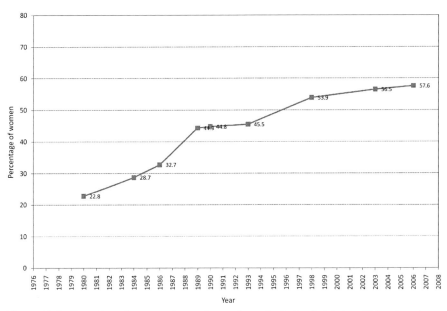

Figure 19.7 Percentage of women using modern contraception in Egypt; data from El-Zanaty and Way[3,9,12,75] and Sayed *et al.*[23]

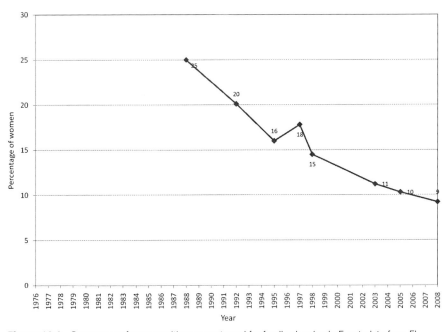

Figure 19.8 Percentage of women with an unmet need for family planning in Egypt; data from El-Zanaty and Way[3,9,12,75]

Huntington *et al.*[24] suggest that abortions are common, at 15 per 100 pregnancies. El Mouelhy's data[25] (including hospital admission case series) on the reported proportions of all abortions that are induced or septic ranges from 60% to 2%, with a median of around 18%, suggesting that most admissions are for uncomplicated abortions. In the 2000 NMMS,[2] abortions contributed to only 2% of all maternal deaths while in the 2006 MMSS[10] they contributed 1%, suggesting that unsafe abortion is not as large a problem in Egypt as in some other countries where it can contribute over 50% of all maternal deaths.[26]

Family planning and abortion care quality

There are data showing improvement in the quality of family planning provision. Among the maternal deaths in 2000, 6% had contraceptive failures.[2] According to the families, 22% of pregnancies were not wanted at all when they occurred and 5% were wanted later, indicating a missed opportunity for contraception.

Huntington *et al.*[27,28] showed that standards in post-abortion care in one large teaching facility in Cairo were poor but amenable to improvements. Only 12% and 41% for government facilities surveyed in SPA2004[5] could provide post-abortion care with a vacuum aspirator or a dilatation and curettage kit, respectively.

What interventions and policies made these changes come about?

Skilled birth attendance

The increase in use of skilled attendants at delivery appears to stem from policies in the late 1960s and early 1970s to expand medical education and increase the number of doctors. These policies did not appear to relate to maternity care specifically. Since 1996, health sector reform efforts have been under way to rationalise (reduce) the number of physicians and increase the number of nurses.[20] There were also maternity care-specific policies, for example to close midwifery schools in the early 1970s. In 1995, a ministerial decree was issued licensing midwifery training once again and pilot programmes were started; more recently, an initiative to provide midwifery training to nurses at the primary healthcare level was initiated and approximately 1700 nurses were trained and allocated to work in nearly one-third of all primary health centres in Egypt.[7] It has not been possible to obtain data on how many deliveries these nurses attend, to identify any policies regarding where births should take place or to determine whether the Ministry of Health wants to encourage private sector deliveries.

Dayas

The policy approach to dayas has also varied. The first daya school was opened in 1912 and, by the 1930s, health centres had daya schools attached to them. However, by 1954, a decree to gradually phase out these schools was issued and all daya schools were closed by 1962.[29] Etman *et al.*[30] have reported that, in 1969, the Egypt Ministry of Health, confident that sufficient numbers of trained nurses and nurse-midwives were available, revoked the licensure of indigenous dayas, even though they attended over 90% of deliveries at that time. However, since the early 1980s, activities aimed at dayas have included training programmes under the auspices of UNICEF and the Child Spacing Program of the Ministry of Health.[31,32] These emphasised the need to avoid harmful practices and the early detection and referral of women with obstetric complications. By 2008, the dayas' role had clearly diminished and they only did 20%

of deliveries.[3] Studies also show that, although most dayas learned their skills from their mothers, few expected their daughters to follow on from them.

Dayas are primarily expected to refer complications, and contributed substandard care to only 8% of maternal deaths in the 2000 NMMS.[2] These results may also indicate that the Ministry of Health and UNICEF may have been relatively successful in training traditional birth attendants to refer women who have complications promptly. Only 6% of government facilities have documented programmes of linking to traditional births attendants (dayas), suggesting that these programmes are not strongly supported.[4]

Private sector

Egypt declared an open economic policy in 1974, allowing for growth of the private health sector. Between 1975 and 1990, the total number of private beds rose significantly.[33] Private care facilities in Egypt range from hospitals that are large, modern and sophisticated to smaller hospitals, daycare centres and polyclinics. Private providers competed for 'business', including by moving in to more rural areas and by conducting home births.

Infrastructure

Factors such as lack of equipment and supplies made a negligible contribution to maternal death in the 1992/93 NMMS[1] and again in the 2000 NMMS.[2] Despite this, the Ministry of Health has been upgrading delivery facilities and, in the late 1990s, Basic and Comprehensive Essential Obstetric Care Services Standards, Essential Obstetric Care Physical Facility Structural Specifications, Essential Obstetric Care Commodity Catalogue, and Comprehensive Essential Surgical Care Physical Facility Structural Specifications were defined.[2,34] USAID has also supported the procurement of commodities. SPA2004[5] suggested there is scope for improvement in supplies and equipment in government facilities that provide delivery care but, in practice, these only carry out a small proportion of deliveries.

Quality of care

The 1992/93 NMMS report[1] drew attention to the substandard care provided by obstetricians, a finding confirmed by the 2000 NMMS.[2] Several efforts have been undertaken to improve the quality of delivery care. The National Child Survival Project (1990–96), the MotherCare Project (1996–98), the Healthy Mother/Healthy Child Project (1998–2004) and the UNICEF project (1996 to date) have targeted maternal and neonatal mortality through interventions to improve the use and quality of antenatal, delivery, postpartum and postneonatal health services. The first project was national while the latter three projects focused on Upper Egypt, where mortality levels were the highest. Currently, the UNICEF project is establishing perinatal care centres of excellence in four governorates in Upper Egypt, targeting 2 million children under 5 years and their mothers. The project supports the national integrated management of neonatal and childhood illnesses and includes training on clean delivery for 11 000 nurses, intensive midwifery for 50 nurses, and neonatal resuscitation for 160 nurses, paediatricians, neonatologists, anaesthetists and obstetricians.

In 1992, it also emerged that there were sometimes no protocols for dealing with obstetric emergencies and most were managed by junior staff, with senior staff usually called too late. The Ministry of Health introduced protocols and standards for managing ten common obstetric emergencies (such as postpartum haemorrhage) in Upper Egypt.[2,34] There is evidence from SPA2004[5] these are, as yet, not widespread, not even in government facilities. Obstetric and core care protocols have also been developed for normal pregnancy and delivery and antenatal and postnatal care.[2,35] Competency-based training modules based on clinical protocols and standards have also been developed and tested. Training programmes have been designed and tested for master and physician trainers.[34,35]

Another problem to emerge is the increasing proportion of deaths where medically trained providers have administered harmful treatments. These appear most marked with the use of oxytocic drugs and increased proportions of ruptured uteruses seen. Also, national caesarean section rates are increasing, suggesting the potential for iatrogenic deaths. There is no evidence of this situation improving.

It is not possible to assess the scale of many of these efforts relative to the need. There is little evidence of improvements in delivery care quality, in part because content has not been systematically measured, but there is evidence of improving antenatal care quality, when judged in terms of improvements in content of care but also coverage of care. Nevertheless, if judged by the reduction in maternal mortality, the quality of care for most women with complications has obviously improved, probably via increased access and use of skilled attendants and emergency care.

Family factors and referral

Referral is one area in need of more research and policy decision making. There are no published data on developments in this area.

Mass-media health education campaigns have emphasised the need to seek medical care for life-threatening obstetric complications.[1,3,35] In Upper Egypt, community efforts in outreach and cooperation with local providers have also tried to mobilise 'birth preparedness' and community resources for such care.[36]

Fertility and abortion

Egypt has had strong population policies since the 1970s, with considerable support from USAID. Fertility decline is likely to have played a role in maternal mortality reduction in three ways. Firstly, it reduces the number of pregnancies, thereby decreasing the number of times women face the risk of maternal death. This is reflected in the declining proportion of female deaths that are maternal, from 10.3% in the 1992/93 NMMS[1] to 5.1% in 2006 MMSS.[10] Secondly, high-risk pregnancies at higher parities can be avoided and, thirdly, women can avoid unwanted pregnancy that may result in illegal abortion or in poorer care-seeking behaviour.[37–39] The biggest impact is likely to be through the first mechanism, although only the latter two have much effect on the maternal mortality ratio.

Abortion in Egypt is restricted to cases of life-threatening maternal health considerations and is surrounded by many social and religious sanctions. Huntington et al.[24] suggested that abortions are common, at 15 per 100 pregnancies, although unwanted pregnancy is low, at 9% of births. Nevertheless, legal provision of safe abortion could reduce deaths further, as could improved access to effective contraception and adequate care for women with complications after abortion or miscarriage.

Other issues

Egypt is fortunate in its underlying epidemiology and geography. Unlike parts of sub-Saharan Africa, for example, malaria is not endemic and nor is HIV an epidemic, and thus there are fewer indirect maternal deaths due to these causes. However, chronic diseases do contribute to maternal deaths, mainly cardiovascular conditions, and a substantial proportion of Egyptian women aged 15–59 years are overweight (28%) and obese (40%); 13% are hypertensive[3] and 39% are anaemic, with 7% being moderately anaemic and 0.3% severely anaemic.[12]

Conducting the national confidential inquiries into maternal mortality in Egypt is a notable feat and it appears that the 1992/93 NMMS,[1] coupled with the international Safe Motherhood Initiative,[40–42] may have drawn attention to the magnitude of maternal deaths in Egypt and stimulated attention to maternal health care. Many of the recommendations made in the 1992/93 NMMS report[1] were adopted. Egypt has also developed the MMSS, which should prove to be a useful source of data on deaths and makes effective use of Demographic and Health Surveys to track key indicators.

Conclusion

Egypt has made good progress in reducing maternal mortality. This decline accompanies statistics indicating increasing access to, and use of, skilled attendants and facility births. Data on access to emergency care and quality of delivery care are harder to come by, although there was an increase in maternal deaths related to access to medical care between 1992/93 and 2000. There is evidence of improvements in coverage and quality of antenatal care.

Some of the policies resulting in these changes were not developed to specifically target maternity care, although others were, such as the effort put into antenatal care, tetanus toxoid coverage and the development of protocols. Reductions in overall fertility and also in unmet need for family planning have also played an important part.

Future declines in maternal mortality ratios are likely to be contingent on taking a health systems approach and tackling system-wide problems.[43,44] These include addressing linkages and continuity between antenatal, delivery and postpartum care, strengthening referral systems, ensuring better oversight and regulation of the private sector, tackling deficiencies in hospital management and hospital systems, developing improved pre-service training, elaborating mechanisms for updating in-service provider skills and knowledge, and strengthening accountability. Also, because obstetricians are the predominant skilled attendants, careful attention needs to be given to avoiding over-intervention and iatrogenic injuries.

Information has an important role to play. Egypt was able to obtain data on levels of maternal mortality from the National Maternal Mortality Studies and the Maternal Mortality Surveillance System and on use of care from the Demographic and Health Surveys. In contrast, data on inputs to services are difficult to come by, such as what policies are in place and what kind of delivery care is being provided for normal births and for emergencies.

The Ministry of Health also needs to conduct policy analyses to plan the future of delivery care. Important features are who should be delivering normal births and where such births should take place. In other words, is the Ministry of Health happy to encourage the trend of increased obstetrician deliveries, even if these were to reach 100%? What is the role of midwifery in Egypt and should it be strengthened? Should births by skilled attendants take place in private clinics or in the public sector facilities?

If in the public sector, should they be in hospitals, maternal and child health units, other health centres with beds or in women's homes? What are the costs associated with these options? To what extent should district hospitals be capable of emergency obstetric care? Given the low volume in some of these hospitals, should resources be put into governorate hospitals instead? Where would women like to deliver if resources were not a constraint?

Egypt should promote good evidenced-based care among health facility births and avoid the overuse of practices such as augmentation, supine position and lack of companionship.[45,46] How can quality of care by private providers be improved? Here the role of professional association needs to be revisited.

In conclusion, Egypt has successfully overcome many challenges in reducing maternal mortality but many others remain, especially the challenges of overcoming poor-quality care for both normal and complicated deliveries, in a largely private sector environment.

References

1.   Ministry of Health and Population. *National Maternal Mortality Study: Egypt 1992–1993.* Preliminary report of findings and conclusions. Cairo: Child Survival Project; 1994.

2.   Ministry of Health and Population. *National Maternal Mortality Study: Egypt 2000.* Cairo: John Snow, Inc; 2001.

3.   El-Zanaty F, Way AA. *Egypt Demographic and Health Survey 2008.* Cairo: Ministry of Health, El-Zanaty and Associates, and Macro International; 2009.

4.   World Health Organization Statistical Information System (WHOSIS) [www.who.int/whosis/en/].

5.   Ministry of Health and Population, El-Zanaty Associates, ORC Macro. *Egypt Service Provision Assessment Survey 2004.* Calverton, MD: Ministry of Health and Population [Egypt] and ORC Macro; 2005.

6.   Sayed HA. *Egypt Service Availability Survey 1989. Availability and Accessibility of Family Planning and Health Services in Rural Egypt.* Columbia, MD: Cairo Demographic Centre and Demographic and Health Surveys IRD, Macro International; 1991.

7.   Ministry of Health, personal communication, 11 October 2009.

8.   Campbell O. Egypt 1992–2000. In: Koblinsky MA, editor. *Reducing Maternal Mortality: Learning from Bolivia, China, Egypt, Honduras, Indonesia, Jamaica, and Zimbabwe.* Washington, DC: World Bank; 2003. p. 93–111.

9.   El-Zanaty F, Way AA. *Egypt Demographic and Health Survey 2000.* Calverton, MD: Ministry of Health and Population [Egypt], National Population Council and ORC Macro; 2001.

10.   Roushdy N. Maternal Mortality Surveillance System. Presented at Scaling Up High-Impact FP/MNCH Best Practices: Achieving the Millennium Development Goals in Asia and the Near East. Technical meeting convened by the Extending Service Delivery Project, 3–8 September, 2007, Bangkok.

11.   Barros FC, Vaughan JP, Victora CG, Huttly SR. Epidemic of caesarean sections in Brazil. *Lancet* 1991;338:167–9.

12.   El-Zanaty F, Way AA. *Egypt Demographic and Health Survey 2005.* Cairo: Ministry of Health and Population, National Population Council, El-Zanaty and Associates and ORC Macro; 2006.

13.   Cherine M, Khalil K, Hassanein N, Sholkamy H, Breebaart M, Elnoury A. Management of the third stage of labor in an Egyptian teaching hospital. *Int J Gynaecol Obstet* 2004;87:54–8.

14.   Darmstadt GL, Hussein MH, Winch PJ, Haws RA, Gipson R, Santosham M. Practices of rural Egyptian birth attendants during the antenatal, intrapartum and early neonatal periods. *J Health Popul Nutr* 2008;26:36–45.

15.   Nabhan A, Ahmed-Tawfik MS. Understanding and attitudes towards patient safety concepts in obstetrics. *Int J Gynaecol Obstet* 2007;98:212–16.

16.   Abd-El-Aziz HM, Zaghloul AA. Job satisfaction and stress among MCH physicians in Alexandria. *J Egypt Public Health Assoc* 2002;77:409–27.

17. El Sherbiny M, El Sobaky A, Sarhan F. Maternal Mortality In Damietta, Egypt (2004). Powerpoint presentation [www.gfmer.ch/IAMANEH_ESMANEH_Cairo_2006/pdf/Maternal_ mortality_Sherbiny_2006.pdf].

18. Abdel-Hady el-S, Mashaly AM, Sherief LS, Hassan M, Al-Gohary A, Farag MK, *et al.* Why do mothers die in Dakahlia, Egypt? *J Obstet Gynaecol Res* 2007;33:283–7.

19. Loza S. *Child Survival: Further Analysis of Baseline KAP Findings.* Draft Report. Cairo: SPAAC (Social Planning Analysis and Administration Consultants); 1994.

20. Sallam I. Health care in Egypt [letter]. *Lancet* 1998;35:1632.

21. Khattab HAS. *The Silent Endurance: Social Conditions of Women's Reproductive Health in Rural Egypt.* Cairo: UNICEF; 1992.

22. Lane SD, Meleis AI. Roles, work, health perceptions and health resources of women: a study in an Egyptian delta hamlet. *Soc Sci Med* 1991;33:1197–208.

23. Sayed HAA, Osman MI, El-Zanaty F, Way AA. *Egypt Demographic and Health Survey 1988.* Calverton, MD: Ministry of Health and Population [Egypt], National Population Council and ORC Macro; 1989.

24. Huntington D, Nawar L, Hassan EO, Youssef H, Abdel-Tawab N. The post abortion caseload in Egyptian hospitals: a descriptive study. *Int Fam Plan Perspect* 1998;24:25–31.

25. El Mouelhy M. Maternal mortality in Egypt. Unpublished. 1987.

26. Royston E, Armstrong S, editors. *Preventing Maternal Deaths.* Geneva: World Health Organization; 1989.

27. Huntington D, Hassan EO, Attallah N, Toubia N, Naguib M, Nawar L. Improving the medical care and counseling of post abortion patients in Egypt. *Stud Fam Plann* 1995;26:350–62.

28. Huntington D, Piet-Pelon NJ. *Postabortion Care: Lessons from Operations Research.* New York: Population Council; 1999.

29. Hefni MM, Kassas E. Daya training program, part I. UNICEF Egypt Working Paper. Cairo: UNICEF; 1985.

30. Etman S, Omran K, Lewis K. Evaluation of TBA program. In: Fayed MM, Ibrahim II, Bayad MA, editors. *Medical Education in the Field of Primary Maternal Child Health Care.* Cairo: Cairo University Faculty of Medicine; 1984. p. 345–71.

31. Ricter A. *Daya Training Programme Evaluation: May 1992.* Cairo: Ministry of Health Child Survival Project, Child Spacing Component; 1992.

32. UNICEF. *Daya Training Programme Trainer'S Guide.* Cairo: UNICEF and Ministry of Health and Population; 1987.

33. Kemprecos L, Oldham L. *Economic Surveys for Health Financing and Sustainability: Final Report.* Cairo: Cost Recovery for Health Project; 1992.

34. Ministry of Health and Population. *The Maternal and Child Health Series.* Cairo: Ministry of Health and Population; (no date).

35. JSI. *The MotherCare Egypt Project, September 1996 – September 1998.* Final report. Arlington, VA: John Snow, Inc, USAID, Ministry of Health and Population, Healthy Mother/Healthy Child Project; 1998.

36. UNICEF. Young Child Survival and Development [www.unicef.org/egypt/immunisation.html].

37. Campbell OMR, Graham WJ. *Measuring Maternal Mortality and Morbidity: Levels and Trends.* Research paper. London: Maternal and Child Epidemiology Unit, London School of Hygiene & Tropical Medicine; 1990.

38. Winikoff B, Sullivan M. Assessing the role of family planning in reducing maternal mortality. *Stud Fam Plann* 1987;18:128–42.

39. Fortney JA. The importance of family planning in reducing maternal mortality. *Stud Fam Plann* 1987;18:109–14.

40. Starrs A, Inter-Agency Group for Safe Motherhood. *The Safe Motherhood Action Agenda: Priorities for the Next Decade.* New York: Family Care International; 1998.

41. Sai FT, Measham DM. Safe Motherhood Initiative: getting our priorities straight. *Lancet* 1992;339:478–80.

42. Mahler H. The safe motherhood initiative: a call to action. *Lancet* 1987;1:668–70.

43. Campbell OM, Graham WJ; Lancet Maternal Survival Series steering group. Strategies for reducing maternal mortality: getting on with what works. *Lancet* 2006;368:1284–99.

44. Goodburn E, Campbell O. Reducing maternal mortality in the developing world: sector-wide approaches may be the key. *BMJ* 2001;322:917–20.

45. Enkin MW, Keirse MJNC, Renfrew MJ, Neilson JP, editors. Pregnancy and childbirth module. *The Cochrane Library*. Oxford: Update Software; 1996.

46. Chalmers I, Enkin M, Keirse MJNC. *Effective Care in Pregnancy and Childbirth*. Volumes 1 and 2. Oxford: Oxford University Press; 1991.

47. El Ghamry A, El-Sherbini AF, Hussein M, El-Tantawi AS, Hamoud E. The feasibility of getting information about maternal mortality from the husband. *Bull High Inst Public Health* 1984;14:195–223.

48. Fortney JA, Saleh S, Gadalla S, Rogers SM. *Causes of Death to Women of Reproductive Age in Egypt*. Working Papers in Development No. 49. East Lancing, MI: Office of Women in International Development, Michigan State University; 1984.

49. Fortney JA, Susanti I, Gadalla S, Saleh S, Rogers SM, Potts M. Reproductive mortality in two developing countries. *Am J Public Health* 1986;76:134–8.

50. El Kady A, Saleh S, Kane T, Stanbeck J, Potter L, Hage M. *Maternal Mortality in Giza, Egypt*. Final report. Cairo: National Population Council; 1989.

51. Abdullah SA, Fathalla MF, Abdel-Aleem AM, Salem HT, Aly MY. *Maternal Mortality in Upper Egypt*. WHO Inter-Regional Meeting on Prevention of Maternal Mortality, 11–15 November 1985, Geneva.

52. Saleh S. Reproductive age mortality survey: Quena governorate, 1989–1990. *Dirasat Sukkaniyah* 1992;14:5–53.

53. Abdullah SA, Aboloyoun EM, Abdel-Aleem H, Moftah FM, Ismail S. Maternal mortality in Assiut. *Int J Gynaecol Obstet* 1992;39:197–204.

54. Stanton C, Abderrahim N, Hill K. *DHS Maternal Mortality Indicators: an Assessment of Data Quality and Implications for Data Use*. DHS Analytical report no. 4. Calverton, MD: Macro International; 1997.

55. Abdel Azeem F, Farid SM, Khalifa AM. *Egypt Maternal and Child Health Survey 1991*. Cairo: Pan Arab Project for Child Development, League of Arab States, Central Agency for Public Mobilization and Statistics (CAPMAS); 1993.

56. Ministry of Health and Population. *Rapid Assessment for the Maternal Mortality in Egypt*. Cairo: Ministry of Health and Population; 1997.

57. Information Decision Support Center Egypt. Statistical Indicators, 2009 [www.eip.gov.eg/nds/nds_view.aspx?id=5313].

58. Stanton C, Abderrahim N, Hill K. *DHS Maternal Mortality Indicators: an Assessment of Data Quality and Implications for Data Use*. DHS Analytical report no. 4. Calverton, MD: Macro International; 1997.

59. Ministry of Health and Population. *Rapid Assessment for the Maternal Mortality in Egypt*. Cairo: Ministry of Health and Population; 1997.

60. Arafa N. *Proposal for a National Study on Perinatal Mortality in Egypt*. MSc thesis. London: London School of Hygiene & Tropical Medicine; 1999.

61. Sarhan AE. Mortality trends in the United Arab Republic. In: United Nations Department of Social and Economic Affairs. *Proceedings of the World Population Conference, 30 August to 10 September 1965, Belgrade, Yugoslavia*. Vol. 2. Selected papers and summaries: fertility, family planning, mortality. New York: United Nations; 1967. p. 358–60.

62. United Nations. *United Nations Demographic Yearbook 1997*. New York: United Nations; 1998.

63. CAPMAS. *Maternal Health and Infant Mortality in Egypt*. Cairo: Central Agency for Public Mobilization and Statistics (CAPMAS), Population Studies and Research Center (PSRC); 1987.

64. El-Zanaty FH, Sayed HAA, Zaky HHM, Way AA. *Egypt Demographic and Health Survey 1992*. Cairo: National Population Council and Macro International; 1993.

65. El-Zanaty F, Hussein EM, Shawky GA, Way AA, Kishor S. *Egypt Demographic and Health Survey 1995*. Cairo: National Population Council and Macro International; 1996.

66. Egyptian Fertility Care Society. *Study of the Prevalence and Perception of Maternal Morbidity in Menoueyya Governorate Egypt*. Final report. Cairo: EFCS; 1995.

67. Egyptian Fertility Care Society. *Community Based Survey of Maternal Morbidity in Assiut Sohag and Quena Governorate Egypt*. Final report. Cairo: EFCS; 1996.

68. Stanton B, Langsten R. *Rates and Factors Associated with Morbidity and Mortality Among Egyptian Neonates and Infants: a Longitudinal Prenatal and Postnatal Study.* Unpublished data. USAID Contract No. HRN-5966-C-00-3038-00. 1999.

69. Aboulghar A, Hussein M. Present status of perinatal mortality in Egypt: a reappraisal. [abstract] In: Fayed MM, Ibrahim II, Bayad MA, editors. *Medical Education in the Field of Primary Maternal Child Health Care.* Proceedings of an international conference, 5–7 December 1983, Cairo, Egypt. Cairo: Cairo University, Faculty of Medicine, Department of Obstetrics and Gynecology; 1984. p. 376–7.

70. Hefnawy F. Pregnancy wastage. *Popul Sci* 1983;4:31–8.

71. Serour GI, Younis NM, Hefnawi F, El-Bahy M, Dagistany HF, Nawar M. Perinatal mortality in an Egyptian maternity hospital. 1981;19:447–51.

72. Younis MN, Bahy M, Serour GI, Daghistany HF, Hefnawi F, Ahmed AK. A study of the biosocial factors affecting perinatal mortality in an Egyptian maternity hospital. *Popul Sci* 1981;2:71–90.

73. Langsten R, Mechael P, Yount K. *Assessment of Care in the Neonatal Units of Luxor and Aswan.* Unpublished data. USAID Contract No. HRN-5966-C-00-3038-00. 1998.

74. World Health Organization. *Coverage of Maternity Care: a Tabulation of Available Information.* 3rd ed. Geneva: WHO; 1993.

75. El-Zanaty F, Way AA. *Egypt Interim Demographic and Health Survey 2003.* Cairo: Ministry of Health and Population, National Population Council, El-Zanaty and Associates, ORC Macro; 2004.

Chapter 20
Learning from the achievements in Sri Lanka

Harshalal Seneviratne

Introduction

Sri Lanka has achieved a high status in maternal and newborn health. This island of $62\,705$ km^2 has a population estimated to be 20.2 million (in 2008), yielding a population density of 322 per km^2.[1,2] Social stratifications, although present, do not affect the delivery of health care to all its citizens. A democratic parliamentary system of government ensures the development of country-specific health interventions. These have been strengthened even more to meet the local health needs following the devolution of power to provinces, districts and divisions.

Since 1947, the government of Sri Lanka has provided education to its people up to university graduation without a fee. Although, by academic selection, fewer than 20% of those qualifying at the General Certificate of Education 'Advanced' level (GCE 'A' level) examination are offered places at the state universities, increasing numbers of the remainder seek higher education at paid courses conducted by non-governmental higher education institutions. All these inputs contribute to the literacy rate of 91.8%.[3]

In a similar manner, the government of Sri Lanka provides a free health service, without a user fee, from birth throughout life. The government health facilities, which are available throughout the country at basic, intermediate and tertiary levels, have also introduced some very advanced therapeutic procedures. For those who wish to obtain curative health services from the non-governmental providers, primary to tertiary care is also available in the private sector establishments. Approximately 4% of total deliveries in the country occur in private sector hospitals.[4]

Sri Lanka's achievement in health for its people has been remarkable. Maternal mortality reached a low figure of 38.1 per 100000 live births by 2005 (Figures 20.1 and 20.2) while the maternal and child health (MCH) coverage had reached 94%.[5] How does its performance in health relate to Millennium Development Goals (MDGs) 4 and 5?

The eight MDGs and the targets to be achieved were set by the United Nations General Assembly in 2000 and were aimed at fulfilling major social and health needs by 2015.[6] New numbering of targets and indicators for monitoring was recommended at the 12th meeting of the Inter-agency and Expert Group on MDG Indicators and noted by the 62nd General Assembly.[7] National-level monitoring, as appropriate for each each country, was recommended.

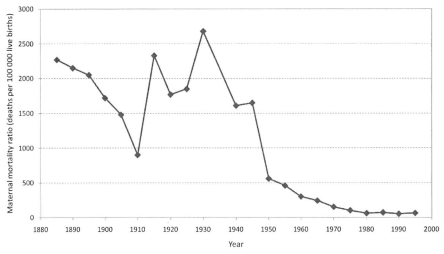

Figure 20.1 Maternal mortality ratio in Sri Lanka, 1895–1996 (maternal deaths per 100 000 live births); data from reports of the Registrar-General on vital statistics and the Family Health Bureau, Maternal and Child Health Unit of the Ministry of Healthcare and Nutrition

Key dates:

1879	First maternity hospital opens
1887	Annual report of Registrar-General
1897	Compulsory registration of births and deaths
1897	Training and registration of nurses and midwives starts
1906–45	Eight malaria epidemics
1921	First antenatal clinic
1926	Community health unit system established and training of public health nurses (PHNs) and public health midwives (PHMs) starts
1931	Universal adult franchise established
1947	Free education introduced
1948	Independence
1953	Family Planning Association formed under the International Planned Parenthood Federation (1952)
1968	Family Health Bureau and Health Education Bureau established
1972	Family planning services integrated with maternal and child health services.

The Sri Lankan success has been achieved by a process of evolution of social and healthcare facilities for well over 100 years.[8] Historically, from ancient times the cultural and religious background of the country encouraged social development by the provision of free health and education to its people under the patronage of the king. This free package for human development operates even today, although, with advancing technology, it has become a financial burden to the state. However, it is of note that the state manages to provide free primary to tertiary education by spending only 2.5% of gross domestic product (GDP).[1] Similarly from basic up to some advanced healthcare facilities are provided by the state throughout life without a user fee at a cost of a mere 1.7% of GDP.[1] Although changes in attitudes and aspirations of the public have led to an increasing shift towards seeking health care in the private sector, free services provided by the state sector are accessible to all Sri Lankans in all parts of the country.

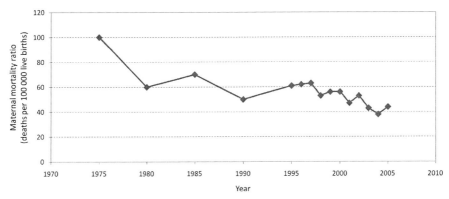

Figure 20.2 Maternal mortality ratio in Sri Lanka, 1975–2005 (maternal deaths per 100 000 live births); data from reports of the Registrar-General on vital statistics and the Family Health Bureau, Maternal and Child Health Unit of the Ministry of Healthcare and Nutrition

Key dates:

1985 Maternal death enquiries launched
1989 Safe Motherhood programmes starts
1994 Maternal death audit implemented
1997 Integrated reproductive health services adopted into government health policy
2000 Maternal death investigation developed

Key interventions

Sri Lanka benefited from the parallel introduction of health and non-health interventions from the 19th century. The administrative, financial, technological and transport infrastructure was established through British colonial rule in the 19th and early 20th centuries. The military and estate (plantation) medical services in the country evolved to provide the current Western type of health care when the Civil Medical Department was established in 1858. Political commitment by local and national leaders gradually emerged within the context of the social, cultural and religious background that was inbuilt in the country from the pre-colonial era. The establishment of the curative health services occurred in the second half of the 19th century, and in the early 20th century the community-based health service was introduced. Key developments in this area were the establishment of the Colombo Medical School (1870), the first maternity hospital (De Soysa Maternity Home; 1879), midwifery training (1897) and the School for Midwifery Training in 1910.[9,10] The first community-based domiciliary health unit was established in 1926,[11] and this widened the coverage of the preventive component of maternity care. Even today, it is the template on which the rest of this service functions countrywide.

Together with these developments, administrative and monitoring systems were introduced. Sri Lanka is unique among developing countries in having maternal mortality records from 1881. Compulsory registration of births and deaths was introduced in 1897.[10] The high status given to maternal health is noteworthy as a separate section on maternal mortality was introduced into the administrative report of the Registrar General in 1921. The progress made is such that today a system of reporting of maternal deaths and their investigation is in place.[11] The maternal mortality ratio has remained below 100 per 100 000 live births since 1976 and during the past decade it has remained at around 50 per 100 000 live births (Figure 20.2). The possible cause for each of the 150–200 maternal deaths per year is determined by an institutional and community-based investigation, following which interventions to prevent such events, together with the persons or agencies responsible for their implementation, are defined.[12] The results from many surveys that have evaluated the components of MCH in the past form the basis for improvement in MCH services introduced over the years.[13] The Sri Lanka Demographic and Health Surveys (SL. DHS) of 1987, 1993, 2000 and 2008 have been key activities in this regard. They provide longitudinal data that show trends in MCH, as well as other important reproductive health and social parameters.[14–17]

Trends towards achieving MDGs 4 and 5 in Sri Lanka

The indicators for MDG 4 to be achieved by 2015 in Sri Lanka are as follows:

4.1   under-five mortality rate of 10.7 per 1000 live births

4.2   infant mortality rate of 6.6 per 1000 live births

4.3   proportion of 1-year-old children immunised against measles to be 100%.

The status of indicator 4.1 is deemed to be on track towards the target for 2015 of 10.7 per 1000 live births as it was already down to 14.0 per 1000 live births by 2005. For comparison, it remained at around 32.0 per 1000 live births from 1983 to 1993 and approximately 20.8 per 1000 live births from 1990 to 2000. The infant mortality rate (indicator 4.2) has a similar status towards a target of 6.6 per 1000 live births by 2015, as a reduction to 11.3 per 1000 live births had occurred by 2003 from 19.8 per 1000 live births in 1990.[18] The prevalence of measles is very low in Sri Lanka. In the preliminary SL.DHS 2006/07 report, the immunisation against measles was 97.1%, and the total immunisation for Bacille Calmette–Guérin (BCG), diphtheria, pertussis and tetanus (DPT; three doses), polio (three doses) and measles was 96.9%.[17]

The indicators for MDG 5 to be achieved by 2015 in Sri Lanka are as follows:

5.1   maternal mortality ratio of 10.6 per 100 000 live births

5.1   skilled attendances at delivery to be 100%.

The target for maternal mortality ratio is to reduce it to 10.6 per 100 000 live births by 2015 from the level of 42.3 per 100 000 live births in 1991. Maternal deaths are individually evaluated in Sri Lanka and, during the period 2001–05, fluctuated between 38 and 53 per 100 000 live births.[12] Although the overall maternal mortality ratio has remained low, the trend towards reaching indicator 5.1 by 2015 has been disappointing. The indicator 5.2 target of reaching 100% skilled attendance at delivery by 2015 has been more favourable. In 1993, 94.1% of deliveries were performed by skilled health personnel and the SL.DHS 2006/07 reported that this indicator had increased to 98.5%.[17]

However, deliveries reported by public health midwives (PHM) or family health workers (FHW) at home numbered 1613 (0.6% of all PHM-reported deliveries) and 1603 (0.5% of all PHM-reported deliveries) in 2004 and 2005, respectively.[5] Although this was a reduction from 12 388 (5.1% of all PHM-reported deliveries) in 1991 and 2550 (1.0% of all PHM-reported deliveries) in 1997, it remains a cause for concern. In Sri Lanka, delivering at home is known to increase the risks to the mother and newborn owing to their emergency nature, inadequate facilities at home in a rural setting and lack of emergency transport to an institution (Figure 20.3). The risk is further enhanced when home deliveries take place with untrained assistance: such PHM-reported home deliveries occurred in 38.1% ($n = 4760$) in 1991, 49.8% ($n = 1270$) in 1997 and 48.1% ($n = 771$) in 2005 (Figure 20.4).[5,19,20] Furthermore, a

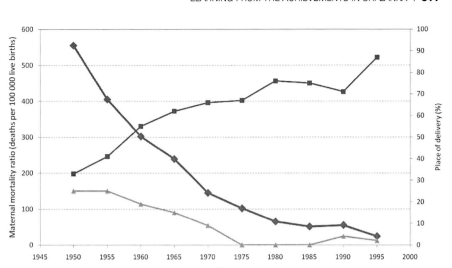

Figure 20.3   Maternal mortality ratio (maternal deaths per 100 000 live births) in Sri Lanka related to place of delivery

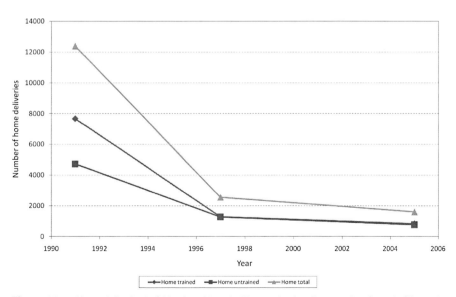

Figure 20.4   Home deliveries in Sri Lanka with and without trained assistance; data from de Silva and Karunaratne,[5] Wickremasuriya and de Silva[19] and Fonseka and Karunaratne[20]

community midwife (PHM or FHW), after her basic training, has only minimal opportunities for regular hands-on participation by attending at deliveries. In Sri Lanka, deliveries conducted at home would therefore place a PHM or FHW who is probably inadequately competent in a situation that is suboptimal in terms of facilities. This issue has been addressed in the *Report of the External Review of Maternal and Newborn Health*[21] in Sri Lanka that was conducted in 2007 by the World Health Organization (WHO) at the invitation of the Ministry of Health and Nutrition. It was recommended that simulated delivery modules should be used in retraining programmes that are to be organised for this purpose.

Health interventions

Very early on in the organisation of MCH services, the importance of human resource development was recognised and implemented, and this has continued for over 100 years. Institutional staffing was ensured first, whereby a hierarchy for medical and nursing care was established. In 1926, with the initiation of community-based domiciliary services, a healthcare provider structure that is comparable to and operates on a parallel basis to the institutional/curative services was established. A significant issue in the success of MCH care in Sri Lanka has been the extent of integration and cooperation between these two services.

The present infrastructure of health care in Sri Lanka ensures that MCH care is provided from basic to the highest level. The three-tiered curative healthcare structure (primary, intermediate and tertiary) is being converted to one with non-specialist (primary care) and specialist facilities. The latter would include institutions ranging from base hospitals to teaching hospitals, with increasing levels of expertise. Some would also have centres of sub-specialisation in various aspects of reproductive health care. The number of deliveries in the provinces (based on population density, with former WHO recommendation being that 5000 deliveries be covered by a specialist unit), the need for Comprehensive Emergency Obstetric Care (CEmOC) (one CEmOC facility for each 500 000 population) and other issues related to coverage for deliveries have been calculated by the author at the request of the Ministry of Healthcare and Nutrition and the Post Graduate Institute of Medicine (PGIM). The result of these calculations is that there is a requirement for 250 specialist units in obstetrics and gynaecology in Sri Lanka by 2015.[22] Each specialist institution would have a minimum of two units in obstetrics and gynaecology. The distribution of new hospitals has been been redesigned to achieve adequate accessibility to services throughout the country.

Curative services are provided by hospitals ranging from non-specialist to tertiary-level specialist institutions.[4] These are well integrated to provide for well-timed referral and transfer of high-risk cases. The preventive services are organised to screen for high-risk situations as well as to promote nutrition, contraception, parent-craft training and immunisation, etc. The recently devolved administrative structure of the country into provinces has maintained the executive component of health care. An important feature of MCH care services of Sri Lanka is the vertical and horizontal integration of the curative and preventive services, thus ensuring adequate coverage as well as extension of care for a range of reproductive health conditions of varying severity.

Another feature that should be noted is the continuity of care on the basis of life-cycle events. The Sri Lankan MCH service ensures that care is provided to the public during infancy, childhood, adolescence, the reproductive years (including pregnancy and the intrapartum, postnatal and neonatal periods) and the postreproductive period of life by the same local healthcare system or providers. Gap-free health care throughout life can be considered a tremendous advantage and is positively exploited now for the prevention of non-communicable diseases such as hypertension, obesity and diabetes mellitus, which are emerging as serious public health problems in Sri Lanka.[4]

Education

A key issue in the experience of Sri Lanka in achieving a high standard of MCH is the education of its public as well as the health service providers. While education has remained very closely built in to the culture that existed from ancient times, the introduction of free education in 1947 ensured that all Sri Lankans had access to learning up to graduation without payment of a fee. This has resulted in a literacy rate of over 90% for both females and males.[3] However, dropout rates of 5–7% from secondary education is a problem as reproductive health education provided at this stage of schooling would be denied to such adolescents. Some other means of providing the reproductive health education and services to these school leavers is urgently needed.

The benefit from education is reflected in the low parity status among the higher educated.[17] Surprisingly, the non-use of contraceptives (34.9%) and the use of traditional methods only (31.7%) were also the highest among those educated beyond GCE 'A' level. In this best-educated group, the use of modern non-permanent technological methods was only 28.1%. These facts present another dimension for consideration during family planning policy development and implementation.

From the late 19th century, the importance of training basic and intermediate-level healthcare personnel with the most current knowledge and skills was realised. The training of midwives, which was hospital based at the beginning, was extended to the community in 1926 by the establishment of the first community health unit. Currently, midwifery training as a PHM/FHW is conducted for 12 months at a school of nursing and 6 months at a field training area. Hands-on skills training for the student PHM/FHW is ensured, as they have to observe ten normal deliveries, conduct 20 normal deliveries under supervision and assist in five 'abnormal' deliveries, as well as provide supervised care for 25 healthy and ten ill neonates to obtain their final qualifications. This comprehensive training is also given to nursing officers and nursing sisters who are selected to obtain midwifery qualifications. Each such trained midwife provides reproductive health services for a population of 3000–5000 within a clearly defined area, where she is given residential quarters with an attached clinic facility.

A direct relationship between the increasing number of staff and increasing skilled attendance at birth and reduction in maternal mortality has been demonstrated in Sri Lanka. The main lesson from the experience of Sri Lanka is the need for any developing country to have primary healthcare personnel who are appropriately trained, provided with adequate facilities, supervised and exposed to continuing professional development. To fulfil MDG 4 and 5, however, the healthcare system also needs to be organised to allow referral when appropriate, which is provided with the availability of the Basic Emergency Obstetric Care (BEmOC) and CEmOC facilities. The assessment of EmOC facilities in Sri Lanka in 2000 reported a 98% utilisation of BEmOC and CEmOC facilities, but the management of complications was at a suboptimal rate of 75.2% at CEmOC institutions.[23]

Newborn and child care

The low levels achieved in infant mortality and under-five mortality are a reflection of the organisation and implementation of the health and non-health interventions in general and the efficacy of field health MCH care in particular. This accounted for the reduction in infant mortality rate from 140 per 1000 live births in 1945 to 19.3 per 1000 live births in 1990.[24] Although 98.5% of deliveries occur in a healthcare facility and the neonatal mortality rate has shown a pleasing decline, further enhancement of the care of the newborn is needed as neonatal deaths account for 67% of the total infant deaths.[17]

A package of good coverage for prepregnancy, antenatal and postnatal care is received by women of reproductive age in Sri Lanka.[4] It is an example of good practices aimed at reaching the targets set for MDG 4. Since 1962, when family planning services were linked to MCH services, an 'eligible couples register' has been maintained by the PHM so that she would be aware of the women of reproductive age in her area who would require these services. This register has also been used to provide for prepregnancy assessment, as well counselling, prophylaxis with folate supplementation and rubella immunisation. It is also well known that adequate spacing of pregnancies improves the survival and wellbeing of the next sibling. The SL.DHS in 2008 demonstrated that up to 33% of women had a fertility preference for another pregnancy but 18% wished to delay their next pregnancy. This tendency was highest, at 44.4%, in women with one child.[17]

The prevalence of low birth weight has been relatively high in Sri Lanka. A study was performed in 1987–88 in a selected area representing all socio-economic groups in Sri Lanka to evaluate the low birth weight status.[24] The study found that 18.6% of live babies who were weighed within 24 hours of birth were less than 2500 g. Although it had declined from 22.8% in 1990 to 16.7% in 1999, the prevalence of low birth weight has remained between 16.1% and 17.6% since then.[17] This is an area that is yet to be evaluated. Exclusive breastfeeding practices have been shown to be at a high level of 83.7% up to the first 3 months of infancy and still remain at 53.4% at 5 months.[17] The postnatal home visits by the PHM are considered to be a key activity that promotes continued breastfeeding. At the same time, there is the opportunity to promote and ensure that immunisation of the newborn is completed and to provide guidance in parent-craft skills.

Conclusion

Based on Sri Lanka's experience, it appears that MDGs 4 and 5 are achievable by developing countries. The strategies to achieve these, however, need to be based on local country-specific needs and logistics. It should be noted that Sri Lanka reached its current MCH status over a period of more than 100 years. Furthermore, Sri Lanka is now faced with new challenges that appear to be based on recent socio-economic needs and concepts.

As a basis for planning, an analysis of health and non-health strengths and weaknesses would be of prime importance, and the main driving force for achieving the MDGs would be commitment by political leaders and policy makers. This would form the basis for encouraging and enhancing the dedication and performance of care providers at all levels of the healthcare system. The focus should be on providing a system of care that is accessible and affordable to all levels of society devoid of bias. Sri Lanka has demonstrated the benefits of conducting a maternal death enquiry. Such a monitoring system enables modifications, which then permit the MCH care system in a country to evolve in a positive manner.

The establishment of a category of healthcare providers (PHMs/FHWs) who seek the recipient and provide care that is of a high level of technical expertise is a basic requirement to achieve MDGs 4 and 5. Sri Lanka has benefited from such a system since 1926. Their tasks are performed while being supervised and supported for referral of high-risk cases by public health nursing sisters, community medical officers and a hierarchy of other healthcare professionals. A parallel curative service has to develop at the same time. Although Sri Lanka developed the curative system first, these should be organised as parallel and integrated services. The many components of MCH as well as reproductive health care could then be added to achieve the MDGs.

Acknowledgements

Professor Lalani Rajapakse, formerly of the Faculty of Medicine in Colombo, and Dr Anoma Jayatilleke, National Professional Officer, WHO country office in Sri Lanka, are thanked for the support given during the preparation of this chapter. The long association with the present and past directors, consultants and programme officers of the Family Health Bureau in the MCH Unit of the Ministry of Health is greatly appreciated in obtaining the material presented.

References

1. Central Bank of Sri Lanka. Annual Report 2008. Part I: Key social indicators [www.cbsl.gov.lk].

2. Department of Census and Statistics of Sri Lanka, 2008 [www.statistics.gov.lk].

3. Ministry of Education. Statistics, 2002 [www.moe.gov.lk].

4. Department of Health. *Annual Health Statistics.* Colombo: Medical Statistics Unit, Department of Health, Ministry of Healthcare and Nutriton; 2006.

5. de Silva C, Karunaratne V, editors. *Annual Report on Family Health 2004–2005.* Vol. 17. Colombo: Family Health Bureau, Ministry of Health, and UNFPA; 2007.

6. United Nations. *Indicators for Monitoring the Millennium Development Goals: Definitions, Rationale, Concepts and Sources.* New York: United Nations; 2003.

7. 12th Inter-Agency and Expert Group Meeting on MDG Indicators, 2007. ESA/STAT/AC.138/19.

8. Seneviratne HR, Rajapakse LC. Safe Motherhood in Sri Lanka: a 100 year march. World Report on Women's Health 2000. *Int J Gynaecol Obstet* 2000;70:113–24.

9. Fonseka C, Kottegoda SR. In: Kottegoda SR, editor. *The Story of the Colombo Medical School in the Colombo Medical School Centenary 1870–1970.* Colombo: Colombo Medical School; 1970. p. 9–20.

10. Chinnathamby S. Perspectives in safe motherhood over the past four decades. *Report on the Inter-Regional Meeting on Safe Motherhood 19–23 August 1991.* Colombo: UNICEF; 1992. p. 10–20.

11. De Silva M. Role of maternal and child health care infrastructure in Sri Lanka. *Report on the Inter-Regional Meeting on Safe Motherhood 19–23 August 1991.* Colombo: UNICEF; 1992. p. 41–2.

12. Attygalle D, Tillekeratne A. *Overview of Maternal Mortality in Sri Lanka 2001–2005.* Colombo: Family Health Bureau, Ministry of Healthcare and Nutrition and UNICEF; 2008.

13. Department of Census and Statistics. *Vital Statistics on Infant, Child and Maternal Mortality 1980–1990.* Colombo: Department of Census and Statistics and the Registrar General's Department of Sri Lanka in Collaboration with UNICEF; 1993.

14. Department of Census and Statistics. *Sri Lanka Demographic and Health Survey 1987.* Westinghouse, Columbia, MD: Department of Census and Statistics, Ministry of Plan Implementation and Institute of Resource Development; 1988.

15. Department of Census and Statistics. *Sri Lanka Demographic and Health Survey 1993.* Colombo: Department of Census and Statistics, Ministry of Finance, Planning, Ethnic Affairs and National Integration in collaboration with the Ministry of Health, Highways and Social Services; 1995.

16. Department of Census and Statistics. *Sri Lanka Demographic and Health Survey 2000.* Colombo: Department of Census and Statistics in collaboration with the Ministry of Health, Nutrition and Welfare; 2002.

17. Department of Census and Statistics. *Sri Lanka Demographic and Health Survey 2006/7*. Colombo: Department of Census and Statistics in collaboration with the Ministry of Healthcare and Nutrition; 2008.

18. Ministry of Finance and Planning. *The MDG Strategy Consultation for Sri Lanka, 20th–21st June 2009*. Colombo: Ministry of Finance and Planning in collaboration with the United Nations Development Programme; 2009.

19. Wickremasuriya KP, de Silva M, editors. *Annual Report on Family Health, Sri Lanka 1991*. Colombo: Family Health Bureau and Ministry of Health and Women's Affairs; 1993.

20. Fonseka A, Karunaratne V, editors. *Annual Report on Family Health, Sri Lanka 1997*. Colombo: Family Health Bureau, Ministry of Health and Women's Affairs and UNFPA; 1998.

21. Ministry of Healthcare and Nutrition. *Report of the External Review of Maternal and Newborn Health: Sri Lanka*. Colombo: Ministry of Healthcare and Nutrition supported by UNFPA, UNICEF and WHO; 2008.

22. Seneviratne HR. *Cadre Projections for Specialist Services By 2015*. Colombo: Post Graduate Institute of Medicine and Ministry of Healthcare and Nutrition; 2007.

23. Women's Right to Life and Health Project Sri Lanka, *Needs Assessment Study, 2000–2001*. Colombo: The Family Health Bureau in collaboration with The Sri Lanka College of Obstetricians and Gynaecologists (SLCOG) and UNICEF, with funding from the Bill and Melinda Gates Foundation; 2003.

24. Wickremasuriya KP, Alahakone KS, de Silva JKM. *Study of Low Birth Weight and Neonatal Morbidity and Mortality, Sri Lanka 1987*. Three country study (India, Sri Lanka and Nepal) on low birth weight and infant morbidity and mortality in collaboration with WHO/SEARO. Colombo: WHO; 1992.

Section 6

Consensus views

Chapter 21

Consensus views arising from the 58th Study Group:
Maternal and Infant Deaths: Chasing Millennium Development Goals 4 and 5

The study group identified many gaps in the evidence required to achieve the Millenium Development Goals 4 and 5. The three most important pieces of research in each area that would address these deficiencies are described below.

Assessing the problem

Audit of maternal deaths

1. All countries should actively enumerate and audit maternal and perinatal deaths.

Disease issues

Postpartum haemorrhage

Prophylaxis

2. Research is needed into the most appropriate components of the active management of the third stage of labour, including the role of controlled cord traction, the role of universal prophylaxis with oxytocics and the most appropriate prophylactic drug in each healthcare setting.

Management of retained placenta

3. Research is needed into the optimal management of retained placenta, including timing of therapeutic interventions.

Treatment of postpartum haemorrhage

4. Research is needed into the most clinically and cost-effective combination of medical and surgical therapy for the management of postpartum haemorrhage, including the role of the non-pneumatic shock garment.

Puerperal sepsis

Disease burden

5. Research is needed to quantify the disease burden related to puerperal sepsis.

Interventions

6. The effectiveness of interventions, particularly those that comprise multiple components related to influencing behaviour and creating improvements in the health system, should be rigorously tested. Research should ideally be conducted in settings where the risk of introducing infection is high.

Cost effectiveness

7. Evaluation of interventions should include analysis of cost effectiveness.

Hypertensive disease in pregnancy

Detection

8. Research is needed into innovative methods of detecting pre-eclampsia in women who do not present for antenatal care. Strategies worthy of exploration include home urine protein testing and community-based blood pressure testing and education.

Prevention

9. Methods of incorporating calcium supplementation into health programmes and the efficacy of community-level food fortification with calcium in preventing hypertensive diseases in pregnancy deserve further evaluation.

Treatment

10. Research is needed into strategies to ensure that magnesium sulphate reaches the settings in which it is needed. Since intravenous administration is not always available, research is needed into alternative routes of administration.

Obstructed labour

The partogram

11. Randomised controlled trials of the partogram are required in sub-Saharan Africa to determine their efficacy.

Maternity waiting homes

12. Randomised trials of use versus non-use of a maternity waiting home where women can stay for the last few weeks of pregnancy while waiting for labour to start should be conducted in sub-Saharan Africa.

Symphysiotomy

13. Randomised trials of symphysiotomy versus alternative methods of delivery should be evaluated in sub-Saharan Africa in women in obstructed labour.

Patient, provider and service issues

Care-seeking patterns at delivery

14. Research is needed into the patterns, co-variates and determinants of healthcare-seeking at the time of delivery, given that delivery is the time of greatest risk for the mother.

Training

15. The effects of training of healthcare workers in Essential Obstetric Care and Newborn Care need to be evaluated and lessons learnt documented.

Packages of care

16. More research is needed in determining quality models of care – mid-level providers, midwives and doctors, and facilities.

Human resources

17. Studies are needed to establish what kinds of human resources are required in specific settings, and how this can be developed and sustained. Specifically, research is needed to systematically review the evidence for techniques and processes leading to the effective planning, delivery and sustainability of a functional workforce for maternity care, using techniques such as realist review that account for contextual factors. Where staffing levels are appropriate and sustained, and outcomes are good, ethnographic work and/or social network mapping should be undertaken to find out what underpins these success stories.

Country issues

Achieving Millenium Development Goals 4 and 5 in Afghanistan

Obstructed labour

18. Research is needed into the role of vitamin D deficiency in the aetiology of obstructed labour and, if a link is proven, whether vitamin D therapy is effective therapeutically.

Obstetric morbidity

19. Research is needed into the prevalence of major obstetric morbidity, including obstetric fistula.

Family medicine practitioners

20. Research is needed into the clinical and cost effectiveness of family medicine practitioners, in comparison with the traditional model of a separate clinician in each specialty, in providing care in rural Afghanistan.

Index

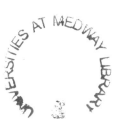